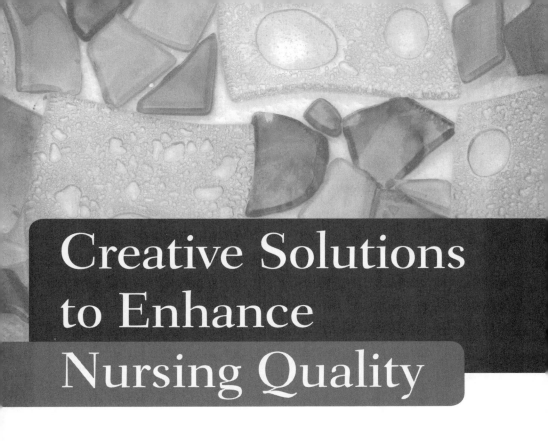

Creative Solutions to Enhance Nursing Quality

Edited By

Bruce Alan Boxer, PhD, MBA, RN, CPHQ

Director of Nursing Quality/Magnet Program Director
South Jersey Healthcare
Vineland, New Jersey

Ellen Boxer Goldfarb, MSN, CRNP

Cardiology Nurse Practitioner
Penn Presbyterian Medical Center
Philadelphia, Pennsylvania

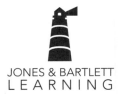

JONES & BARTLETT
L E A R N I N G

D1416660

World Headquarters
Jones & Bartlett Learning
40 Tall Pine Drive
Sudbury, MA 01776
978-443-5000
info@jblearning.com
www.jblearning.com

Jones & Bartlett Learning
Canada
6339 Ormindale Way
Mississauga, Ontario L5V 1J2
Canada

Jones & Bartlett Learning
International
Barb House, Barb Mews
London W6 7PA
United Kingdom

Jones & Bartlett Learning books and products are available through most bookstores and online booksellers. To contact Jones & Bartlett Learning directly, call 800-832-0034, fax 978-443-8000, or visit our website, www.jblearning.com.

Substantial discounts on bulk quantities of Jones & Bartlett Learning publications are available to corporations, professional associations, and other qualified organizations. For details and specific discount information, contact the special sales department at Jones & Bartlett Learning via the above contact information or send an email to specialsales@jblearning.com.

The authors, editor, and publisher have made every effort to provide accurate information. However, they are not responsible for errors, omissions, or for any outcomes related to the use of the contents of this book and take no responsibility for the use of the products and procedures described. Treatments and side effects described in this book may not be applicable to all people; likewise, some people may require a dose or experience a side effect that is not described herein. Drugs and medical devices are discussed that may have limited availability controlled by the Food and Drug Administration (FDA) for use only in a research study or clinical trial. Research, clinical practice, and government regulations often change the accepted standard in this field. When consideration is being given to use of any drug in the clinical setting, the health care provider or reader is responsible for determining FDA status of the drug, reading the package insert, and reviewing prescribing information for the most up-to-date recommendations on dose, precautions, and contraindications, and determining the appropriate usage for the product. This is especially important in the case of drugs that are new or seldom used.

Production Credits
Publisher: Kevin Sullivan
Acquisitions Editor: Amy Sibley
Associate Editor: Patricia Donnelly
Editorial Assistant: Rachel Shuster
Associate Production Editor: Katie Spiegel
Marketing Manager: Rebecca Wasley
V.P., Manufacturing and Inventory Control:
 Therese Connell
Composition: DataStream Content Solutions, LLC,
 Absolute Service Inc.
Cover Design: Scott Moden
Cover Image: © Maxfx/Dreamstime.com
Printing and Binding: Malloy, Inc.
Cover Printing: Malloy, Inc.

Library of Congress Cataloging-in-Publication Data
Boxer, Bruce Alan.
 Creative solutions to enhance nursing quality / Bruce Alan Boxer, Ellen Boxer Goldfarb.
  p. ; cm.
 Includes bibliographical references and index.
 ISBN 978-0-7637-8185-9 (pbk.)
 1. American Nurses Credentialing Center. Magnet Recognition Program. 2. Nursing services—United States—Administration. 3. Nursing services—United States—Quality control. I. Goldfarb, Ellen Boxer. II. Title.
 [DNLM: 1. American Nurses Credentialing Center. Magnet Recognition Program. 2. Nursing—organization & administration—United States. 3. Evidence-Based Nursing—United States. 4. Organizational Innovation—United States. 5. Quality Assurance, Health Care—methods—United States. 6. Quality Assurance, Health Care—organization & administration—United States. WY 105 B788c 2011]
 RT89.B72 2011
 362.17'3068—dc22

                                    2010018276
6048
Printed in the United States of America
                        4 3 2 1

For Sandy and Bill Boxer, mom and dad.

You gave us everything.
We give you this humbly,
With our love and deepest gratitude.

Table of Contents

Foreword

TRANSFORMING HEALTHCARE ENVIRONMENTS TO IMPROVE CARE QUALITY

The most enduring and motivating observation of my entire career was the surprise and dismay I experienced as a new nurse when the institution that I was so proud to be a part of undermined my very best efforts to give the high standard of nursing care that I was personally capable of providing. I came well prepared to hospital nursing practice. I was highly motivated. I was very fortunate to have had a great education and wonderful clinical nurse role models. My classmates and I thought we were entering nursing practice with the expertise, intelligence, and motivation to tackle the most challenging clinical problems. Then we encountered a very big problem that was beyond the capacity of any single nurse to fundamentally change: an organizational context that was not consistent with or supportive of clinical nursing excellence. As my career progressed, I was exposed to many hospitals and other healthcare settings, and the organizational context of nursing practice in almost all of them was far from ideal and, too often, downright hazardous to patients and caustic to nurses.

When I was elected president of the American Academy of Nursing in 1979, I urged the fellows of the academy to make the transformation of the nurse practice environment in hospitals a major priority (Aiken, 1981). The resulting academy study identified 41 hospitals nationally that nurses ranked good places to work. The study led to the use of the term *Magnet hospitals* because these 41 hospitals were successful in attracting and retaining nurses whereas other hospitals in their local labor markets were experiencing nurse shortages (McClure, Poulin, Sovie, & Wandelt, 1983). Research confirmed that these 41 institutions had in common organizational features that promoted and supported professional nursing practice.

Even though hundreds of thousands of bedside care nurses have made similar observations to mine—that the organizational context of professional nursing practice is deficient—not much sustainable progress was made toward transforming the organizational context of care until the academy's national study confirmed that certain organizational attributes of hospitals were associated with better outcomes for nurses. That empirical finding motivated researchers like me to undertake additional studies to show that these hospitals not only experienced better nurse satisfaction and retention, but that their patients were more satisfied with their care and mortality rates were lower (Aiken, Sloane, Lake, Sochalski, & Weber, 1999; Aiken, Smith, & Lake, 1994).

It took 20 years for the findings of the American Academy of Nursing's landmark study on nurse work environments to be formally operationalized through the American Nurses Credentialing Center's (ANCC) Magnet Recognition Program. The ANCC provided a blueprint for replicating the successful organizational features common to the original reputational Magnet hospitals. The Magnet Recognition Program grew slowly for almost a decade before gaining momentum and more recently experiencing exponential growth in the United States and capturing significant attention abroad. Interest in improving nurse work environments was stimulated in 1999 by evidence that medical errors and preventable complications of medical care were widespread, and that care outcomes were better in hospitals with work environments that supported professional nursing practice (Institute of Medicine, 2004).

Through our program of research at the University of Pennsylvania, we estimate that about one quarter of hospitals in the United States have Magnet-like qualities, even though only about 5% currently have ANCC Magnet Recognition. Additionally, about 50% of hospitals have some Magnet-like features but not all, and about 25% have poor nurse practice environments. The differences in nurse practice environments across hospitals are a significant predictor of hospital mortality rates (Aiken, Clarke, Sloane, Lake, & Cheney, 2008) and patient satisfaction (Kutney-Lee et al., 2009).

International initiatives have offered opportunities to test whether the Magnet journey is transformative in the sense that care environments can be shown to improve after, as compared to before, hospitals begin the ANCC Magnet application process. Two international initiatives, one in England (Aiken, Buchan, Ball, & Rafferty, 2008) and one in the countries of Russia and Armenia (Aiken & Poghosyan, 2009), both show that nurse work environments and predictors of quality of care improved in participating hospitals following the introduction of organizational features consistent with Magnet principles. We also have new (yet unpublished) research findings documenting that nurse work environments in Pennsylvania hospitals that did not have Magnet recognition in 1999 but had achieved Magnet status by 2006 improved significantly more over the period than was true of other hospitals in the state. Evidence is growing that the forces of magnetism, when implemented, foster improved work environments for nurses and improved outcomes for both patients and nurses.

When I review the evidence base showing that improved nurse work environments are associated with better outcomes, practically minded executives and clinicians often ask me how they should proceed to improve their institution's work environment. A simple answer is to refer them to the materials produced by the Magnet recognition program to use as a guide for how to proceed whether or not they seek formal Magnet recognition. However, I have observed and collaborated now with enough nurses who have been successful in creating professional nurse practice environments to realize that true transformations in organizational culture are tremendously challenging to achieve. Change requires unfailing leadership, great creativity and ingenuity, organizational savvy, and persistence. That is where this inspiring and practical book by Bruce Alan Boxer and Ellen Boxer Goldfarb is invaluable.

Boxer and Goldfarb provide the evidence and concrete examples of what works to successfully transform an institution's work environment under real-life circumstances. Nurses on the Magnet journey will find the book immensely useful in planning and implementing a successful Magnet application. However, this book has a broader audience that includes all of us who yearn for organizational transformations that will enable nurses to be successful in consistently providing a high standard of care. I found this volume intriguing because it makes the previously impossible seem achievable. The book provides tested ideas and practical implementation strategies that hold great promise for restoring joy to clinical nursing practice and confidence that our vision of safe, patient-centered care can be achieved.

Linda H. Aiken, PhD, RN, FAAN, FRCN
University of Pennsylvania
February 2010

REFERENCES

Aiken, L. H. (1981). Nursing priorities for the 1980s: Hospitals and nursing homes. *American Journal of Nursing, 81*(2), 324–330.

Aiken, L. H., Buchan, J., Ball, J., & Rafferty, A. M. (2008). Transformative impact of Magnet designation: England case study. *Journal of Clinical Nursing, 17*(24), 3317–3323.

Aiken, L. H., Clarke, S. P., Sloane, D. M., Lake, E. T., & Cheney, T. (2008). Effects of hospital care environments on patient mortality and nurse outcomes. *Journal of Nursing Administration, 38*(5), 223–229.

Aiken, L. H., & Poghosyan, L. (2009). Evaluation of "Magnet Journey to Nursing Excellence Program" in Russia and Armenia. *Journal of Nursing Scholarship, 41*(2), 166–174.

Aiken, L. H., Sloane, D. M., Lake, E. T., Sochalski, J., & Weber, A. L. (1999). Organization and outcomes of inpatient AIDS care. *Medical Care, 37*(8), 760–772.

Aiken, L. H., Smith, H. L., & Lake, E. T. (1994). Lower Medicare mortality among a set of hospitals known for good nursing care. *Medical Care, 32*(8), 771–787.

Institute of Medicine. (2004). *Keeping patients safe: Transforming the work environment of nurses*. Washington, DC: National Academy Press.

Kutney-Lee, A., McHugh, M. D., Cimioitti, J. P., Flynn, L., Neff, D. F., & Aiken, L. H. (2009). Nursing: A key to patient satisfaction. *Health Affairs, 28*(4), w669–w676.

McClure, M. L., Poulin, M., Sovie, M. D., & Wandelt, M. A. (1983). *Magnet hospitals: Attraction and retention of professional nurses*. Washington, DC: American Academy of Nursing (ANA publication G-160).

Introduction

Are you a Magnet Program Director (MPD), performance improvement coordinator, and/or quality manager? Are you a nursing administrator looking for creative and sound ways to enhance patient care delivery within your institution? Are you a nurse manager trying to better the patient care on your unit? Are you a staff nurse leading an initiative to better your unit's quality? Are you a healthcare instructor/educator either at the university or the bedside needing to pragmatically teach principles of quality improvement? If you have answered "yes" to any of these questions, this book is for you. This book is designed to provide instruction and ideas to better patient care and the hospital work environment. It is also designed to delineate the most crucial elements in achieving and sustaining any quality initiative. Through insight and example, we will take you through the process of quality improvement without all the theoretical mumbo jumbo.

The purpose of this book is to:

- Offer instruction in bettering patient care and patient satisfaction;
- Provide guidance to those working to achieve Magnet designation;
- Advance the engagement, knowledge, satisfaction, and professionalism of the institution's nursing staff; and
- Recommend valuable creative solutions to achieve institutional, departmental, and unit goals.

This book is for:

- Nurse leaders at any level: Nurse Executives, Nurse Managers, Nursing Council Leaders, Staff Nurses, and Nurse Educators;
- Magnet Program Directors;
- Nursing Faculty at the Diploma, Associate, Bachelor, and Graduate level;
- Nursing Students at the Diploma, Associate, Bachelor, and Graduate level; and
- Nursing Quality/Nursing Performance Improvement Professionals.

The main goal of this volume is to assist readers to better patient care. This volume will explain the need for creative solutions to solve today's nursing problems by addressing:

- The fast pace of health care, the slow pace of knowledge, and the need for innovation.
- The need to involve the staff in the creation of care, not just its delivery, to promote ownership of care, ownership of nursing practice, and facilitate engagement.

- The need to properly utilize evidence-based practices to individualize patient care.
- The need to understand that there is a slippery slope, going from randomized, controlled research to we "will try anything."

Beyond explaining the need for creative solutions, this volume will act as a guidebook for tackling the initiation, implementation, and enculturation of principles in and components of the Magnet program, an evidence-based framework to promote nursing quality, through the application of creative solutions designed to facilitate the adoption of these Magnet principles and components. We are in no way telling you that you must do it the way we say or the way others have done it. Each institution is unique, with a unique culture, workforce, patient population, and service community. To suggest that one size fits all is ludicrous. Instead, we provide guidance, tips, and ideas to integrate into your projects to achieve the excellent nursing care and exemplary patient outcomes we all seek. We believe creative solutions can take the best of evidence-based practice, its proven efficacy, and overcome one of its main limitations, overlooking the need to individualize practice to institutional culture and patient need. Creative solutions take a practice typically proven to work and find inventive ways to make its implementation easy, providing a degree of flexibility so that tweaking is expected, not frowned upon. In this resource-limited, fast-paced healthcare environment, the information this volume provides is critical. And who knows . . . Magnet designation or redesignation just might be a bit easier to achieve if you are armed with this knowledge!

This volume can be read from cover to cover, or chapters can be used as needed. Each chapter is intended to stand alone. You may be referred to other chapters, but we have tried to keep this to a minimum to create chapter-specific guides to each particular topic. Of course, synergy will most likely occur if more than only one chapter is utilized as the topics are more symbiotic than mutually exclusive. You might also find topics revisited in various chapters. This is a consequence of attempting to make each chapter its own entity. Take it as reinforcement. If you feel you do not need the reinforcement, just skip the section. It is your choice. We hope this volume will assist you in bettering patient care and improving your work environment.

Acknowledgments

From Ellen:

I would like to thank my coauthor and mentor, my brother Bruce, for giving me such a wonderful opportunity to help create this important publication and for his personal and professional guidance and encouragement throughout my life. Were it not for him, I would not be where I am today professionally.

I would like to thank my parents, Sandy and Bill Boxer, for their truly unconditional love and unmatched support; my brother, Ron; and my sister, Randi, for always offering an ear and invaluable words of advice.

I would like to thank my husband, Josh, for always standing by me and for being my rock.

I would like to thank my two amazing sons, Jake and Brody, for being my daily inspiration. All I do, I do because of them.

I would like to thank Jones & Bartlett Learning for their assistance through the publishing process and for allowing us to relay this information to our peers with a goal of improving healthcare quality.

I would like to thank Linda H. Aiken for her enlightening contribution to and endorsement of this work.

From Bruce:

I first want to thank my parents, Sandy and Bill Boxer, for listening to my out-of-the-box ideas with interest, love, and approval. They always show belief in my ability and intellect—making me feel that there is nothing I cannot accomplish. Mom would listen for hours as I explained my ideas about nursing projects (she is not a nurse), giving input and encouragement. Dad beamed after each and every accomplishment, allowing me to feel that I was giving something to him as well as expressing my own voice. I love them very much.

I also want to thank the rest of my family. Their excitement and interest sustained this project. I could not have completed this book and all my schooling without their support.

I want to thank all of my colleagues at South Jersey Healthcare. Many of them contributed to this volume, and others gave me the support I needed to complete it. I want to single out one individual, Joanna Galletta, my friend and coworker. She is a talented lady and totally a class act. Her input and assistance truly empowered and enabled me to feel confident in my writing.

I want to thank all the people at Jones & Bartlett Learning and Dr. Linda H. Aiken for their belief in this project and their assistance in its creation.

A huge thank you to the professors and my colleagues at Holy Family University in Philadelphia, PA, especially Dr. Kathleen McMullen and Honour Moore. Their support, encouragement, and promotion of my endeavors and accomplishments helped propel me along in my academic studies, as well as in writing this volume.

I want to especially thank my nephew, Jake Goldfarb. As his mother (my sister) and I spent countless hours pouring over the research for this manuscript, he wrote his own volumes entitled *Spiderman Defeats the Green Goblin* and *Word World*. I am certain his are more interesting than ours.

And to my beautiful and brilliant sister and coauthor of this volume: I could not have done this without you. Writing this book was just an excuse to spend more time with you and the family. I love you very much.

I would also like to applaud all nurses that believe it is an honor to care for someone—to be allowed an intimate connection to the patient's world and the potential to positively affect patients' lives. As a nurse, I feel privileged. However, this privilege comes with an enormous amount of responsibility to patients, society, myself, and the profession of nursing. I hope this volume helps nurses meet this responsibility head on, achieving some amazing patient outcomes; personal and professional growth; and, ultimately, satisfaction, empowerment, and pride when proclaiming, "I am a nurse."

Contributors

Samantha Abate, RN, BS, CCRN
Assistant Nurse Manager, Cardiac ICU
and Cardiac Step Down
South Jersey Healthcare
Vineland, New Jersey

Linda H. Aiken, PhD, RN, FAAN, FRCN
Claire M. Fagin Leadership Professor
in Nursing, Professor of Sociology,
and Director of the Center for
Health Outcomes
University of Pennsylvania
Philadelphia, Pennsylvania

Bonnie Becker, RN, BSN
Perinatal Data Center Coordinator
Sanford USD Medical Center
Sioux Falls, South Dakota

Marie Bosco, BSN, RN, IBCLC
Lactation Consultant
Royal Oak Beaumont Hospital
Royal Oak, Michigan

Megan Bynoe, RN, BSN, CCRN
Assistant Nurse Manager
CentraState Healthcare System
Freehold, New Jersey

Roseanne M. DeFrancisco, MSN, RN
Clinical Outcomes Manager
South Jersey Healthcare Elmer Hospital
Elmer, New Jersey

Patricia Dysthe, RN, BA
Clinical Care Coordinator
Sanford USD Medical Center
Sioux Falls, South Dakota

Ruben D. Fernandez, PhD(c), MA, RN
Vice President, Patient Care Services
Palisades Medical Center
North Bergen, New Jersey

Sheri Fischer, RN, BSN
Nursing Unit Director
Sanford USD Medical Center
Sioux Falls, South Dakota

Joanna Galletta, BA(c)
Magnet Program Assistant,
Administrative Assistant, and
Nursing Project Coordinator
South Jersey Healthcare
Vineland, New Jersey

Susan Langin, WHNP-BC, MSN, RN
Advanced Practice Specialist
Holland Hospital
Holland, Michigan

**Bonnie Michaels, RN, MA, NEA-BC,
FACHE**
Vice President, Chief Nursing Officer
Mountainside Hospital
Montclair, New Jersey

Patricia A. Sanchez, RN, BSN
Nurse Manager, Medical Acute
South Jersey Healthcare
Vineland, New Jersey

**Lorna Schneider, MSN, RN, APN, BC,
CS, CCRN, CCNS**
Clinical Coordinator
Palisades Medical Center
North Bergen, New Jersey

Bette Schumacher, RN, CPN, MS
Clinical Nurse Specialist
Sanford USD Medical Center
Sioux Falls, South Dakota

Daniel J. Singleton, RN, BSN
Nursing Performance Improvement
    Coordinator
Aria Health
Philadelphia, Pennsylvania

Terri Spoltore, RN, MSN, CCRN
Director, Medical Care Center and
    Transitional Care Unit
South Jersey Healthcare
Vineland, New Jersey

**Fay Spragley, DNP, RNC, APRN, BC,
    CCRN**
Clinical Coordinator and Nurse
    Practitioner
Palisades Medical Center
North Bergen, New Jersey

Emily Turnure, RN, MSN, NEA-BC
Administrative Director Education and
    Joint Commission Coordinator
South Jersey Healthcare
Vineland, New Jersey

The Legend

Each creative solution will have an overall evaluation for its appropriateness with respect to where a hospital is on the journey to nursing excellence (subsequently referred to as "the journey"). Utilizing Patricia Benner's classification system for the stages of nurses' clinical competence, the novice-to-expert framework (Benner, 1984), we will provide nurse leaders with insight into how well the specific creative solution matches their stage of the journey. These ratings are not absolute, nor are they mutually exclusive; they are a continuum. Any institution can consider any creative solution. The ratings are merely meant as a guide to assist nurse leaders in evaluating the sophistication of their institution with respect to the specific creative solution topic.

A **NOVICE** creative solution is for hospitals/institutions that are just starting the journey, and may have not yet decided to seek Magnet designation, but can also be utilized by those on more advanced stages. The novice hospital may not have many processes or procedures yet in place to support the journey, but are diligently working to establish what is needed.

An **ADVANCED BEGINNER** creative solution is for hospitals that have begun the journey and might have decided to seek Magnet designation, but are not yet ready to apply, and have identified gaps in their processes and practices with best practice standards. They generally are more process focused.

A **COMPETENT** creative solution is for hospitals that are well on their way on the journey, possibly seeking Magnet designation in the near future or have recently been designated, and have processes and practices in place, but are seeking to be more outcomes focused.

A **PROFICIENT** creative solution is for hospitals that have been on the journey for a while, and have probably achieved Magnet designation and are now looking toward redesignation. They are typically outcomes focused and looking to achieve even greater advances in nursing quality; and might be looking more globally to create a local environment of nursing excellence, sharing best practices and participating in multi-institutional learning opportunities.

An **EXPERT** creative solution is primarily for hospitals that are leading the journey to nursing excellence and have probably achieved Magnet designation and possibly redesignation; have been outcomes focused and have this focus enculturated into their institutional practices beyond just the nursing discipline. They are looking globally to create a regional milieu of nursing excellence, sharing best practices and coordinating research activities with other institutions; and are innovative and are continually creating standards of care.

FINANCIAL RESOURCES REQUIRED

$ = virtually no cost

$ $ = minimal financial resources (easily within budget)

$ $ $ = moderate financial resources (should be within budget, but may require reallocation of budget resources)

$ $ $ $ = substantial financial resources

$ $ $ $ $ = may require capital budget request

TIME RESOURCES REQUIRED

= requires virtually no time allotment

= requires minimal time allotment

= requires moderate time allotment

= requires substantial time allotment

= may require allotted FTE(s)

PERSONNEL RESOURCES REQUIRED

 = only nurse leader needed

 = nurse leader and small group of staff needed

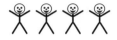 = nurse leader and possibly large or multiple groups of staff needed

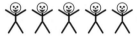 = requires nurse leader, possibly large or multiple groups of staff, and possibly additional personnel outside the unit (possibly other disciplines)

 = requires nurse leader, possibly large or multiple groups of staff, possibly additional personnel outside the unit, and possibly personnel outside the institution

OTHER RESOURCES REQUIRED

 = requires senior leadership backing

 = requires having an expert consultant or an expert on staff

 = requires special machinery

 = requires buy-in and approval of nursing management and leadership

 = requires ancillary department buy-in and approval

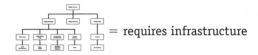 = requires infrastructure

 = requires special skill(s)

 = requires staff buy-in and approval

 = requires direct nurse leader and manager support

Grades for efficacy, transferability, malleability/adaptability, and ease of implementation:

A = excellent/easy

B = good/straightforward

C = fair/complicated

D = questionable/difficult

E = poor/very difficult

REFERENCE

Benner, P. (1984). *From novice to expert: Excellence and power in clinical nursing practice.* Menlo Park, CA: Addison-Wesley.

## CHAPTER 1

Creativity and Innovation

"To be creative you have to contribute something different from what you've done before. Your results need not be original to the world; few results truly meet that criterion. In fact, most results are built on the work of others."
—LYNNE C. LEVESQUE
BREAKTHROUGH CREATIVITY

"The best way to have a good idea is to have a lot of ideas."
—DR. LINUS PAULING

CREATIVITY AND INNOVATION

Ideas for free! Who would not want ideas for free? Well, they might not be all good ideas, but with a little scrutiny and development, you might have a winner—an idea that could change the way things are done, possibly improving patient care and the work environment; maybe even saving some money. This is what a hospital in northeast Philadelphia, PA, did to get free ideas. They realized they had a virtually untapped resource for great ideas: their bedside caregivers. Their goal was to find a way to harness this resource.

The hospital has an effective shared governance structure implemented and thought, "why not use what's already here and working?" A little brainstorming and they came up with something called the *Idea Line*. The Idea Line is actually a form on the hospital's intranet that anyone can fill out and submit with an idea, whether it be an idea to solve a problem or an idea to make something even better. The true innovation comes from the process they developed, from utilizing what was in place and realizing that technology could help.

The goal was to allow everyone to be able to submit ideas and to have these ideas placed in one repository. Suggestion boxes were considered, but for system-wide access, they were deemed impractical. So with the help of the Information Technology Department, they utilized internal e-mail for this idea form, which is accessible from any computer in the institution and after completed arrives at a specific e-mail address that the Chair of the Professional Development Council has access to. The Chair brings all ideas submitted to the Coordinating Council for review and consideration.

The Coordinating Council is made up of the chairs of all of the shared governance councils (all bedside caregivers) as well as nursing leadership. All ideas submitted are reviewed. Those that are considered impractical or unnecessary are noted, and the persons who submitted are thanked for their submissions and notified of the reasons their suggestions could not be implemented, thus closing the communication loop (an important consideration when designing a process such as this). If an idea is implemented, the person submitting it receives recognition and a small stipend as a thank-you. The Idea Line is well publicized internally with recognition and incentives to entice and achieve engagement. The Idea Line is a creative and innovative way of helping to change a culture of complaining about what is wrong to one of finding ways of solving problems. It is also a creative and innovative way to integrate creativity and innovation.

WHAT EXACTLY IS CREATIVITY?

Creativity is one of those terms that is easy to conceptualize, but a bit more difficult to define. We all know someone who is creative; someone who can create a culinary masterpiece from baking soda and a banana, or make an infection control poster that would make Martha Stewart proud. But what exactly are the skills, talents, abilities, or whatever you want to call them, that make up creativity? Can you teach someone to be creative, or is it innate and in one's genes? And, what does creativity have to do with nursing and quality patient care?

Our old friend Webster defines creativity as ". . . creative ability; artistic or intellectual inventiveness" (Agnes & Guralnik, 2008, p. 340). This definition makes creativity clearer, but still does not provide the skills or abilities to know whether we can teach, facilitate, or develop creativity. Webster then leads us in a circle by defining inventive as "creative" (p. 751). Inventiveness as we see it is seeing what could be, not what is (i.e., seeing new uses for things to solve problems and fulfill needs). It is taking some tape and a wooden spatula to make an impromptu splint when your neighbor falls and fractures her arm in your kitchen. It is using the technology available to automatically generate a reminder to practitioners to reevaluate a patient's need for the Foley catheter that has been in for 2 days to help prevent a urinary tract infection.

Creativity and innovation are by no means mutually exclusive. Instead, they overlap and are somewhat hierarchic. You can be creative without being innovative, but not vice versa. Innovation is defined as ". . . something newly introduced; new method, custom, device, etc." (p. 737). Innovation pushes creativity one step further. Innovation enables one to manipulate things and see new uses or processes that have never been tried before. Creativity is inherent in innovation. Because of this relationship, creativity and innovation seem to require the same basic skill set and abilities.

Nurses use creativity and innovation daily in their practice. If a nurse cannot get medications fast enough from the pharmacy, he or she might stash extras in a drawer for later use. Is this practice legal? No. Is it safe and appropriate? No. So why is it done? It is a work-around, a creative and sometimes innovative practice that bypasses an institution's established policies and practices to fulfill a patient care need not met through traditional channels. Every work-around is a manifestation of creativity, and may be truly innovative. Nurse leaders need to take this creativity and innovation and channel it into appropriate venues. Formal venues such as shared governance councils and informal venues such as staff brainstorming sessions can help to provide the structure necessary to make creativity and innovation productive for both nurses and the institution, ultimately improving patient care and solving problems with usable and safe solutions that meet regulatory, professional, and evidence-based standards.

In the book *Mavericks at Work*, authors Taylor and Labarre (2006) discuss how individuals have creatively developed frameworks that promote creativity and innovation, leading to ideas with lucrative solutions to seemingly unconquerable problems. As CEO of Goldcorp, Inc., Rob McEwen had a failing gold mine in the Red Lake district of northwest Ontario. From exploratory drilling, geologists estimated that there was a rich concentration of gold ore, but could not say how big the deposit was nor where drilling should occur to unearth the deposits. Placing this dilemma on the back burner for a bit, McEwen spent some time learning about trends in information technology at MIT. There he serendipitously learned about open-source software, software that is written by programmers, which no one owns the rights to, that many programmers use as a foundation to creatively develop innovative applications. McEwen then did something completely innovative. He saw this framework as one that he could use to spur the creativity and innovation needed to find the drilling strategies he needed to make the Red Lake district gold mine profitable.

McEwen then posted 50 years worth of the company's data on the mine on the Internet to entice scientists from all over the world to come up with practical drilling plans, harnessing the intellectual power of scientists from all over the world to creatively and innovatively solve Goldcorp's problems. As an incentive, McEwen created a contest. Judges would evaluate the submissions and choose the best, dividing prize money of $500,000 among 25 semifinalists and 3 finalists. Over 140 applications from 51 countries were received, which resulted in detailed drilling plans identifying twice the number of possible drilling sites than the Goldcorp geologists originally identified. In 2006, the Red Lake mine was considered the richest gold mine in the world. The creativity involved in finding a structure to facilitate creativity and innovation is exactly what nurse leaders need. Fortunately, you do not have to reinvent the wheel or develop a drilling prospectus; we are here to help.

Facilitating creativity and innovation in nurses may also help to enhance their critical thinking skills. And who does not want to enhance the critical thinking skills of nurses? Everyone from nurse educators to nurse administrators look for ways to enhance the critical thinking of nurses under their charge. The need for the ability of nurses to critically think is exemplified in the Rapid Response Team initiative recommended by the Institute for Healthcare Improvement's (IHI) "Saving 100,000 Lives" campaign (IHI, n.d.-a). Studies found that adult patients often show subtle signs of physiologic deterioration hours before a cardiopulmonary arrest (Buist et al., 1999; Hillman et al., 2001; Schein, Hazday, Pena, Ruben, & Sprung, 1990). The ability to act on these subtle signs quickly is at the heart of the Rapid Response Team initiative.

The Rapid Response Team is most commonly a team of nurses, physicians, and respiratory therapists who can be notified immediately to evaluate a patient if the nurse caring for that patient feels there is something that is "just not right," attempting to correct whatever may be happening with the patient before it escalates into a fatal event. Of course this process only works if the nurse recognizes and realizes that these subtle and nuanced signs are meaningful. This is where critical thinking is so important. It can truly make the difference between life and death.

THE ABILITY OF ORGANIZATIONS TO ADAPT

The ability of an organization to adapt is crucial to the organization's survival. As a whole, the organization or hospital, in this case, uses creative strategies and innovative methods to implement adaptation strategies. But adaptation does not merely occur as an overall hospital initiative. It trickles down, in some way, to every corner of the institution, affecting some areas more than others. As the hospital implements adaptation strategies, each department will also need to find strategies to adapt to the changes the hospital initiates. So as adaptation needs to enter every corner of the hospital, creativity and innovation are required as well.

Nurses are used to adaptation as it pertains to individual patients, how they adapt to their illnesses, and the strategies they use. Joan, recently diagnosed with diabetes, had to adapt to changes in diet and lifestyle, including checking her blood glucose before meals and taking medicines as scheduled. The need to adapt to diabetes outweighs her desire to continue the status quo, eating as she pleases without regard for the effect it has on her body. Joan knows that not adapting to the illness could be fatal. How she adapts, however, could minimize the impact of the illness on her life. Creative and innovative strategies and products like the medicine bottle that beeps as a reminder and scheduling work breaks around her blood glucose testing schedule can help.

We all remember Biology 101, where we learned about biologic adaptation in response to environmental changes i.e., survival of the fittest. The moth that has the wing color and pattern most like the pattern of tree bark has the best chance at camouflage to avoid predators, thus enabling it to pass the same genes on to its progeny. Anyone looking at the various patterns of wing colors and patterns and the advantages they provide to the different species of moths would have to admit that creativity and innovation is apparent. But unlike biologic adaptation, which seems to occur without intention, organizational adaptation requires planning, creativity, and innovation. This planning, creativity, and innovation needs to occur everywhere in the organization if adaptation is to be successful.

HOSPITALS ARE BUSINESSES

As much as healthcare providers try to ignore it, we cannot avoid the fact that hospitals are businesses. And as businesses, hospitals are just as susceptible to changes in the economic environment as other businesses. Granted, there are differences. Most hospitals are nonprofit, and most people do not pay for their health care out-of-pocket like we do for food or clothes. But these differences do not make the business of health care any easier to understand. Many times these differences actually make the economic environment more complex and adaptation to changes in this environment becomes more difficult. And, of course, in health care, economics affects everything, from staffing to the products and technology used to deliver care.

Creativity and innovation can have a huge impact on the financial outlays of a hospital and can affect its ability to adapt to environmental changes. The "Call to Action" program at a southern New Jersey hospital saved hundreds of thousands of dollars by developing creative and innovative ways to cut hospital costs by creating less waste and by maximizing productivity. In one project, a nurse noticed that most nurses took too many supplies into each patient's room when performing wound care. Further investigation determined the reason: Nurses did not have the time to travel back and forth to the supply closet if more supplies were needed. The solution that was developed was simple, creative, and innovative: a wound care cart to mobilize supplies, making them readily available for each patient. From this single project, nurses reduced both the cost of health care and the time they spend hunting and gathering supplies, saving the hospital money and allowing more time for direct patient care (Matlack, 2009).

THE FAST PACE OF HEALTH CARE

Within the past 40 years, health care has changed drastically. The 1970s saw years of excess: Health care as a business was booming and consumers could get care when and where they wished. Hospitals made money, physicians made money, and consumers received care. Everyone was happy, with the exception of those paying for health care, the insurers, and the federal government. In 2001, the US national health expenditures rose to 14.1% of the nation's gross domestic product (GDP), with healthcare spending reaching $1.4 trillion (Levit et al., 2003). But we are paying for the best health care in the world, are we not? Well, before the World Health Organization started ranking the quality of nations' healthcare systems in 2000, we really did not know. So throughout the 1970s, 1980s, and 1990s we were paying a lot for health care, and did not know if we were getting our money's worth. Furthermore, costs were not stable; they were increasing at an alarming rate. Something had to be done.

The past 4 decades have been devoted to trying to lower costs and ensure quality in health care. This effort continues today, and there is no real sense that we have made many improvements. In 2007, the total spending for health care in the United States was $2.4 trillion, 17% of GDP (Keehan et al., 2008). The World Heath Organization (WHO, 2000) states, "The US health system spends a higher portion of its gross domestic product than any other country but ranks 37 out of 191 countries according to its performance . . ." (para. 4). But the news is not all bad. There is a new paradigm in tackling this problem. The thought was that a top-down approach could solve the problem, that national policy could deliver the cost-effective care we sought.

Some of the most significant changes over the last 40 years have come from grass roots efforts started by local organizations and institutions that took the challenge of developing cost-effective care personally. These organizations used creativity and innovation to create and develop new processes to deliver cost-effective care. We see pockets of this cost-effective health care within our nation. The Cleveland Clinic in Ohio and the Mayo Clinic in Minnesota are two healthcare systems that demonstrate that we can achieve cost-effective and quality health care (Naymik & Tribble, 2009). These pockets of cost-effective, quality health care provide encouragement and hope, but also guidance that can assist other healthcare institutions in creatively adapting principles, processes, and innovations to deliver more cost-effective health care.

Technology

The increase in technology use and advances in technology have made a huge impact on healthcare delivery and the incredible pace with which changes occur. Technology impacts quality of care, quality of life, and the cost-effectiveness of health care. Improvements in diagnostic capabilities and treatments have led to increases in longevity and decreases in morbidity. For example, laser technology has been used to perform surgery with less trauma than the typical manual surgery and has a shorter postsurgical recovery time (American Society for Dermatologic Surgery, 2008). Technology has allowed many of those with disabilities to lead better lives. It has allowed treatment of previously untreatable terminal illnesses such as diabetes, end-stage renal disease, and AIDS. Technology has permitted pharmaceutic breakthroughs to treat heart disease, cancer, and AIDS. New, creative, and innovative technologies have resulted in new ways of delivering treatments like transdermal patches infused with opiates, which have significantly increased our ability to manage chronic pain (Applied Data Research, 2009).

Technology is growing by leaps and bounds, not just within health care, but in other disciplines as well. To a moderate extent, technology within other disciplines drives changes in health care. For example, bar coding has been around for quite a while in the retail market. Its creative and innovative use, applied in health care to deliver inpatient medications and enhance patient safety, is an example of the transferability of technology and the need to look at all new technology with innovative eyes, seeing how it can benefit patient care (Hook, Pearlstein, Samarth, & Cusack, 2008).

Regulations

Ask anyone currently working in health care about The Joint Commission and the Centers for Medicare and Medicaid Services (CMS) and they will most likely become contemplative and use politically correct speech. They may also become a little more emotional and decry the multitude of regulations that grow in number each year by leaps and bounds. The core measures, a measure of hospital process compliance with specific evidence-based protocols implemented by CMS, began as a trial project to enhance hospital compliance through payment incentives. The core measures now consist of 30 compliance measures (indicators) and the list is expected to grow larger (Eramo, 2008). Compliance is no longer rewarded, it is expected. Hospitals that do not report these quality measures are financially penalized.

Regulatory requirements were not created to simply make life miserable for healthcare administrators, but sometimes it seems that way. We all acknowledge that these requirements are meant to enhance patient safety and the quality of patient care, although sometimes the connection between these requirements and patient care seem vague. However, regulatory requirements cannot be ignored. And with the growth in regulatory requirements comes the need to meet more and more operational and practice standards. Unfortunately, with each new standard there is no new revenue source, which means hospitals have to meet these requirements with the same fiscal resources. To do this, hospitals need to be creative and innovative. Many have redesigned processes and realized greater efficiency in the need to meet these requirements. Meeting these requirements has also enhanced the quality of hospital care.

Since the Institute of Medicine's (IOM) groundbreaking report, *To Err is Human: Building a safer health system* (1999), the elusive formula to ensure healthcare quality has been sought. What has been found is not so much the formula for quality, but the realization that there might be many formulas for achieving quality.

This is a new paradigm, a view that says there is not only one way of doing something to achieve desired quality outcomes. This view should not be taken to mean that anything goes, or to forget the need for evidence-based practices. It merely says that standards and evidence-based practices can occur in a variety of processes and practices, thus asserting that there are many paths to quality care. This paradigm has fostered the need for creativity and innovation to construct a formula for quality within the various constraints of the healthcare system and the limitations and considerations imposed by an institution's own resources and culture.

Expectations

Patient expectations are also rapidly changing. With the drive for transparency in hospital information and the accessibility of this information to the media and the public, patients are aware of the quality of care in specific institutions and its variability among institutions. Many realize that they now have a choice of where to receive their care, not based solely on their physician's or their family's recommendations, but based on objective measures of compliance with quality indicators such as the core measures, which is easily obtained from the web at www.hospitalcompare.hhs.gov.

Unanticipated healthcare needs can also call for creativity and innovation. Many nurses become like MacGyver when faced with unanticipated healthcare needs, creating new processes and innovating new uses for common materials to meet whatever needs arise. On a larger scale, from experiences such as Hurricane Katrina, we know that mass emergencies rarely play out as practice drills do. There are so many variables and factors involved that anticipating, addressing, and preparing for each one would be impossible and unmanageable. We can prepare for the probable, and facilitate creativity and innovation to meet unexpected needs. That is not to say that we should not try to prepare for every possible scenario, it is just doubtful that everything possible can be anticipated. The immediacy of healthcare emergencies makes creativity and innovation necessary skills.

There are also the expectations of nursing from society, which has led to some very creative and innovative academic degrees and job descriptions. Society expects nursing to play the role of coordinator of care to a greater extent than ever before. To help nurses fulfill this expectation, a new course of study and job description has been developed, the Clinical Leader. The Clinical Leader program is a master's degree program designed to educate nurses on the coordination of care throughout a patient's stay, emphasizing quality of care, appropriateness of treatment, and expected length of stay through interdepartmental coordination and collaboration. As a job, the Clinical Leader takes a leadership position within their designated unit, providing clinical care and ensuring each patient's care is managed appropriately (American Association of Colleges of Nursing, 2008).

INITIATIVES INTEGRATING CREATIVITY AND INNOVATION

The Magnet Recognition Program

The Magnet program has been around since 1994, administrated by the American Nurses Credentialing Center (ANCC), an affiliate of the American Nurses Association (ANA) (ANCC, 2009). For those of you unaware or unfamiliar with the Magnet program, here is a brief overview. The Magnet program uses an evidence-based framework to evaluate healthcare institutions as environments where quality health care is provided. The program is based on research done in the 1980s, which sought to determine the factors common to hospitals that retained and even attracted other nurses during the devastating nursing shortage. These hospitals had some distinct similarities, and their characteristics were analyzed and grouped into 14 categories. These categories are known as the Forces of Magnetism, and provide the framework and standards for evaluating the quality of a healthcare institution's people, processes, and outcomes. Currently, only approximately 6% of hospitals nationwide have earned Magnet designation.

Although distinct, the 14 forces are not mutually exclusive. Forces overlap, demonstrating the interconnectedness of healthcare practices. In an effort to decrease redundancy in the application process and create a simple overarching framework, in 2009, the ANCC created a new Magnet model, grouping the original 14 forces in 5 components: Structural Empowerment; Transformational Leadership; New Knowledge, Innovations, and Improvements; Exemplary Professional Practice; and Empirical Outcomes (ANCC, 2008). Creativity and innovation are infused throughout the Magnet framework, featured most prominently in the New Knowledge, Innovation, and Improvements component. Here, the importance of creativity and innovation are emphasized through specific standards such as "(d)escribe and demonstrate (i)nnovations in nursing practice" (ANCC, 2008, p. 33) that institutions under evaluation must demonstrate to meet designation requirements. Creativity and innovation are not merely encouraged by the Magnet program, they are expected.

Transforming Care at the Bedside

Transforming Care at the Bedside, or TCAB as it is affectionately known, is an initiative originated by the Robert Wood Johnson Foundation to promote creativity and innovation at the bedside, where care is provided. Through this model, all caregivers are challenged to incorporate quality improvement methodology into their daily bedside care, making small creative, and innovative process and practice changes that can lead to large improvements in patient care. TCAB uses a rapid-cycle PDSA (plan, do, study, act) methodology to provide a framework for the change process (Rutherford, Lee, & Greiner, 2004; Robert Wood Johnson

Foundation, 2008). Both the speed of the process and its ease of use make the rapid-cycle PDSA the ideal framework for the TCAB initiative. However, some caution must be taken. In some ways, the rapid-cycle PDSA process sacrifices rigor for speed and ease of use, so one must be careful to find a balance among utility, facility, and rigor, always keeping the desired outcomes in mind.

Creativity and innovation are at the heart of TCAB. Their motto, "steal shamelessly," speaks volumes about their goal to have bedside nurses creatively find and adapt innovative practices to better patient care, no matter where the ideas originate. Use the ideas to your advantage. Do not recreate the wheel. It appears that the authors of this book and the TCAB initiative creators have much in common.

Other National Initiatives

Many other national initiatives have focused on specific goals and outcomes, challenging institutions to come up with their own processes and practices for achieving them. The Institute for Healthcare Improvement's (IHI) 100,000 Lives campaign charged healthcare institutions with creating innovative practices to save the 100,000 lives annually lost to medical errors and failure to rescue. "Based on data collected over several years from multiple partner institutions, IHI estimates that nearly 15 million instances of medical harm occur in the US each year—a rate of over 40,000 per day" (IHI, n.d.-b, para. 3). Based on this data, one of the initiatives, the "rapid response" team, was developed and is now an industry standard. Although the rapid response team takes many different forms in different institutions, its goal is the same, to ensure the safe and timely care of the patient. The various forms of the team represent the creativity that institutions demonstrate in meeting the goal. IHI estimates that 122,000 lives have been saved in 18 months of the campaign (IHI, n.d.-b). Ahhh, the power of innovation!

National Patient Safety Goals, created and endorsed by The Joint Commission, are additional examples of using the creativity and innovation of each hospital to achieve specific outcomes, in this case, national goals to enhance patient safety (Agency for Healthcare Research and Quality, 2008). The goals were established, but each hospital has free reign in developing the policies and practices it implements to meet these goals. Luckily there are some methods that work for a number of hospitals. These are sometimes called best practices and are similar in concept to the creative solutions found in this volume. Best practices can guide hospitals in the process of achieving desired outcomes, again eliminating the reinventing the wheel situation, which wastes both time and money.

One might say the ultimate in incentivizing creativity and innovation comes from the federal government, specifically the Centers for Medicare and Medicaid Services (CMS). CMS defined what are known as "never events." These are nosocomial events that CMS believes should never occur such as patient falls, hospital-acquired pressure ulcers, and surgery on the wrong part of the body. These are only of a few of those proposed. Although many of those proposed are hotly debated by healthcare administrators as to their classification as never events, CMS will no longer reimburse hospitals for the additional hospital care of Medicare and Medicaid patients who acquire many of these conditions (CMS, 2006).

Hospitals are frantically trying to lessen or eliminate these events from occurring in the patients to whom they provide care. Of course, eliminating these events will increase the quality of patient care, just what CMS is hoping to do. Some hospital administrators also believe health care may be negatively affected. By decreasing reimbursement for these events, hospitals will have that much less fiscal resource to provide quality care to patients. The decreased reimbursement could mean a death sentence to hospitals on the edge of bankruptcy. Where does the creativity and innovation come into play? Well, how do you think hospitals are going to reduce and hopefully eliminate these never events? There is no magic formula, and current strategies are not enough. Creativity and innovation are needed to use each hospital's resources to the fullest and to find methods that work with each hospital's distinct culture.

Partnerships with Manufacturers

More and more institutions are partnering with manufacturers and suppliers to create innovative products that specifically meet institutional needs. This relationship is beneficial to the institution in a number of ways. Most apparent is that the institution gets a custom-made product, designed with the institution's distinct needs in mind. Secondly, nurses become intimately involved in the process of innovation using evaluative and critical thinking skills throughout the process. Suppliers and manufacturers benefit in various ways as well. Now known as a nurse-friendly company, word of mouth in the healthcare community may increase their business and allow them to parlay the innovative product changes into a product that dominates the market in essence, using this partnership as a mini research and development (R&D) department, again, a creative and innovative way to ultimately better patient care with a product that enhances and facilitates patient care delivery.

TOOLS, TECHNIQUES, AND RESOURCES FOR FACILITATING CREATIVITY AND INNOVATION

Brainstorming

Brainstorming is probably the most recognized technique for finding creative and innovative solutions to specific improvement opportunities. It is pretty much a self-explanatory process. Get a group together. Present them with a problem, and ask them to creatively solve it. Now you can make this session as formal or casual as you would like. If you have members of the group who are shy, you may want to require each member of the group to provide some input and assure, through appropriate facilitation, that members feel comfortable voicing their opinions and ideas. There are some more specific techniques for more specific needs.

How to Facilitate Brainstorming

- Know the Four Ground Rules for Brainstorming (Osborn, 1963).
- Focus on the quantity of submissions, not the quality. The more ideas generated, the greater the probability that a plausible, creative, and innovative solution will be found.
- Do not criticize ideas. Anything is acceptable and up for consideration. Later in the process, the group will help eliminate implausible ideas.
- Welcome the "out of the box" ideas. These ideas may demonstrate new ways of thinking about the problem at hand. Participants should feel free and uninhibited to submit ideas.
- During the process of facilitating brainstorming, consider combining and improving ideas. Many times combining ideas and interventions can lead to synergy, "(t)he interaction of two or more agents . . . so that their combined effect is greater than the sum of their individual effects" ("Synergy," n.d.).
- Set the stage. Tell the group the process of what you are going to do and the goal—to get as many ideas as you can. All ideas are welcome. Tell the group the background of the issue and explicitly define the problem. Assure the group that their ideas will not be criticized. You are looking for the most ideas possible.
- Pass out slips of paper and ask participants to write each idea, no matter how plausible, on one piece of paper anonymously. Here you may want to require a minimum number of submissions to nudge those shy individuals and facilitate participation.
- Collect the papers and write each idea on a flip chart and with the help of the group, eliminate repetitive ideas and consolidate similar submission.

You now have a set of creative and innovative ideas to address the problem presented. You can then facilitate the choice of which idea(s) to implement by using one of many techniques, such as multivoting.

Multivoting

Multivoting is a technique to reduce the number of plausible solutions after a brainstorming session. First, decide on the number of solutions you want to be left with. Number each solution submitted. Decide how many choices each member can vote for. The usual number is five. Now, on a piece of paper, each member individually selects the five items he thinks are most important and ranks the choices in order of merit (1 = greatest merit). Write all the rankings next to each choice. Look for a consensus of items that are most important and those that a majority of the group feels has the most merit. Shorten the list to the top choices. If still too many choices are listed, use multivoting again, but reduce the number of choices each member has until the number of desired solutions are obtained.

Asking Questions

Asking the five Ws and H: **W**ho, **w**hat, **w**hen, **w**here, **w**hy, and **h**ow is a common technique for initiating thoughts and conversation about a topic, issue, or problem. It probes the breadth of the issue and creates the framework in which the issue exists. This technique is a creative way of gathering information about a problem or situation to be explored. From this information, it might be easier to identify the cause of a problem and help in finding the solution. Another technique is asking your group "Wouldn't it be nice if . . .?" and "Wouldn't it be awful if . . .?" These are two ways of identifying desirable outcomes and obstacles that you need to overcome. Asking "In what way might . . ." can be useful in identifying various things that could occur if an idea were put into practice.

Mind Mapping/Concept Mapping

Mind mapping is another technique that can be used to generate, visualize, structure, and classify ideas to help with organizing, problem solving, and decision making. Some may be familiar with the term concept mapping, an analogue of mind mapping, which is relatively popular in nursing. Concept mapping is used in nursing to "promote critical thinking, improve problem-solving skills and foster understanding of the interrelationships among patient's health concerns . . ." (Hicks-Moore, 2005, p. 348). A concept map is just what it implies, a map that visually displays the relationships among a set of related concepts and ideas. When constructing a concept map, the group can reflect on things they know and things they do not know, determining what may be needed to better understand the problem under consideration. There are five steps to creating a concept map:

- The first step requires that the group involved is given a topic or problem to consider and the group then makes a list of facts, terms, and ideas that are in any way associated with the topic or problem. Do not worry about how important the item is. Just write all contributions on individual note cards. You want to generate the most facts, terms, and ideas as you can.
- In the second step, spread out your many note cards and organize them with the help of the participants into groups and subgroups of related items. You can still collect more ideas, if more are realized during the organization

process. Some of the concepts may fall into more than one group, and that is okay.

- In step three, you and the group try to come up with an arrangement that best represents the relationships between and among the identified groups. Put the most important concepts in the center and work outward, placing the most closely related groups and subgroups near to each other. There is no one right map. This is dependent on your participants, their understanding, and their insight.
- The fourth step consists of a final agreement on the arrangement and drawing lines with arrows to correct the groups and subgroups showing the relationships between connected items. You can have more than one arrow start or end on a group or subgroup; it depends on your relationships.
- The last step is simply a matter of finalizing the concept map by achieving agreement that the arrangement of items conveys your participants' understanding of the initial concept or problem. You can now make the concept map permanent so that others may use and discuss it, possibly igniting their creativity and innovation in finding possible solutions to the problem posed.

Other Techniques

In his book *Thinkertoys*, Michael Michalko (2006) describes various techniques for unleashing creativity. Many of his techniques may be useful for nurse leaders attempting to enhance creativity and innovation. One technique in particular seems a good fit. He calls this technique *Cherry Split* and describes the process as follows. State the problem in two words. Then, split each of the words in two separate concepts. For example, the problem "prevent UTIs (urinary tract infections)" is split and then each word or concept is split further. No two people will split the concepts the same way. That is where creativity plays a key role. You continue splitting concepts further until you feel there are enough concepts to spark some thought. Then look at each concept and brainstorm for ideas. Think about how some of these concepts might be addressed and what possible interventions might help. What you are attempting to do here is a type of controlled word association and help group members see a problem in a new way, making the problem appear fresh and new. A new problem may lead to a new solution (Figure 1-1).

FACILITATION

This is probably the most useful place to discuss facilitation. The 'nurse leader as facilitator' is by no means a radical new idea. The whole concept of transformational leadership, a style of management many nurse leaders aspire to achieve

Figure 1-1   Example of "Cherry Split."

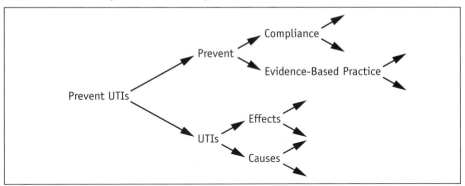

is founded on nurse leaders as facilitators. It is difficult, however, to get many nurse leaders to buy into the facilitator role with any more than a superficial nod. Most seem unable to easily adapt to facilitator role, possibly because most nurses are hands on, used to having significant control over most situations. Also, most nurses were educated in a transactional environment; do this, this, and this and you get an A. Facilitation skills are rarely taught in nursing education, yet they are so necessary for working in a multidisciplinary, multihierarchical environment such as a hospital or healthcare system.

There are distinct principles and actions for facilitation, but more so, facilitation is a frame of mind, a paradigm for problem solving, playing a role where control is achieved through indirect influence and mediation. The goal is not to get a group to do what you want them to do, but more globally, to help the group through the problem-solving process, reaching consensus on a viable and palatable solution. This frame of mind is often contrary to the overwhelming need to just get things done, and done correctly (depending upon what your view of correctly is). Nursing occurs in a fast-paced environment and as anyone working in health care can attest to, constant change has become the norm. The increasing pressure for nurse leaders to get things done sends a message that transactional methods are needed. Yet, most senior nursing leadership and nursing scholars verbalize the merits of becoming a transformational leader, definitely giving mixed messages to an audience looking for prescriptive advice. Of course, experienced nurse leaders know that you cannot be transformational without being transactional to some extent. You just need to find a balance.

We believe the discomfort with business concepts in nursing comes from the history of nursing as a vocation, a calling, and the core of nursing as pure altruistic caring. Business is characterized by many, if not totally uncaring, more like an indifferent series of mechanical transactions. The heat of the passion of pure caring in nursing, when combined with the coldness of indifference in business, causes some to fret that the combining will produce a lukewarm environment of nursing as a business, negatively affecting the nurse–patient relationship.

Most nurse leaders have little, if any, formal education in management and leadership. This was always the realm of the discipline of business, not nursing. The realization that health care is a business and nurses are a part of this business has caused distress to some, and to others, a new realization for the need to integrate business skills and concepts into nursing practice. Facilitation is one of those skills. Facilitation is necessary in a shared governance environment and any environment where decisions affecting many disciplines are made. So to recap, facilitation skills are necessary. Facilitation skills are needed. Facilitation skills are not typically taught in nursing school, so do not feel like you are the only one without these skills. And, the good news is that understanding the purpose of facilitation, its goals, and the role of the facilitator, is the most crucial ingredient for becoming a good facilitator.

Volumes have been written on the art and science of facilitation. As a science, there are structural practices necessary for facilitation to occur as well as practices shown to enhance the process. As an art, the facilitator brings his/her personality, culture, language, knowledge, and skills to the facilitator role, enhancing or detracting from the experience. For simplicity's sake, we have decided to group the components of facilitation into a few categories. See if this helps you understand facilitation a bit better.

Components of Facilitation

The first component involves those structural and procedural dos and don'ts that are common in many articles and books about facilitation (Shepard, 2003).

These are things like:

- Help everyone to participate in the discussion.
- Ask good open questions that get the participants thinking.
- Keep discussion on track and keep to the agenda and goal.
- Create a safe place for discussion; there is no hierarchy.
- Mediate situations when needed. Stop a discussion before escalation occurs.
- Develop trust in the process and in each other.
- Keep team members aligned with previous agreements made.
- Use creative and innovative ways to encourage everyone to participate
- Pay attention to body language: 90% of communication is nonverbal.
- Make clear what group members are saying. Restate what the group is saying to make it clear to everyone.
- Do not lecture others.
- Do not just consider facts alone. Emotions are important.

- Do not dominate the discussion.
- Do not answer the questions yourself. Allow the group to come up with answers.
- Do not permit personal criticism. The issues discussed should never solicit personal attacks (Sanderbeck, 2006/2007).

The second component of facilitation is the specific techniques used to reach your goals. We have given a sampling, such as brainstorming and concept mapping. We suggest that you go down to your local bookstore and check out the business section. You will most likely find volumes on group facilitation that will provide various tried and true techniques, and maybe some that are a bit experimental. Try what feels comfortable. Everyone has a different style. One way to learn new facilitation techniques is to observe others when they facilitate. When we attend meetings or conferences, we are always bringing back some techniques to try. Not every technique works for everyone with every audience in every situation, so you need to critically appraise what you will feel comfortable using, and what looks like it might be successful. Then, try it out in a situation and with a group it would be most favorable. Do not confuse technique with style. You may see a very demonstrative and gregarious facilitator that uses techniques you thought good, but you are not a demonstrative and gregarious facilitator. Try the techniques anyway; just modify them for your style. They may not all work, but facilitation is as much an art as a science, and with the art, a level of unpredictability is natural.

Reflection and debriefing are the third component of facilitation and possibly the most important. Debriefing in this situation consists of utilizing someone in the audience, possibly a friend or colleague who can give you constructive feedback. Spend a little time as soon as possible after the meeting to discuss what went well, and what did not go so well. The next step is using their information in self-reflection to contemplate how to better facilitate next time, possibly discontinuing ineffective techniques and employing some new techniques. Of course you will not always be able to have a friend or colleague in the audience. As you get more experience with facilitation, you will be able to better read the audience and better determine through self-reflection what facilitation techniques did and did not work, minimizing the need for debriefing with a colleague. However, if a colleague is available, it is always preferential to ask for a debriefing session.

STRUCTURES AND PROCESSES FOR FACILITATING CREATIVITY AND INNOVATION

There are many ways to facilitate creativity and innovation within a healthcare institution, but without the appropriate structures and processes, the creativity and innovation will never be encultured into your institution and become a regular part of how things are done. The culture of an institution is key to setting standards and establishing norms, and an institution's culture can affect patient and staff satisfaction as well as the quality of patient care. Establishing appropriate structures and processes are essential to promote and enculturate creativity and innovation.

Culture as defined in *Webster's Unabridged Dictionary* (2001) is "the quality in a person or society that arises from a concern for what is regarded as excellent . . ." (p. 488). To make creativity and innovation regarded as excellent, it needs to be valued, promoted, and integrated. Only then will it grow and eventually become enculturated. There are many creative and innovative ways to integrate creativity and innovation into your institution's culture. (Sounds a bit repetitive, we know!) The following are but a few.

Job Descriptions

Integrating expectations for creativity into formal processes and institutional documents emphasizes their importance to the institution and demonstrates that it is expected of its employees. What better place to start than the job description, and not just the nursing job description, but every employee's job description. This expectation then becomes a standard for all employees. Let us not forget that any set standard must have a corresponding evaluation to assure individuals are meeting the standard. To assure employees are meeting the standard set forth in the job description for creativity and innovation, it must be a part of their periodic evaluation, linked to a merit salary increase or merit bonus. Linking creativity and innovation to merit increases sends a clear message that, in Webster's words, creativity and innovation are ". . . regarded as excellent . . ." (2001, p. 488). We are not being judgmental or demeaning when we say that, in general, what is linked to money (salary, bonus, etc.) is what gets noticed. Not to say that there are not those employees for whom money is secondary and the fulfillment they get from their work is their primary motivation. However, we believe this is not the norm, and one would be wise to believe that linking a standard such as the expectation for creativity and innovation to salary and bonus will help to get buy-in from employees as well as help to enculturate the standard. So how do you do this? The first thing that needs to be done is to operationalize the standard. How will you measure if employees are being creative and innovative? You might require them to submit a specific number of creative and innovative suggestions for bettering patient care or improving the work environment. Possibly add an additional incentive if one of their ideas is implemented.

The Clinical Ladder

Most nurses are familiar with the clinical ladder, a program that encourages bedside nurses to expand their skills and acquire new ones while maintaining their presence at the bedside. Typically, clinical ladders have various levels, graduated in difficulty and commitment with corresponding monetary incentives. It is touted by many as a way to increase the professionalism in nursing and encourage the professional development of nurses (Loyola University Medical Center, n.d.; NYU Lagone Medical Center, 2009; University Medical Center, n.d.). By its nature, the clinical ladder is an excellent venue to integrate creativity and innovation. For example, a community hospital in northeast Philadelphia has a requirement that nurses applying for a certain level of the clinical ladder complete one patient care or workplace related improvement project on their unit. The project must be creative and innovative, required only to be practical and show positive outcomes. In this exemplar, the clinical ladder program serves as both a mechanism to integrate creativity and innovation and a way to incentivize it. The clinical ladder program itself can be as creative and innovative as one would like. Using it strategically, however, can assist the nursing department in meeting its strategic goals, possibly one is Magnet recognition, and help to set the standard and enculturate the expectation.

Employee Meetings

Employee town hall meetings are another venue where creativity and innovation can be emphasized and its expectation within the institution strengthened. Employee town hall meetings are typically intermittent meetings open to all staff, led by senior leadership, to update staff on the institution's financial status and strategic plans. Staff questions and concerns are voiced, rumors clarified, and opportunities for improvement noted.

Senior leadership can ask that meeting attendees come prepared with creative and innovative solutions to the problems they see or ask, at the meeting, for creative and innovative suggestions to concerns voiced; thus, giving staff a voice in how the institution better meets its mission by meeting the needs of patients and employees. Underlying these requests from senior leadership is a subtle message that creativity and innovation are welcome and expected; sending a message that everyone's ideas are important, and that if you find an opportunity for improvement, you have also found an opportunity to be creative and innovative.

Having staff involvement in strategic planning sessions and retreats sends a clear message that their creative and innovative input is expected and necessary for the institution. Ownership seems to be an impetus for action and engagement. It is the phenomenon seen by many; for example, the difference between owning or renting a home. A homeowner is much more likely to fix up their home than a renter and keep it maintained, partly so it will retain its value, but also for the pride that comes with a well maintained home. It says something about the owner,: that he or she cares about the house. It is a reflection of his or her tastes and his or her priorities. It is the same with one's employment. Creating a sense of ownership in employees will increase their engagement in the hospital's accomplishments. Soliciting creative and innovative ideas will help develop this sense of employee ownership. It gives employees a belief that they can make change and add value to the institution. They then feel empowered and valued, which may promote additional creative solutions and innovations, truly a self-perpetuating cycle.

Performance Improvement

The performance improvement (PI) department in your hospital can also facilitate creativity and innovation. The PI department is constantly looking at quality indicators for trends, both good and not so good. A quality indicator trending in the wrong direction is the perfect impetus for tapping the creativity and innovative abilities of those staff affected. After PI identifies a need to improve a quality indicator, they can then solicit ideas from staff to creatively implement an evidence-based practice or, if no best practice exists, solicit innovative ideas for intentions to improve quality indicators gone awry. Throughout the PI and evidence-based practice (EBP) processes, creativity and innovation are necessary for the development of interventions and the translation and implementation of these interventions to meet the institution's needs and match its culture. The more this creativity and innovation can be developed, the easier the process of translation and implementation will be, developing critical thinking skills along the way.

Ideas from the Bedside

Cannot nursing leadership just generate the ideas? Do we really need to involve staff nurses? Nursing leadership is removed from the bedside, and rightfully so. They play a key role in facilitating patient care. They assure that necessary resources are available and allocated appropriately, that standards of practice are met, that fiscal stewardship is considered, and that the environment is safe for patients, families, and employees. They are specialists in management, but no longer specialists in patient care. These specialists are the bedside caregivers. The bedside caregivers know the needs of their patients, and they are the ones to carry out whatever is necessary to achieve quality patient care. It is only logical then that these caregivers are the ones to help construct and implement creative and innovative processes and practices that continually improve care and the work environment. Their creativity and innovation is already present, seen frequently in what we healthcare workers know as work-arounds, those creative and innovative process and practices not sanctioned by nursing leadership, but to the bedside caregiver, necessary to deliver appropriate care under current working conditions. Many nurse leaders see work-arounds as a negative, a blatant insubordination, directly counter to established policies and practices. Maybe we need to change this paradigm. Work-arounds are a clear message to nurse leaders that a policy or practice does not work in the current environment and needs to be reconsidered. It also shows that creativity and innovation are alive and well at the bedside. So we have turned the negative work-around to a positive opportunity to create effective policy and funnel the demonstrated creativity and innovation into more appropriate endeavors.

Involving bedside caregivers in creating, developing, and implementing quality initiatives also enhances buy-in because the ones who developed the new practices are the ones who will perform the new practices. It is their idea, and they own it. They now have a vested interest in its success. It is no longer a mindless following of directions, but a planning of what will work to achieve the goal and facilitate the workflow. This is the bottom-up approach. Many are more familiar with the typical top-down approach where senior leaders meet and decide on a policy or just one leader, possibly the chief nursing officer (CNO) or director of nursing creates the policy with little input sans his or her own anec-dotal experience and forces everyone to comply, no matter how inane the policy might be or how badly it meshes with current policy and practice or culture. The bottom-up approach has a number of advantages over the top-down approach. Aside from the increased buy-in as stated previously, bedside caregivers can cre-atively achieve better results than the top-down directive through the input and experience of many, providing a richer database, if you will, for what works and what does not. Bedside caregivers see not just the typical situation where the directive or policy would apply, but also the possibility of deviations from the typical, providing variant situations for consideration. Considering the pos-sible variant situations and accounting for them prior to implementation can save time, money, effort, and staff buy-in. A clinically or culturally unworkable policy invites work-arounds, just the thing the policy is trying to prevent. When it comes to developing practices and policies to enhance quality, the more input from bedside caregivers, the better, and not just input. Allow them to own the policy and procedure. With leadership guidance, facilitation, and support, the product (policy, program, practice) developed from the bottom-up approach will far surpass top-down direction.

With all of the benefits the bottom-up approach can bring, why then is the top-down approach used? We will answer briefly, saying that the historic paradigm of management is extremely hierarchic: Those in higher positions know better and make better decisions. This paradigm also proclaims that control should and must be in the hands of those high in the management hierarchy. Over the past few decades, this paradigm is shifting. The benefits of the bottom-up approach have been demonstrated time and time again. In this new paradigm, leaders are seen not so much as decision makers but more as facilitators who help their staff to make decisions that are best for their clients as well as for the work environ-ment. The belief is that those who interact frequently with clients know best what clients need and want, and what policies and procedures create a work environment conducive to achieving company goals. You might say, "Okay, I believe you and will gladly heed your advice." We would say, "Wow, we're more convincing than we thought." But, do not just take our word for it. It is advice that is found in many quality enhancing programs and initiatives.

The Magnet program is built on a foundation of shared decision making, typically through a shared governance framework. This framework prescribes that decision making in most circumstance occurs through a structure where bedside caregivers are well represented and drive the decision-making process. Of course there are decisions that only senior leadership can and should make, but typically decisions concerning patient care, patient care delivery, and workforce satisfaction can be made through the shared-governance frameworks with leadership support and guidance. If this all sounds like some utopia, trust us, it is not. It is incredibly difficult to achieve a state where staff engagement is rampant and consistent. But from all reports, when achieved, it can have major effects on enhancing quality and bettering patient outcomes. Many look at the financial resources necessary to achieve this and cringe. Currently, studies are investigating the relationship between shared decision making and patient outcomes. Although anecdotal evidence abounds, statistical analysis will eventually demonstrate, we believe, the benefits to patient outcomes of creative innovation from the bedside.

We cannot emphasize enough the benefit of obtaining these creative and innovative ideas from nurses at the bedside. Bedside practitioners are closest to the point of care delivery and know and understand what patients want and need. These practitioners are faced daily with situations where there is no established policy, no best practice procedures; situations where it is necessary to think on your feet. Creativity and innovation are daily nursing practices, necessary to perform in today's complex healthcare environment.

CREATIVE SOLUTIONS

Creative Solution Title: *Idea Line*

Creative Solution Author: **Bruce Alan Boxer, PhD, MBA, RN, CPHQ**
Director of Quality/Magnet Program Director
South Jersey Healthcare, Vineland, NJ
Former Evidence-Based Practice Coordinator
Aria Health/Frankford Hospitals
Philadelphia, PA

Purpose: The goal of this project is to create a mechanism to facilitate and encourage creativity and innovation, and utilize creative and innovative ideas to better patient care and the work environment.

Legend

Overall Rating: **ADVANCED BEGINNER**

Financial:

Time:

Personnel:

Other Resources: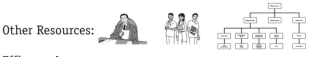

Efficacy: **A**

Transferability: **A**

Malleability/Adaptability: **B**

Ease of Implementation: **B**

Synopsis: See Chapter Introduction

Description of Organization: Aria Health (formerly Frankford Hospitals) is a healthcare system consisting of three hospitals and various outpatient services located in northeast Philadelphia, PA. They are currently not a Magnet-designated facility.

The Case Study: Aria Health has a mature shared-governance structure and has been on the journey to nursing excellence for a while. The nursing department embraces the voice of bedside caregivers and wanted to provide a venue where bedside caregivers could submit creative and innovative suggestions to better patient care and the work environment. Specific units had suggestion boxes, which were successful, but only on the unit level. Many times, a unit would implement a creative and innovative new practice that was successful in achieving its goal, yet other units were unaware of the new practice or its success. Also, many suggestions were unit specific, and not geared to the system as a whole.

The next step was to find a system-wide mechanism to facilitate submission and consideration of these creative and innovative ideas. The idea that was implemented combined technology already accessible with a creative and innovative process, using the shared-governance structure to collect, review, evaluate, and possibly implement ideas from bedside caregivers. Actually, anyone in the institution, irrespective of position, could submit an idea. Some ideas were geared toward operations, submitted by those that worked with those processes. It was all about having those working with the processes find ways to better the processes, no matter what specifically the processes were, clinical, operational, or whatever.

The Nursing Department worked with the Information Technology Department to develop a process where a form was placed on the system's intranet that could be filled out and submitted electronically. The submission would go to a specific e-mail address where someone, namely the Chair of the Professional Development Council, could easily retrieve and collect all the forms submitted. The form could be submitted anonymously, but was developed to encourage the person submitting to provide his or her name and unit to close the loop on the communication and assure the submitter knew their voice was heard. This encouragement was accomplished by offering recognition and a reward as an incentive if the idea was implemented.

The Chair of the Professional Development Council brings all forms submitted to the monthly Coordinating Council meeting, where all council chairs are present as well as nursing leadership. All ideas are presented, discussed, and evaluated for merit and feasibility. After a consensus is reached on the fate of the idea, the submitter is then notified. If the idea is implemented, the submitter is given recognition through the monthly nursing newsletter and a small stipend to show appreciation. The program is successful, with many ideas implemented. Anecdotally, submitters say they are very satisfied with the feedback received from the process. When the number of submissions decreases, an awareness campaign keeps the program in the staff's consciousness.

Outcome Measures:

Formative/Compliance: Anecdotal staff awareness of the Idea Line; submission process operating as designed.

Summative/Outcome: Number of Idea Line submissions; number of ideas from Idea Line implemented; number of those submitting notified of the status of their submission; satisfaction of submitters and staff.

Evidence Supporting this Creative Solution: This is an electronic version of the suggestion box incorporating a communication feedback loop, which is thought essential in achieving buy-in with an intervention such as this (Heathfield, 2009).

Recipe for: *Idea Line*

Ingredients:

CNO support

Incentives

Venue for publicizing initiative and those submitting ideas implemented

Staff buy-in

One Council Chair to coordinate initiative and one nursing administrator to monitor the program

Small group to create the online form and to promote the initiative

Information technology support and resources

Shared-governance structure to support the initiative

Step-by-Step Instructions (see Figure 1-2 for Step-by-Step Instruction Timeline):

Step 1: Obtain support from CNO.

Step 2: Establish small group including coordinator to work with information technology staff to write form and establish submission and feedback processes.

Step 3: Publicize the Idea Line and incentives.

Step 4: Review and evaluate every submission at the Coordinating Council meeting.

Step 5: Provide feedback to all who submit. Have the person responsible for this defined in your process. If the idea is to be implemented, make sure your process defines who is responsible for seeing that the implementation occurs. This should be someone in nursing leadership.

Step 6: Publicize implemented ideas. Reward and recognize the person submitting.

Step 7: Monitor formative and summative measures.

Figure 1-2   Timeline for "Idea Line."

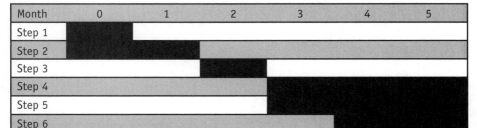

Additional Outcomes to Consider Measuring:

Formative/Compliance: No additional measures.

Summative/Outcome: Cost of implementation and upkeep of Idea Line vs savings from ideas implemented; more formal staff and submitter satisfaction measures.

Insights from Original Implementation:

- Include an information technology representative from the beginning. He or she will guide you on what is feasible and what is not.
- Place the topic "Idea Line Submissions" as a standard item on Coordinating Council's monthly agenda.
- Although the Chair of the Professional Development Council is responsible for retrieving and bringing the ideas submitted to the Coordinating Council meetings, have a nurse leader/administrator designated to mentor or assist and monitor the entire process.

For Further Guidance Contact:

Bruce Alan Boxer, PhD, MBA, RN, CPHQ
bruceboxer@ymail.com

Creative Solution Title: *The Staff Retreat*

Creative Solution Author: Patricia A. Sanchez, RN, BSN
Nurse Manager, Medical Acute
South Jersey Healthcare, Vineland, NJ

Purpose: The goal of this project is to integrate creativity and innovation into the staff-driven process of annual goal development for a hospital unit.

Legend

Overall Rating: **NOVICE**

Financial:

Time: 🕐🕐

Personnel: 👤👤👤

Other Resources: (optional)

Efficacy: **A**

Transferability: **A**

Malleability/Adaptability: **A**

Ease of Implementation: **B**

Synopsis: The Staff Retreat is a strategic planning meeting held outside the workplace to enable staff to create annual goals and use creativity and innovation to develop interventions to achieve these goals. The venue should eliminate the stress of the working environment and have a casual atmosphere where staff can develop camaraderie and cohesion as a team. This environment helps to facilitate creativity and innovation by reducing stress and allowing free-flowing ideas. Staff is able to focus on one mission, the unit's goals and how to meet them.

Description of Organization: South Jersey Healthcare (SJH) is a Magnet-designated, multiple-hospital system. The health system encompasses two full service inpatient hospitals consisting of approximately 350 inpatient beds, comprehensive health centers and outpatient and specialized services such as a Bariatric Center of Excellence, Wound Care Center, Sleep Center, and Balance Center. In 2008, SJH performed over 18,700 surgeries and the Emergency department visits topped 97,400. The health system also serves as clinical site for nursing students from a number of local colleges and maintains a professional relationship with Cumberland County College, which is adjacent to the Regional Medical Center (RMC) campus.

The Case Study: An effective leader realizes that they cannot do anything significant on his or her own, and involves the team that provides value and promotes ownership in achieving the outcomes. A team is more than a group of people; they are a group of people working toward commitment of a shared vision or goal. They support each other and the vision to create a positive atmosphere. An effective team together with effective leadership can come up with creative and innovative interventions to develop and meet the unit's goals and produce quality outcomes and provide quality patient and family care. Nursing leadership determined the need to designate a set time and place without interruption to brainstorm, develop unit goals, realign our unit goals with system and department goals, and creatively develop innovative interventions and action plans to meet our unit goals.

At South Jersey Healthcare, quarterly retreats and workout sessions that start at the leadership level and extend to the unit staff level are used to create and achieve the goals for the nursing department. These retreats are key in developing and achieving unit goals and creating a synergistic effect, integrating creativity and innovation through the use of Participative Management and Transformational Leadership techniques.

As a new manager in 2006, I realized there was a need to created shared expectations and goals with my staff. Having the staff actually create and develop the unit's goals, with my facilitation, will gain buy-in and will foster the staff's engagement with improvement initiatives. I recognized that they have a wealth of experiential knowledge and creativity that I was not using.

Together with my clinical director, Terri Spoltore RN, BSN, MSN, CCRN and the support of Senior Nursing Leadership, we began having quarterly staff retreats facilitated by myself (manager) and including the assistant nurse managers, and occasionally the Clinical Outcomes Manager and Performance Improvement Manager.

The only costs were the hourly time of the attendees to attend the event and the cost of the food (usually shared among the team or even provided by the team in a pot luck style). I used my house as the venue for the retreat, so there was no cost, just cleaning-up time. I used PowerPoint for communicating the data to the staff, but had my personal laptop and borrowed a projector from work. I also used Excel for some of the data analysis. The only true skills required are skills in planning events and skills in facilitating. The retreat lasts until all goals are met. I schedule a full day, but some of that time is spent on team building and motivation. Approval for the retreat was obtained from my director and Senior Nursing Leadership for the paid time out of the building to attend the retreat. Occasionally I have presented information from seminars I attended, and have invited members of other disciplines to give presentations (e.g., Case Management and Social Services came to explain their role and how we can work together as a team to decrease length of stay through creative and innovative strategies). Baseline data used was a pre-retreat data analysis on the quality indicators, employee opinion survey, performance appraisals, and fiscal budget. We have shown an improvement in all areas. Anecdotally, I believe we have also improved communication, problem solving, and the fulfillment of expectations throughout the unit.

Outcome Measures:

Formative/Compliance: Number of staff committing to attend vs number who did attend.

Summative/Outcome: Staff satisfaction with retreat; number of usable goals/interventions developed; monitoring outcomes of creative and innovative interventions such as monthly and quarterly quality indicators data, annual review of employee opinion survey, annual performance appraisals with higher goal setting, and more job satisfaction; fiscal responsibility maintained within the budget allowance.

Evidence Supporting this Creative Solution: The synergistic effect of a team implies that people work together to produce extraordinary results that could not have been achieved by any one individual (Mears, 1997; Walters, 2006; Kerfoot, 2006).

Recipe for: *The Staff Retreat*

Ingredients:

CNO/Director support

Staff buy-in

Facilitation skills

Team-building activity

Time allowance for staff with salary

Laptop and projector for PowerPoint (optional)

Flipcharts, whiteboard, markers (optional)

Venue to hold retreat and food

Step-by-Step Instructions (see Figure 1-3 for Step-by-Step Instruction Timeline):

Step 1: Obtain support from CNO/Director.

Step 2: Discuss retreat with staff and schedule staff as necessary so that as many as possible can attend. Obtain commitment from staff members and assistant manager to attend. If you have many staff members, choose or ask for volunteers to obtain a sampling from each shift to represent those not in attendance. Be creative with how you get commitment from staff, and be fair on how the choice of who is invited is made.

Step 3: Plan the retreat: find venue (outside of institution), plan food, reserve laptop/projector (if necessary).

Step 4: Identify and collect data to review at retreat (i.e., employee opinion survey, nurse-sensitive indicators, budget, staffing, patient satisfaction, staff competency, and educational needs). Bring system and department annual goals to review.

Step 5: Designate someone in attendance as minute-taker (possibly assistant nurse manager).

Step 6: Find a team-building activity to do at beginning of retreat (look in business section of bookstore).

Step 7: Create agenda with specific goals for the retreat. Gather and integrate supplies and techniques to facilitate creativity and innovation such as brainstorming, asking the five Ws, etc. (See Creativity and Innovation chapter). You may want to use a flipchart or whiteboard.

Step 8: Facilitate retreat. Be explicit in communicating the goals of the retreat as well as the desire for creativity and innovation in meeting these goals. Goals should include developing unit goals, developing creative and innovative interventions as well as creating action plans to meet these goals with time-sensitive milestones.

Step 9: After the retreat is completed, review and analyze minutes, identifying unit goals and interventions developed. Type up these goals and interventions and distribute to all staff. Discuss at staff meetings. Proceed with action plans as developed.

Step 10: Monitor interventions according to action plans. Encourage feedback from retreat participants; possibly use an anonymous survey. Tweak retreat as necessary to meet unit and staff needs.

Figure 1-3   Timeline for "The Staff Retreat."

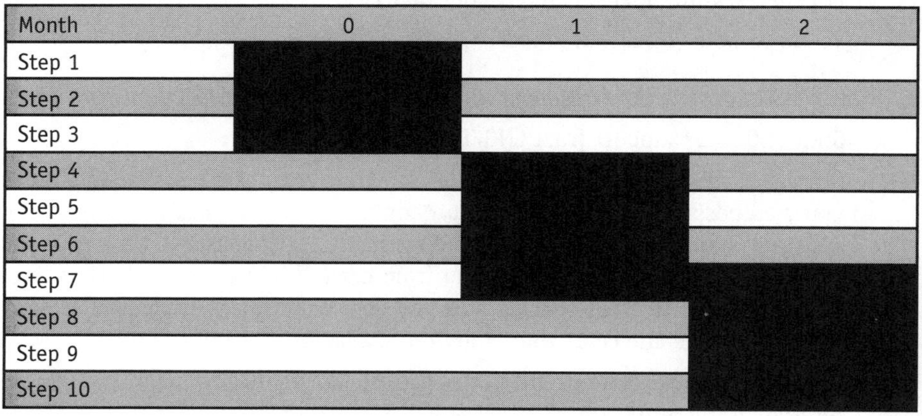

Month	0	1	2
Step 1			
Step 2			
Step 3			
Step 4			
Step 5			
Step 6			
Step 7			
Step 8			
Step 9			
Step 10			

Additional Outcomes to Consider Measuring:

Formative/Compliance: No additional measures.

Summative/Outcome: No additional measures.

Insights from Original Implementation:

- Listening and clarifying to understand what is being said and allowing for feedback and positive communication are critical to achieving results.
- Bring system/hospital and nursing department strategic goals down to the unit level. This allows for the shared vision of the organization to be successful.
- Commitment of the staff is essential.

For Further Guidance Contact:

Patricia A. Sanchez, RN, BSN
sanchezp@sjhs.com

REFERENCES

Agency for Healthcare Research and Quality. (2008). *National patient safety goals.* Available at: http://www.psnet.ahrq.gov/resource.aspx?resourceID=2230. Accessed July 27, 2009.

Agnes, M., & Guralnik, D. B. (Eds.) (2008). *Webster's new world college dictionary* (4th ed.). Cleveland, OH: Wiley Publishing, Inc.

American Association of Colleges of Nursing. (2008). *CNL frequently asked questions.* Available at: http://www.aacn.nche.edu/CNL/FAQ.htm. Accessed July 27, 2009.

American Nurses Credentialing Center. (2008). *Application manual. Magnet recognition program.* Silver Springs, MD: Author.

American Nurses Credentialing Center. (2009). *History of the Magnet Program.* Available at: http://www.nursecredentialing.org/Magnet/ProgramOverview/HistoryoftheMagnet Program.aspx. Accessed July 28, 2009.

American Society for Dermatologic Surgery. (2008). *Laser surgery information.* Available at: http://www.asds.net/LaserSurgeryInformation.aspx. Accessed July 27, 2009.

Applied Data Research. (2009, May 14). *Global pain management set to drive transdermal patches and gels to $8 billion in 2012.* Available at: http://www.medicalnewstoday.com/ articles/149977.php. Accessed July 27, 2009.

Buist, M. D., Jarmolowski, E., Burton, P. R., Bernard, S. A., Waxman, B. P., & Anderson, J. (1999). Recognising clinical instability in hospital patients before cardiac arrest or unplanned admission to intensive care: a pilot study in a tertiary-care hospital. *The Medical Journal of Australia, 171*(1), 22–25.

Centers for Medicare and Medicaid. (2006, May 18). *Eliminating serious, preventable, and costly medical errors—Never events.* Available at: http://www.cms.hhs.gov/apps/media/ press/release.asp?Counter=1863. Accessed July 27, 2009.

Culture. (2001). In *Webster's Unabridged Dictionary* (2nd ed.). New York: Random House, Inc.

Eramo, L. (2008). *CMS proposed rule could significantly expand quality measures.* Available at: http://www.healthleadersmedia.com/content/209564/topic/WS_HLM2_ QUA/CMS-proposed-rule-could-significantly-expand-quality-measures.html. Accessed July 27, 2009.

Heathfield, S. M. (2009). *Harness the power of an employee suggestion program: Beyond the suggestion box.* Available at: http://humanresources.about.com/od/quality/a/ suggestion_pro_3.htm. Accessed July 31, 2009.

Hicks-Moore, S. L. (2005). Clinical concept maps in nursing education: An effective way to link theory and practice. *Nurse Education in Practice, 5*(6), 348–352.

Hillman, K. M., Bristow, P. J., Chey, T., Daffurn, K., Jacques, T., Norman, S. L., et al. (2001). Antecedents to hospital deaths. *Internal Medicine Journal 31*(6), 343–348.

Hook, J. M., Pearlstein, J., Samarth, A., & Cusack, C. (2008). *Using barcode medication administration to improve quality and safety. Findings from the AHRQ health IT portfolio.* Available at: http://healthit.ahrq.gov/images/dec08bcmareport/bcma_issue_paper.htm. Accessed July 27, 2009.

Institute for Healthcare Improvement. (n.d.-a). *Overview of the 100,000 Lives Campaign.* Available at: http://www.ihi.org/IHI/Programs/Campaign/100kCampaignOverviewArchive. htm. Accessed July 25, 2009.

Institute for Healthcare Improvement. (n.d.-b). *Protecting 5 million lives from harm. Overview.* Available at: http://www.ihi.org/IHI/Programs/Campaign/Campaign.htm?TabId=1. Accessed July 27, 2009.

Institute of Medicine. (1999). *To err is human: Building a safer health system*. Washington, DC: National Academy Press.

Keehan, S., Sisko, A., Truffer, C., Smith, S., Cowan, C., Poisal, J., et al. (2008) Health spending projections through 2017: The baby-boom generation is coming to Medicare. *Health Affairs, 27*(2), w145–w155.

Kerfoot, K. (2006). Authentic leadership. *Dermatology Nursing, 18*(6), 595–596.

Levit, K,. Smith, C., Cowan, C., Lazenby, H., Sensenig, A., & Catlin, A. (2003). Trends in U.S. health care spending, 2001. *Health Affairs, 22*(1):154–164.

Loyola University Medical Center. (n.d.). *Nursing clinical ladder*. Available at: http://www.luhs.org/feature/nursing/clin_ladder.htm. Accessed July 27, 2009.

Matlack, J., (2009, March). *Reducing supply waste to maximize patient bedside care*. Poster presentation presented at The Organization of Nurse Executives (ONE)/NJ Research Day, New Jersey.

Mears, P. (1997). *Healthcare teams: Building continuous quality improvement*. Boca Raton, FL: St. Lucia Press.

Michalko, M. (2006). *Thinkertoys* (2nd ed.). Berkeley, CA: Ten Speed Press.

Naymik, M., & Tribble, S. J. (2009, July 23). *President Barack Obama's Cleveland Clinic visit highlights role model of health care*. Available at: http://www.cleveland.com/medical/index.ssf/2009/07/president_barack_obamas_visit.html. Accessed July 27, 2009.

NYU Lagone Medical Center. (2009). *Clinical ladder program*. Available at: http://nursing.med.nyu.edu/become-a-nurse/clinical-ladder-program. Accessed July 27, 2009.

Osborn, A.F. (1963) *Applied imagination: Principles and procedures of creative problem solving (Third Revised Edition)*. New York, NY: Charles Scribner's Son.

Robert Wood Johnson Foundation. (2008, June 4). *Chapter 3: How to test changes*. Available at: http://www.rwjf.org/pr/product.jsp?id=30073. Accessed July 27, 2009.

Rutherford, P., Lee, B., Greiner, A. (2004). *Transforming care at the bedside. IHI Innovation Series white paper*. Boston: Institute for Healthcare Improvement.

Sanderbeck, A. (2006/2007). *Building leadership skills: Leading teams*. Available at: http://www.infopeople.org/training/past/2007/BLS-leading-teams/Dos_and_Donts.doc. Accessed July 28, 2009.

Schein, R. M., Hazday, N., Pena, M., Ruben, B. H., & Sprung, C. L. (1990). Clinical antecedents to in-hospital cardiopulmonary arrest. *Chest, 98*(6), 1388–1392.

Shepard, M. (2003, March 10). *Facilitating "do's" and "don'ts."* Available at: http://www.smallgroups.com/departments/biblestudyextras/facilitatingdosanddonts.html. Accessed July 28, 2009.

Synergy. (n.d.). The American Heritage Dictionary of the English Language, Fourth Edition. Retrieved March 14, 2010, from Dictionary.com website: http://dictionary.reference.com/browse/synergy

Taylor, W. C., & Labarre, P. (2006). *Mavericks at work. Why the most original minds in business win*. New York: Harper.

University Medical Center. (n.d.). *UMC's clinical ladder*. Available at: http://www.umcarizona.org/workfiles//fornurses/UMC_Clinical_Ladder_Program.pdf. Accessed July 27, 2009.

Walters, S. R. (2006, September). The benefits of holding a staff retreat and how to do it well. *Journal of Financial Planning*. Available at: www.britannica.com/bps/additionalcontent/18/22334896/The-Benefits-of-Holding-a-Staff-Retreat. Accessed March 5, 2010.

World Health Organization. (2000). *World Health Organization assesses the world's health systems*. Available at: http://www.who.int/whr/2000/media_centre/press_release/en/index.html. Accessed July 24, 2009.

## CHAPTER 2

People, Processes, and Structures for the Magnet Journey

"Individually, we are one drop. Together, we are an ocean."
—RYUNOSUKE SATORO

"Too often, effective ideas get rejected because they have to travel too far in an organization filled with fiefdoms and inevitable roadblocks."
—MITCH THROWER

PEOPLE

Of course, everyone needs to be involved in the journey to nursing quality, but there are some who are more essential than others. Although Magnet is an institutional achievement and designation, it is ultimately a validation of nursing's ability to provide quality patient care in a healthy, nurturing work environment. This affects those whom you involve and how you structure your journey. The individuals you want to deeply involve are those who see beyond the explicit benefits of the journey to implicit and secondary advantages such as the personal satisfaction and self-development that comes with the journey, not to mention the pride in knowing and demonstrating that they are delivering excellent patient care. You want critical thinkers, independent problem solvers: individuals who are driven to deliver specifics, but who also understand how the specifics combine to reach the overarching goal. You also need to consider each individual's availability and flexibility. Everyone has a life outside of what they do as a profession: family, friends, education, and commitments. Understand each person's availability and flexibility and you will be seen as a considerate and pragmatic leader. Realize that the goal of the Magnet designation is achievable, but you need to understand that as driven as you might be to achieve the goal, others might not share your intensity. Do not discard them just because they are not quite as passionate about the goal as you are. Instead, accept what they can offer and push for just a little bit more. It keeps the bar high and keeps people on their toes. Now it is time to find out who these individuals are.

Magnet Program Director (MPD)

We have tried to categorize the individuals you will need to involve in the journey to nursing quality (Magnet journey). These categories are by no means mutually exclusive, and you may find that an individual wants to be more involved than you need. That is great. Give them as much responsibility and accountability as you feel possible. Just ensure that there is one person coordinating all the efforts (Drumm, 2005). That person is the Magnet Program Director (MPD) or the Director of Nursing Quality. Individuals responsible for coordinating nursing quality initiatives have various titles, but they are all known as MPDs in the Magnet community. Typically this person is a master's degree prepared nurse, although many MPDs have master's degrees in disciplines other than nursing. If you are fortunate enough to hire a PhD, RN, this individual can function as both the MPD and the Research Consultant as well (two for the price of one). Because the gist of the Magnet Program or Journey to Nursing Quality is patient care outcomes and workplace justice, equity, and satisfaction, the MPD will truly need many different but complementary skills, such as statistics and data analysis, project management, vision, leadership and fiscal responsibility, presentation and team development, writing and communications ability, etc. Where do you find such a person? You may have him or her already in your institution, or you may be this person. If you are the MPD or the Director of Nursing Quality, we are certain you already know some of the skills necessary to facilitate and coordinate the Magnet journey.

The typical job description of an MPD can be generally summarized by the phrase "all activities necessary to meet and maintain Magnet designation"; to denote the many things that the MPD will need to do, that at the present, cannot be enumerated. It is a dynamic and enjoyable position, constantly learning and envisioning a better process, a new opportunity, and a way to raise the bar on patient care and workplace satisfaction. We cannot list here all the activities the MPD will be involved in and responsible for. We can say that the MPD needs to have the capacity for self-learning and integrating and evaluating data, processes, and initiatives.

In our attempt to categorize personnel necessary for the journey to nursing excellence, the MPD or the Director of Quality is the lynchpin, the one that holds all the pieces of the journey together, and in our opinion, in a category alone. We have categorized other personnel with respect to their day-to-day involvement in the planning and implementing of strategic initiatives for the journey.

Nursing Leadership

The most involved will be nursing leadership: directors, managers, and assistant managers. We call these individuals "managers" collectively. They need to be involved right from the start and should have input into the decisions on what, when, where, and how to implement initiatives. They should be frequently educated on the journey and what changes to old processes and creation of new processes are needed. Initial involvement will help to get buy-in to the Magnet designation vision, as well as help to keep everyone on the same page. Although you may decide to have certain individuals work on specific pieces of the journey, integration is the key to success, and the more you inform nursing leadership of how their piece fits into the big picture, the greater success you will have.

Nursing leadership will be the "worker bees" for the Magnet journey. They will be responsible for completing whatever projects and initiatives are necessary. Some of the skills that are important for these individuals to have are some of the same skills necessary to be an effective manager, mostly delegation and project management skills. If an individual is known to be a poor delegator, do not use this time to challenge his or her abilities. Give tasks and projects that match the strength of the person to whom you are delegating. At one institution on the Magnet journey, it was decided to have all nurse managers take part in writing the application. Of course this is fair and equitable; everyone has a piece to complete. The problem is that writing is a skill, and not all nurse managers had the same skill at writing. What happened was a mishmash of writing styles, with pieces left incomplete as a result of the procrastination of many of the nurse managers, no doubt, due to their fear of writing. Fairness does not mean everyone must do the same thing, just that everyone does his or her part.

First, assess the strengths of your managers and delegate strategically, playing to each manager's or director's strengths. If a manager is particularly good at team building, give him or her the responsibility of helping to mentor shared decision making (shared governance) councils. If a manager is particularly adept at data analysis and data communication, delegate the responsibility for nurse-sensitive indicator presentation and analysis to him or her. And just a word of caution: Never give responsibility without authority. A staff nurse cannot be given the responsibility to educate the medical staff. Why? Because they have no authority or credibility to do so. As much as we would like to believe that we are all one big happy team working together without an administrative hierarchy, the result of that thinking is that no one would be accountable and nothing would get done. So work within the hierarchy you have. Typically, the CNO has credibility and authority in the eyes of the medical staff. He or she is the one that should educate the medical staff (with assistance if necessary, of course).

Consultants

You may decide to hire a consultant to work with your team to develop strategic plans to meet your goals. Consultants are common when an institution decides to begin the Magnet journey. The consultant should be someone with appropriate credentials and experience to help guide you through the journey. Typically, consultants will perform a gap analysis to show you where your organization is strong and where there is opportunity for improvement. The consultant should be involved in, and help plan, the initiatives necessary to meet the requirements for Magnet designation.

You may initially look to other similar institutions that have attained Magnet designation for consultation. This will be a more informal way to identify needs. It will definitely be less intense than a professional consultant. An institution has only their own experience to relate. A professional consultant has usually seen and possibly assisted many institutions in the journey. You must obtain the success rate the consultant has in assisting institutions through the journey. Check references. Make sure the consultant is right for your type of institution. The Magnet program office offers professional consultation (American Nurses Credentialing Center, 2010). It is definitely something to consider.

PhD, RN

One of the requirements for Magnet designation is ongoing nursing research. If you already have an established nursing research department, you most likely have a PhD, RN at the helm. If you are just beginning your nursing research initiative, you will need an appropriate leader. Now, one of the authors is a bit biased (can you guess which?), but having a PhD, RN on staff is definitely a worthwhile investment. Would you go to a family physician to have your gallbladder removed? We did not think so. You would want a specialist, such as a surgeon to do it. Well that is what a PhD, RN is: a specialist in research. If you cannot afford or cannot find a PhD, RN, you can get some help from your nearby university. Frequently, institutions begin their nursing research initiative with a part-time PhD, RN. This could be a consultant or a faculty member from your local university. It is best if they are familiar with Magnet program requirements (for those of you seeking Magnet designation). However, if you have a Magnet consultant, he or she should work with the PhD, RN to make sure Magnet program requirements are met.

As a staff member, a PhD, RN could play a number of roles until the research initiative becomes more established, needing their full-time attention. Professional dissemination (i.e., abstracts and articles, data analysis for quality initiatives, staff education on the research and evidence-based practice [EBP] processes) should all be within the scope of the PhD, RN. There is also the connection and engagement that comes with identification as an employee of an institution. Who invests more, a home owner or a renter? You want an owner.

"Worker Bees"

The next group of individuals is the "worker bees." We have already identified nursing leadership, but you will also need other individuals that may be within the nursing department or might report to other hospital leadership. Crucial to any quality initiative is the Director/Manager of Performance Improvement (PI). He or she will know what data is currently collected and what data can be collected, and will help to determine what data needs to be collected and the best way to accomplish it. Nursing quality is synonymous with achievement in nurse-sensitive indicators. So, in operationalizing nursing quality, the Magnet program looks at both the internal progression of nurse-sensitive indicator metrics as well as the external comparison of these metrics with similar institutions. The PI Director/Manager can determine which metrics have opportunity for improvement.

Bringing the nurse-sensitive indicator data to the bedside nurse is essential for awareness and improvement. The PI Director/Manager can assist in developing a format for disseminating unit-specific, nurse-sensitive data to direct-care nurses. He or she will also be able to teach and mentor the performance/quality improvement process. Institutions typically adopt a performance/quality improvement model or process and use it throughout the institution as their standard. Although the similarities of the various processes outweigh the differences; some do have distinct differences in what they are designed to do. For instance, the DMAIC (Define, Measure, Improve, and Control) process is used to improve and control processes, whereas the plan-do-study-act (PDSA) is focused more on continuous improvement than process control. DMAIC works well with the Six Sigma philosophy. The Transforming Care at the Bedside (TCAB) initiative utilizes a rapid cycle PDSA or test of change. Whichever performance model your institution chooses to use, just be aware of its focus and how well it works with your institution's culture.

Educators

The Director/Manager of Staff Development/Education is another key player in the journey to nursing quality. Nearly all initiatives implemented will require some sort of staff education. Many will require the development of new educational initiatives geared toward nursing professional development in national certification, continuing education, and formal education. The Director/Manager of Staff Development/Education should be involved in the strategic planning of all initiatives and possibly be given responsibility for meeting many of the professional development requirements for the Magnet program. Institutions have various structures, and might utilize advanced practice nurses (APNs) as clinical specialists, overseen by the Director/Manager of Staff Development/Education. APNs are a great resource for direct-care nurses and can act as liaisons between the strategic professional development plan and the direct-care staff: mentoring, providing education, and forming national certification study groups.

APNs are also an important resource for shared-governance councils. Their clinical expertise can guide direct-care staff responsible for developing evidence-based practice and policies. They can also aid in educating about the Centers for

Medicare and Medicaid's (CMS) core measures and nurse-sensitive indicators. They will be important workers in the quest for Magnet designation. We want to stress once again that it is key to strategically assess each person's skills and match your institution's needs with their skills, and do not be afraid to look beyond the nursing department.

Hidden Talent

There is much talent hiding in your institution. One of our Six Sigma black belts was a graphic designer before he became our process improvement expert. We utilized him to assist with mentoring direct-care staff in developing posters for professional presentation. Our night nursing supervisor is a terrific flautist. She played beautifully as we had our graduation celebration to recognize and congratulate staff who completed formal education programs in the past year.

Now, who is the best event planner in your nursing department? Why do we ask? Well, this person will possibly be the most important to the Magnet journey. This is the person who can plan a conference and delegate with skill and grace: the person everyone comes to for assistance because they know he or she will get it done. And if he or she does not know how to do it, the person will know who does and can easily obtain their assistance. Unfortunately, all too often we have seen this person taken for granted since he or she shines as a facilitator for others' initiatives, with others getting most of the credit for success. This person should be valued, even cherished. We suggest when you find this person, try to remove some of their other responsibilities so he or she can focus on the events occurring throughout the Magnet journey. At one of our institutions, one of the authors is privileged to work daily with such an individual. During the past year, she has successfully planned Research Day, Graduation Celebration, Nurse of the Year Celebration, Nurse Aide/Tech Day, the Women's Health Conference, and the Falls Prevention Product and Intervention Fair, to name just a few. She can design invitations, create and maintain an Excel database, facilitate meetings, and facilitate projects using various project management tools. Find this person in your institution and you will have a true keystone for the Magnet journey. If you cannot find one, hire one quickly.

Champions

Another group of workers you might decide to amass are typically called the Magnet Champions. These are direct-care nurses who meet monthly as a group, usually one representing each unit. They act as workers, communicators, and motivators; initiating and facilitating unit-based Magnet initiatives, disseminating the latest Magnet information to their unit staff, and championing the efforts throughout the Magnet journey (University of Iowa, 2007).

It pretty much goes without saying that you need to pick the right person from each unit for this group. This is not a group to win over, but a group that is cheering the team on, a group that believes in the goal and truly enjoys the engagement the journey brings. The Magnet Program Director leads this group, and members will definitely need to use some nonproductive (nonstaff) time to complete the work that needs to be accomplished. Many hospitals are staffing with 12 hours shifts, so a full-time nurse typically works 36 hours. This allows 4 hours per week more without using overtime pay. Of course you cannot mandate that they work an extra 4 hours, but it might be a real incentive for those who want the additional salary to do something other than direct patient care. Herzberg's motivation-hygiene theory (1968) posits that true motivation comes from expanding employees' work roles, and providing an opportunity to learn and practice new skills. Of course, earning a little more money does not hurt either.

Physician Champion

There is another champion you will need for the journey. This champion may be a bit more difficult to recruit. Although we have called this the Journey to Nursing Quality, it is rarely all about nursing. For nursing to do quality work, efforts must be interdisciplinary, and the discipline other than nursing most directly involved in patient care outcomes is medicine. The sometimes elite status physicians typically enjoy in healthcare institutions and society as a whole can work for or against the Magnet initiative; you definitely want them on your side. You will need to identify one or possibly a few physicians that are seen as supporters of nursing: true collaborators in patient care. Now you will need to make your case. Considering the hospital hierarchy, this may be a job for the CNO. He or she should use the literature on the quality difference between Magnet and non-Magnet-designated institutions as well as the notoriety that comes from Magnet designation to convince these physician(s) to be a part of and champions for the Magnet journey. Focus on excellence in patient care.

A little name-dropping also might be effective. The old saying goes, "You're judged by the company you keep." If this is true, then achieving Magnet designation would put your institution in some pretty good company with Cedars-Sinai Medical Center in Los Angeles, CA; the Hospital of the University of Pennsylvania in Philadelphia, PA; Georgetown University Hospital in Washington, DC; the Cleveland Clinic in Cleveland, OH; and Robert Wood Johnson University Hospital in New Brunswick, NJ—hospitals known for their excellence in patient care (American Nurses Credentialing Center, 2008b). It should not be difficult to convince physicians that the journey will be beneficial. But you need more than their agreement that this is a good idea; you need their commitment to act as a driving force for the initiative, informing physician colleagues of new initiatives and garnering support within the medical hierarchy for the journey. They need to be participative, not just supportive. After the CNO gains their commitment, the next step is to present it to the medical staff. How this is done is truly dependent upon the medical physician structure in your institution. It may be a presentation at a medical staff meeting or it may be one-on-one sessions with individual physicians. If at all possible, we would make the committed physicians members of the Magnet Steering Committee. This will provide a direct communication link with the medical staff, especially for those initiatives that directly impact physicians' processes. A word of caution here: Use your physician champions wisely. They are powerful assets. In other words, do not ask your physician champion to make a poster or to help arrange a celebration event. Use them mainly for communication and support. They are not exactly worker bees, but their assistance is invaluable.

Ancillary Department Heads

The next group we would like to discuss is the ancillary department heads. Although the Magnet designation is fundamentally a mark of nursing excellence, much of the criteria for meeting designation standards are highly dependent on interdisciplinary cooperation and coordination. Also, much of the data you need for your Magnet application may come from departments other than nursing. For example, the database containing the nurse turnover rate and percentage of nationally certified nurses might be maintained by the Human Resources Department or the Finance Department. They need to know what data you need, and a gap analysis should be performed to determine what data need to be collected that is not currently collected. Have a regular, established way to communicate to ancillary department heads about the progress of the journey. This could be done through quarterly meetings with the group of ancillary department heads or through e-mail updates, newsletters, or a combination of methods. Just remember that communication needs to be regular and tailored to the audience. There is nothing more annoying to someone than to be told "we need this from you" at the last minute without having involved them in the timeline and planning. Base your communication on interdisciplinary cooperation, not on the demanding customer (nursing) and unprepared supplier (ancillary department) paradigm (Havens & Johnston, 2004). This merely creates animosity and negative feelings, which might taint the plans for establishing interdisciplinary cooperation in patient care, and thus achieving Magnet program standards.

Finance

And so now we come to the department that always seems to get a bad rap when nursing is contemplating any new initiatives: finance. I feel a measure of sympathy for those in the finance department. While I am sure there are other words in their vocabulary besides "no," that is the one we seem to hear and fear the most. We have found that the best way to get what you need is to involve the Finance Department from the beginning. Of course, they will most certainly be involved in the decision to take the Magnet journey, but many times the cost of initiatives necessary to achieve quality goals cannot be foreseen. Therefore, it would behoove you to have someone designated as your finance liaison for the Magnet journey. This person could and probably should be a member of your Magnet Steering Committee. In this way, prior to the full development of an initiative, you will know if it is fiscally appropriate or if you need to look for a less costly intervention, which will ultimately save you time and trouble. This finance liaison should also be accountable to communicate pertinent information about the journey to those in the Finance Department who need to be made aware. The budget for the journey should take into consideration that there might be unforeseen initiatives and should apportion a sum for such an event.

There are many others that could be included, depending upon the specific structure of your organization. We will leave that to your discretion. Keep the same strategic focus: Involve them as much as you need to, based on their role in the Magnet journey. Remember that everyone (and we do mean everyone) should know about the journey: what it is, and what it can do. And do not forget new hires. Orientation is a great time to indoctrinate them to the journey for nursing quality.

Board on Board

The Board of Directors of the institution (assuming it is a nonprofit) should also be well informed and approve the Magnet journey. Relate the benefits of the journey to the institution and the community it serves. The board should also be regularly updated on the progress of the journey, since they will most likely want to see that the journey's financial impact is offset by its impact on quality patient care; that the rewards of the journey are well worth the cost.

PROCESS

Gap Analysis

There are far too many processes necessary for the Magnet journey to list here, but we would like to cover some of the essential ones. We will start with a process we mentioned in the previous section: the gap analysis. The gap analysis is really quite straightforward. It is a matter of knowing where you are and comparing it with where you want to be, noting the things that are missing. You do not fix things in a gap analysis. Leave that for later. The purpose of the gap analysis is to note what is missing. After you perform the gap analysis, you can then concentrate on how to "fill in" these gaps. The gap analysis is a real way to focus everyone on what is specifically needed to meet the goal, in this case, Magnet designation. A gap analysis may be a very formal process where an expert consultant is hired to perform the analysis with respect to a specific initiative. Many institutions hire consultants to perform a gap analysis for the Magnet journey. Typically, these consultants were either Magnet program appraisers or nursing leaders intimately involved with the Magnet journey. A huge benefit of hiring a consultant to perform a gap analysis is their expertise in interpreting ambiguous requirements and their understanding of the gestalt, the way everything should come together. When you dissect an initiative into pieces, you can lose the ability to evaluate the synchronicity, synergy, and symbiosis of all the elements that are only able to be evaluated as a whole system. Also, consultants are external to the institution and might see things missed by employees. In the same vein, this may also be a limitation in that there is limited familiarity with the organization and the consultant might miss what employees would not. Therefore, it is best if the gap analysis is a cooperative process between the consultant and a nursing leader who is very knowledgeable about the institution. A consultant may also have a better idea of the relative weight or importance of each requirement, and also knowledge of the interdependence of specific requirements, providing the institution with a hierarchy of areas for improvement.

Readiness Survey

In addition to a gap analysis, you may want to do a readiness survey. This is usually a survey of staff, leadership, or both, to determine staff perceptions of where they feel their unit and the organization are on meeting the Magnet program components. This can be done as a paper and pencil survey, but we recommend using an electronic or Internet-based survey like SurveyMonkey. This service will guide you through survey construction, distribution, and will even tabulate statistics. If you are not well versed in surveys, SurveyMonkey or a comparable service is a must.

Our advice when surveying:

- Make it anonymous; just require the participant's unit if using unit-specific questions. You will get a better response rate and a truer evaluation.
- If you are using a strongly disagree-to-strongly agree Likert scale, use four choices (strongly disagree, disagree, agree, strongly agree). This forces participants to make a choice. Using an undecided choice will lessen the value of the survey.
- Make it easily available for the target audience. Make sure the target audience has the skills (computer, language, etc.) to complete the survey.
- The survey should be voluntary, but highly publicized. You want the highest response rate you can get. Know beforehand how many are in your

target audience. You will then be able to track your response rate, noting if more time or more publicity is needed. When evaluating your results, the response rate is crucial. The better the response rate, the more believable the results.

- Track the response rate frequently during the survey and publicize it to your target audience. This may help drive the need to elicit more participation.
- Keep the survey as short a possible while still obtaining the information you need.
- Have others who are familiar with the content read over the questions. This will help validate the survey. Have them critique the questions for clarity and grammar.
- Resurvey your targeted audience periodically throughout your quality journey to compare the progression on meeting your goals. Use the survey results, along with other available data, to create action plans specific to areas with opportunities for improvement.
- Have a definite end date for the survey and publicize it. This will help create a sense of urgency to participants.
- Make sure you provide enough time so that your target audience has sufficient opportunity to complete the survey.
- If your response rate is poor, consider extending the end date. Possibly allow an additional week and publicize the extension and the new date. After one or two extensions, you need to evaluate your process for publicizing the survey. A poor response rate may signify apathy in your audience, something that will need to be addressed separately before you can proceed on your journey.

Employee Opinion Survey

More formally, you will need to administer an employee opinion survey (EOS) that you can benchmark nationally. There are a number of companies that offer the EOS service. The EOS process is very similar to the survey process discussed previously, but the specifics of the process are determined by the specific survey provider. The survey is a standard format, typically with standard questions, so that benchmarking is possible. The survey provider may have some ability to customize your EOS. Have an internal committee composed of leaders and staff to preview the survey prior to committing to it. You want the survey to be meaningful to your institution. When you review the survey, think about what you can do with the information. You will need to use this information to create action plans, which will address opportunities for improvement in employees' perceptions of the work environment. For guidance in interpreting perception data, see Chapter 5: Measuring Outcomes. The Magnet program requires institutions to survey staff at least annually (American Nurses Credentialing Center, 2008a), but some institutions might do it more frequently. When you resurvey staff, you will want to use the same survey so that you can compare results with previously administered surveys to determine the progress you are making. The result of the EOS should be shared with your employees, as well as the action plans designed to address opportunity for improvement. Their input into these action plans is important and should be encouraged. The more frequently you survey employees, the better you can determine if your interventions are working. But be realistic. Do not survey staff too often or you will tax their desire to participate. Also, it takes time for perceptions to change, so allow enough time between surveys to be able to realistically evaluate your efforts.

Patient Satisfaction

If you are not already doing so, you will need to measure patient satisfaction. There are various companies that will survey your patient population. The key is to provide meaningful questions that provide meaningful information and the ability to benchmark nationally. If you are a recipient of Medicare funds, your patient population is already being surveyed by the Center for Medicare and Medicaid (CMS). This survey is known as Hospital Consumer Assessment of Healthcare Providers and Systems (HCAHPS), and aggregate hospital data is available to anyone at www.hospitalcompare.hhs.gov (HCAHPS, 2009). You may want to use the HCAHPS as your patient satisfaction survey. There are services such as HealthStream Research that can assist you with data acquisition and interpretation (HealthStream® Research, 2009).

Performance Improvement

Action Plans, Goals, and Objectives

As discussed in Chapter 5, there are various models you can utilize for the quality improvement/performance improvement (QI/PI) process. Choose the one that best fits your institution. From the QI/PI processes, you can then develop action plans. Action plans define what is there to do, who will do it, and by when, and are typically broken up into goals and distinct objectives to meet these goals. A sample action planning form is provided in Chapter 3.

To write an action plan, you first need to define your goals. Goals are sometimes interchanged with objectives, but there is truly a hierarchy. Goals should come first and are overarching statements of intent, like "to better the health of the community this year." Commonly, the SMART goals format is used to help guide the writing of meaningful goals. SMART stands for specific, measureable, attainable, realistic, and timely (Goal Setting Guide, n.d.). If you consider these factors when writing goals, you can hardly go wrong. This is where, at times, goals and objectives are confused. It is not essential that you draw a distinct line in the sand defining which is a goal and which is an objective. The important part is assuring that goals meet the SMART criteria and that objectives are specific, operationalized, and are designed so that if all objectives are met, the goal is achieved.

From the goal, objectives are derived and are designed to meet the goal. The objectives are like the steps of a ladder necessary to reach new heights. But really, objectives are meant to narrow down the goal further, often cleaving it into manageable pieces (actions) that can be assigned to an accountable individual or group and to be completed by a certain time. The action plan is a logical dissection of a goal into manageable and measurable pieces that are delegated and scheduled, ensuring accountability and timely completion.

Evaluation

Defining goals, writing objectives, and developing action plans lead you to the process of evaluation. Evaluation can take many forms, dependent upon the situation in which you find yourself. Evaluation is a process, not just a metric. There are many elements that go into an appropriate evaluation. Using outcomes and compliance data in evaluations are discussed in Chapter 5. Further evaluation can occur with benchmarking, also discussed in Chapter 5. The process of benchmarking relates your data to a standard, whether it is a national average of like institutions or a historic measure that you are trying to better. Evaluation might also consider a cost/benefit analysis, a process again discussed in Chapter 5. The extent of the evaluation should match the need. If you are evaluating a very costly and complex initiative that affects the institution's entire workforce, you definitely want as much and as precise data as you can get. If you are evaluating something like a new time to hold meetings, a simple percent attendance may be adequate. Who does the evaluation is as important as what data is considered. The person or persons evaluating need to understand the initiative, the process, or the product that they are evaluating, the decision the evaluation will determine, and have the ability to analyze the data used in the evaluation (McNamara, 2008).

Shared Decision Making

A crucial and necessary process for the Magnet journey is the shared decision-making process where nurses have a venue to share in the decision-making process and have a voice on issues that affect their practice and work environment. This process is explained in much more detail in Chapter 9: Institutionalizing Nursing Autonomy and Professional Development.

Budgeting

Now we finally discuss what no one really likes to talk about: money. You will need to budget for the Magnet journey. From all anecdotal accounts we have heard, the journey is not cheap. However, it truly depends on what is already in place and what resources you might be able to easily access. There are many costs to consider aside from the application fee. First you will need to consider the personnel needed to coordinate the journey. Costs that might be difficult to quantify are the time and supplies of leadership to implement the specific initiatives necessary for the journey, as well as planning and educating. Of course, one could argue that part of leadership's job is to ensure quality, so the journey is not necessarily additional work. More directly, costs will arise from the need for additional personnel, consultants, and direct-care nurses' participation in quality initiatives. If you already have a shared decision-making structure in place, you would not consider staff participation a cost of the Magnet journey. If not, it will be somewhat costly to establish the structure in addition to the costs of participation of direct-care nurses. For example, if you establish a shared decision-making councilor structure and you have four councils with 20 members each, meeting monthly for 1 hour, that is: 4 councils × 20 members each × 1 hour × $25/hr (example salary rate) × 12 months = $24,000. That is $24,000 a year, just for salary costs for staff participation. Frequently, chairs and cochairs of these councils are provided additional time to do council work such as creating agendas, typing minutes, and implementing initiatives. There will also be costs derived from the previously discussed processes, such as the Employee Opinion Survey and the Patient Satisfaction Survey. Employee recognition is also a process that needs funding. The establishment of mostly all of the processes necessary for the journey will require financial outlay. Again, how much depends on what is already in place, and what is needed. Your gap analysis should help you greatly in the budgeting process. Remember, budgets are typically done annually and the journey is a multiyear commitment, so you may be able to spread out costs over multiple annual budgets.

The year the application is sent and the appraisers visit will most likely be the most costly. This is when the final application fee is due as well as the preparation for the site visit. (They can occur in consecutive years). The preparation for the site visit can include everything from painting and furniture replacement to sprucing up the lobby to a possible hospital-wide celebration if Magnet designation is achieved. There are ways of narrowing down what should be included in the budget. A consultant should be able to help you determine the specific events. Plotting the journey on a Gantt chart should provide a basic timeline for budgeting coinciding with the projects to be implemented. We also recommend reaching out to a similar local Magnet-designated institutions and speaking to their Magnet Program Director (MPD). He or she should be able to help guide you.

So you now have a few tools to help you budget for the journey: the gap analysis; the Magnet program consultant; your Gantt chart; and the MPD in a local Magnet-designated institution. We also suggest giving a little padding to the budget for unexpected needs and events. As stated before, some costs will be explicit, like additional personnel and supplies, and some will be hidden, like leadership's time and effort in planning and implementing initiatives. Explicit financial outlays should definitely be included. How much of the hidden costs you include is up to you and your leadership's discretion.

Other Processes

Communication

As we have previously stated, there are many other processes involved in the Magnet journey that we discuss throughout this book, such as the performance improvement process, the evidence-based practice process, the research process, the process of creating and establishing nurse autonomy, the process of disseminating project and research results, etc. There are just a few more we need to touch on here. We discussed a bit about the communication process as we listed the people necessary for the journey. We want to expand, just a little, on this truly important topic. We have all heard the mantra "communicate, communicate, communicate." We agree with it, but we would like to add "strategically." What we mean by this is that you need to think and plan before you talk. Should you tell all your staff exactly how much the journey costs? Should you tell ancillary department heads about the nurse theorist you have chosen as a foundation for your nursing practice? Maybe, but we think you will need to show some discretion and consideration. Not everyone needs to know everything. You need to tailor your message to your audience. The thing we stress most of all is that communication should be regular, whatever your venue and whomever your audience. Regular communication promotes inclusion and a feeling of belonging to the journey (Pierson, Miller, & Moore, 2007).

Venues for Communication

Now you need to think about venues for communication. Staff meetings are good, but rarely do you get a large audience, and managers may need to have three or more sessions monthly to capture as much of the night, day, and weekend staff as possible. E-mail and newsletters are other good venues. It might be beneficial to provide monthly updates to nurse managers and ancillary department managers, and ask if your Magnet journey update could be a standing item on their monthly staff meeting agenda. Managers could then relate this update to their staff. Be creative in your communication. You might have a bulletin board outside the cafeteria where you post updates: Whatever works for your institution. As stated previously, if you are a nonprofit institution, you will also need to consider regular updates to the board members to demonstrate your progress on the journey.

Education

The process of educating staff about the Magnet journey can be challenging. New employees should be indoctrinated during their orientation and preceptorship. That means working it into their current curriculum, and not just nurses, all new employees. As for current employees, there are a number of ways we have seen education occur. If you have computer-based training, you may be able to incorporate a module on the Magnet framework and journey. We suggest making it mandatory and tracking compliance. Another method might be to create a self-learning packet that requires employees to complete a test after reading the Magnet information framework. Again, make the assignment mandatory and track it by collecting tests. You may also want to reinforce learning through contests, puzzles, posters, pamphlets, or badge cards. Prior to the Magnet program appraiser visit, one hospital took their show on the road, going unit to unit, playing self-created Magnet Jeopardy with any available staff. The more fun you can make it, the more staff you will attract. You will need the assistance of your staff development department or whatever structure you have in place for implementing educational initiatives and assuring clinical competence. Incorporate a Magnet minute into the agendas of all standing committee and council meetings, and provide committee and council chairs with monthly updates to present. Celebrate achievements as you progress through your journey. This progression validates all of the efforts and resources put forth, and celebration recognizes and rewards these efforts.

Collecting Evidence for the Magnet Application

The next to last process we will discuss here is the process of collecting evidence for the Magnet application. Evidence supporting your narrative will be mainly in five forms: policies, meeting minutes, anecdotal exemplars, outcome data, and miscellaneous supporting documents. Policies should be available to all staff and can probably be accessed through your institution's intranet or by perusing your policy binder. Meeting minutes may be a bit more difficult to find. Minutes are usually kept by the person running the specific meetings or the division's administrative assistants. They are rarely kept in one central location. Which minutes you will need to submit will, of course, depend on what empirical outcome you want to demonstrate.

We recommend adopting a standard format for meeting minutes including the name, credentials, position, and department of everyone in attendance. This way it will be easy for you and the Magnet appraisers to know who was in attendance and note the presence of direct-care nurses in decision-making venues. It would also be an asset to keep all meeting minutes in one location. SharePoint, a Microsoft Office application, has the potential to create virtual workspaces and each council or committee could have its own workspace. Within each workspace, an area could be defined for meeting minutes. This level of standardization is rarely achieved, but would be an MPD's dream.

One more word about minutes: Include the minutes that provide the evidence for your exemplar. There is nothing more confusing than evidence that does not support what you state. Make the connection clear to the reader. Anecdotal exemplars are necessary to demonstrate Magnet standards. These examples will be varied. There are two standard ways of proceeding: You could collect every story possible and fit them in where you think they belong, or note what exemplars you need from the Magnet application and then strategically advertise throughout your institution for these anecdotes. Make sure you capture all the information you need to write your exemplar. Noting just the gist of the story and trying to recreate it a year later when writing the application will be difficult, if not frustrating. It would be best to develop a form for each exemplar and create a file for which empirical outcome it addresses. If you take our advice and do this, you will find the application process much less stressful. Outcome data is discussed in Chapter 5. When you do find out who keeps the data you need, use a spreadsheet and note the type of data, who manages it and in which department, and the lag time in obtaining it, so that the next time you need to submit something, you will know who has it and how long it will take to get it.

The Change Process

Last, but not least, is the process that permeates all other processes: the change process. It is interesting how we all learn the grieving process in nursing school (Kübler-Ross, 1969), which we apply in many patient situations to understand our patients' reactions, yet we are not typically taught the change process, which we could use nearly every day, in nearly every aspect of our lives. Understanding this process and its natural progression can help to normalize our reactions and set up the expectation for the typical feelings of uncertainty, anger, and concern experienced during change (ChangingMinds.org, 2009). We strongly recommend that all staff be taught the change process and the expected reactions that accompany each stage. You may even want to integrate the change process in planning initiatives requiring change. For example, plan the creation and implementation of a shared governance structure in accordance with who will need to change and how implementations can be staged in accordance with their stages of change. Awareness and acknowledgment of the stages of change make feelings real and able to be attended to. We discuss the change process in greater detail in Chapter 4: Motivation, Buy-In, and Enculturation.

Structure

A structure, as defined by the *Oxford American Dictionary* (Structure, 2006, p. 120), is nothing more than a framework or a way of organizing something. In a hospital, as in most any institution, structures are ubiquitous. We tend to think of structures as large, physical entities, like distinct buildings or units. We want you to expand your concept of structure to think of it as anything with an organizing framework. The Magnet program is a structure. It is not as physical as a building, but it is an evidenced-based organizing framework designed to create an environment for quality patient care and a safe and satisfying workplace. So when you look around at your institution, you can see that structures abound, from the structure of your hospital's campus, to how to structure your patient care.

We want to talk about structure for a bit because it is crucial to obtaining your goals. Structures are typically static and need to be built upon. A structure's existence does not necessarily imply that there is a reason for its existence or a purpose to the structure. Sometimes we do not fully understand the purpose of a structure, such as our solar system, an ancient complex structure which may have been created as a great design or may have merely happened by chance. These designed structures, we believe, should have a purpose. When we see a designed structure that appears to have no relating outcomes or is ineffective, we need to ask, "Who designed the structure and for what purpose?" Many times you will find that what you supposed was a designed structure actually happened by chance, and no one has yet questioned its existence. Keep this in mind when you look at the structures in your institution. You may be surprised at the number of chance structures you find. The quality mantra "structure, process, outcome" (Donabedian, 1966) really says it all. You need a solid structure before you can develop processes to achieve your outcomes. When you think about it, it is a no-brainer, yet frequently you will find inappropriate or nonexistent structures when you begin to analyze initiatives with unrealized outcomes. An optimal structure may give rise to synergistic processes that actually enhance outcomes. The Magnet framework is a perfect example. For instance, the Magnet framework promotes nursing research, quality improvement, and evidence-based practice processes, which are interrelated in many ways, and can actually work together interactively to better desired outcomes. Let us look at an example. Consider that you are caring for a woman with poorly controlled diabetes. She has a Stage II pressure ulcer. Each day you see her, the ulcer looks worse. You and your colleagues are adhering to the care protocol stringently. The clinical specialist on the unit has been consulted and thinks that there may be a better wound treatment protocol for patients with uncontrolled diabetes. She utilizes the evidence-based practice (EBP) process and searches database after database, coming up with nothing except literature that recommends performing research studies to determine the best treatment. So, without an evidence base for the treatment of uncontrolled diabetic patients with pressure ulcers, there is little the clinical specialist can recommend besides the standard treatment protocol, which leaves the original query unanswered. Now here is where the EBP process hands over the inquiry to the research process. With a research nurse (PhD, RN) to assist, the clinical specialist and the direct-care nurse design a research study in the hopes of determining the best treatment for pressure ulcers in patients with uncontrolled diabetes. The study produces a revised treatment protocol with demonstrated efficacy for patients with uncontrolled diabetes, thus bettering patient care. The Magnet framework (structure) relates the two processes, and EBP and research (process) work together in sequence to ultimately enhance patient care (outcome).

Structures Already in Place

Rarely, if ever, are you able to structure things as you would like for your particular purpose. You cannot simply change your institution's organizational structure to suit your needs for the Magnet journey, although I am sure some have tried. That is not to say that you cannot modify structures. With that said, the key to success is to use the structures you have already in place to your advantage, all the while attempting to integrate similar structures. For example, a hospital we visited has structure for performance improvement consisting of about a dozen teams, each working on a specific indicator, such as catheter-associated urinary tract infections (CAUTI), nosocomial pressure ulcers, patient falls, etc. They also have shared governance structures that include a practice council and a quality council. The two structures work toward similar purposes, basically to achieve better patient outcomes. Yet, there was really no integration of the two structures. The councils are not aware of what the quality indicator teams are doing and vice versa. You can imagine how much work is replicated and how teams and councils might implement contradictory interventions all in an effort to improve their specified indicator. Without integration, you have muddled productivity at best, chaos at worst. The key is to integrate, integrate, integrate. Oh, and do not replicate. There are enough opportunities for improving patient care to go around. If a group or team is working on an initiative and is not successful, tweak the team or tweak their methodology, do not just start another team. It is a waste of time, money, and resources.

Gap Analysis and Evaluation

First, look at the structures you will need for the Magnet journey (some of the necessary structures are discussed later in this chapter). Then, familiarize yourself with the structures currently in place in your institution that will affect the Magnet journey. Are they working? Can they, in their present state, fulfill the requirements of the Magnet journey? Can you tweak the structure to make it more effective? Does the structure serve a purpose that adds value to both the institution and to the journey? If you find that a structure is obsolete and ineffective, can you dismantle the structure without negative repercussions? If you can, do it with the appropriate leadership backing, of course.

Perform a gap analysis on the structures that are necessary for the journey. You might want to work with a consultant on this. Again, are the structures you have in place sufficiently able to meet the requirements? What are the new structures you need to put into place? You might want to categorize structures into those that are sufficient, those that need tweaking, those that need to be dismantled, and those that need to be created. This classification system is a good way to describe the structures from your gap analysis and communicate your assessment to senior nursing leadership.

Creating New Structures

So, how do you create a new structure? Some of what you will need to do will be specific to your institution, but we will talk about some of the things that are mostly universal. The first step is to know what you need to create and then find the best practice to do it. This means searching the literature, not necessarily the research literature. You will most likely find this type of information in quality improvement literature, or in one of our forthcoming books. For example, you want to create a shared decision-making structure. After a bit of searching through the pertinent literature, you find that there are various models of shared decision-making structures to choose from. What you want to know is which types of structure would be a best fit with the culture and structures already in place. Your best bet is to look for similar institutions and see what types of structures they use. Did it work for them? What issues did they have when they implemented the structure?

You can learn a lot through published case studies. The problem is, not many institutions publish their experiences. That is why we feel this book and forthcoming volumes are so necessary. So, when you do create and implement your shared governance structure, take notes and be sure to write about and publish the experience. You will make it easier for other institutions to help them achieve quality nursing care. Now you have found a structure and literature that shows it has worked in institutions like your own. Next you have to make a plan and sell it to leadership (first) and to staff (second). Once your plan is laid out, you can then approach leadership for support and resources to begin implementation. Your plan should spell out what you are going to do, how you are going to do it, who will be involved, a timeline for implementation, and costs. You may want to do a cost/benefit analysis, but a structure such as a shared decision-making system might not produce a quantifiable benefit (at least not right away). The benefit will be mostly in staff engagement, but you may see a decreased turnover rate and decreased vacancy rate as more long-term benefits.

After you have the green light from senior leadership, you will need to work on obtaining support from middle management and staff. First, assemble your implementation team. This may be your Magnet Steering Committee or a different team. We suggest using your steering committee, since they have already bought in to the journey. If you are able to obtain the necessary resources, we suggest using a consultant to help guide you through the implementation process. You will not necessarily need a consultant for every structure you create, but creating and implementing a shared decision-making structure is quite an undertaking. Sometimes the voice of an outside consultant or expert is accepted more easily than an internal voice. While in the planning stage prior to implementation, consider what would constitute a successful implementation. How will you know you have achieved what you set out to do in measurable terms? If one of our colleagues makes a statement to the effect of: "We've had a successful implementation." We ask, "Is there staff representation from each unit on the councils? How many decisions did staff participate in?" In other words, what is your definition of success? It should be measurable and relate to the purpose of your initiative. If your purpose is staff engagement, then a measure of success might be the number of staff participants. If your purpose is staff involvement in decision making, then your measurement might be the number of decisions made with staff input. Metrics help demonstrate your success to others and provide an operational definition to the purpose of your initiative. Plan ahead what you will need to measure. When you are planning the new structure, make sure you consider how the structure will integrate with existing structures in your institution. You will want to avoid competing structures, such as two teams working on improving the same nurse-sensitive indicator. If you have two structures with similar purposes, try to separate and delineate their roles, creating as much mutual exclusiveness as possible.

Structure for Communication

Facilitate communication between the groups using one or two common members. This will provide each group with a sense of what the other is working on and how it meets the overall goal. This is an example of one of the three principles to keep in mind when creating a structure. Consider communication: how communication will flow to, from, and within the structure. Sure, you can call communication a process, but we know structure affects process, so considering communication when planning your structure will allow you to plan better, to consider other interdependent structures, and the way information will flow. Part of this communication should be the reporting structure within the organization. Who will oversee this structure? How will communication flow to facilitate oversight and accountability?

Structure for Cost-Effectiveness

The second principle to consider is to structure for cost-effectiveness. What we mean by this is that when you create the structure, consider all the costs involved and try to minimize these costs as much as possible. Consider a shared governance structure. One organization we visited had two of their five councils requiring membership from each nursing unit. It was very costly and cumbersome to replace direct-care staff for two different 2-hour meetings, as the minimum managers could schedule a replacement each time was 4 hours. So, two different meetings meant 8 hours of extra staff salary. What they did was to structure the two council meetings back-to-back at the same location. They also had mostly the same membership on both councils. This structure allowed unit managers to schedule a single 4-hour replacement shift to cover both meetings, saving 4 hours of salary multiplied by 25 units each month. Attendance at both meetings soared, and council members and unit managers were more satisfied.

Structure for the Least Amount of Change Possible

The third principle is to structure for the least amount of change possible. In general, most people do not welcome change. It is a process that can be quite time consuming and can absorb much energy. Instead, try to structure using things that are familiar and will not require a huge upheaval. It may mean building your structure as an extension of an existing structure, at least in the beginning. Then gradually, you can introduce more change. Let us go back to the shared governance structure. The same institution we told you about in structuring for cost-effectiveness wanted to implement unit-based practice councils (UBPC) for each of their inpatient units, bringing performance improvement processes and empowerment to the direct-care nurses. Creating these councils on all units is somewhat of a daunting task. Scheduling staff; recruiting members, chairs, and cochairs of the councils; establishing regular meeting schedules, especially with staff working various shifts; and assuring member representation from all shifts require a considerable amount of change and buy in from staff and leadership. In order to lessen the amount of change, they structured the unit-based practice councils as an extension of mandatory staff meetings, making sure to delineate one meeting from the other. This structure facilitated the adoption of the unit-based practice councils, ultimately buffering the effect of the change process by decreasing the novelty. Familiarity lessens change and expedites acceptance. As time progressed, the UBPC membership became more committed and the goals of the council became more distinct. Eventually, the council meetings were divorced from the staff meetings, and the structures of the two meetings matured into distinct forms. This is what we mean when we recommend structuring for the least amount of change possible. The initial change was minimal, and the implementation progressed with contoured incremental change so that the implementation never became overwhelming or burdensome.

Some of the Structures You May Implement

Teams

There are numbers of other structures you will need to create and implement on the Magnet journey. The most common structures you will implement are teams. Teams are utilized for a number of purposes, everything from planning the journey to implementing quality improvement initiatives. You are probably quite familiar with structuring teams. Just a repetitive word of advice, consider the flow of communication and how you are measuring the effectiveness of the team. This will depend on the purpose of the team and if the team is permanent or just a temporary task force assigned to a specific purpose. Evaluating a team is a lot like evaluating an initiative: You have compliance measures (process) and outcome measures. It is the same with a team. Compliance measures might be the number of times the team has met out of how many times it was supposed to meet and how many attended the meetings out of how many should have attended. Outcome measures are metrics that show if the team achieved its goals. For a Patient Falls Prevention Team, an outcome measure might be the rate of patient falls or the number of interventions successfully implemented. It depends, as we have said, on the purpose of the team. We could go on and on about teams, creating, facilitating, and motivating, but we will leave that for another time.

Professional Development

Some kind of professional development structure will need to be implemented, one that will allow direct-care nurses a path for professional development, with graduated incentives to achieve higher levels and continued professional growth. Many know this structure as a clinical ladder, and it can take many forms. Take a look at the literature on clinical ladders and adopt one that will work with your institution's culture. Ask other neighboring institutions if they have a clinical ladder and how it works. There are some things to keep in mind at this stage. First, do not make professional development so complex that you need a PhD to decipher its requirements. Also, look strategically for what you want to get from the ladder. Most want to increase the number of nationally certified nurses and the educational level of the nurses. You may want to tie in incentives, such as tuition reimbursement or reimbursement for the cost of certification fees as well as a discretionary incentive, typically a monetary bonus. Funding for attending conferences and continuing education credits are also perks that will help you achieve your goals for professional development. Make the process user friendly for nurses and be cognizant of the time commitment necessary for achieving each level of the ladder. We have seen hospitals incorporate quality improvement projects, requiring a unit-based project to fulfill ladder requirements.

Remember, this professional development program will cost money. If your institution already has incentives for education and certification, you may just need to restructure them into levels with graduated requirements. It is relatively easy to do a cost/benefit analysis on the program. Estimate how many nurses are expected to achieve each level. Calculate the cost and look at what the institution gets: more certified nurses, more educated nurses, and quality improvement projects. As for structure and process, you will need a way to apply to the program, someone for oversight and evaluation of the program (this may be a committee), a timeline from application to decision, a process for communicating the decision, and a process for administering incentives and monitoring cost-effectiveness. We think the best way to get started on this structure is to list what the institution wants to get out of the program. Then, survey your nurses and see what they want to get out of the program. Perform and use a gap analysis of the demographics of your current staff and where they need to grow for Magnet consideration (i.e., education, levels, percent nationally certified, number belonging to professional organizations, number with professional publications, professional speaking engagements, and professional presentations, etc.). This gap analysis can also help to establish a realistic timeline for meeting goals for the Magnet journey.

Employee Recognition

You will also need some type of employee recognition structure. You may be able to utilize your institution's Human Resources Department for this. There needs to be a structure where employees can recognize each other and leadership can recognize staff for exceptional contributions or milestone achievements. Some recognition may be annual, some may be continuous, and some may be a one-time acknowledgment. Whatever it is, it is beneficial to have a structure where an individual or group can develop and administer programs for employee recognition. In many institutions, these structures are decentralized by department, in others, they are centralized under one umbrella, and frequently there is some combination of publicity both internal and external. This is crucial, and we believe internal and external publicity should be formulated in a strategic plan for the promotion of nursing. The benefits may be far reaching: the reputation of your nursing department in the professional community, the reputation of your nursing department in your public community, the satisfaction of your patients, and the pride and esteem your staff feel as members of your nursing department. It is difficult to put a price on an empowered and trusted staff, and an adoring community. That is exactly what your promotion should strive for.

Strategic Plan to Promote Nursing

Do you have a strategic plan to promote nursing? Do you have a structure and process for disseminating nursing's professional accomplishments internally and externally? If not, it is something you should really consider. It can significantly raise the self-concept of your nursing workforce. In the first year of working at one institution, one of the authors wrote or facilitated the writing of 12 abstracts accepted for professional conferences, one research grant, four research studies, and eight local and one national nursing awards. There is nothing these nurses think they cannot do now. The sky is the limit. These nurses have been doing excellent work all along. They just thought it was what everyone else was doing. Sometimes it takes fresh eyes and a bit of coercion at the beginning to get the staff to see their own potential. Then watch out! There is no stopping them. The motivation builds one nurse at time, so do not get impatient if everything does not happen immediately. Remember, it is a journey, not a destination.

Institutional Review Board

We will ever so briefly mention here some other structures you will need for the Magnet journey which you might already have. For your nursing research initiative, you will need an Institutional Review Board (IRB). If you do not already have one at the start, we recommend utilizing an established IRB at a different hospital, a university, or a privately run IRB. We have no doubt you will find one to use. After your research program becomes enculturated and established, you might then want to think about establishing your own IRB. Make friends with the IRB coordinator, wherever you decide to go. He or she will be a great help in facilitating your submission and might be able to provide some assistance in the construction of nursing research proposals. A word of advice: Try to utilize an IRB that is familiar with nursing research. It can be a grueling process presenting a study when the IRB members are used to seeing only medical and pharmaceutical clinical trials.

Performance/Quality Improvement Structure

Other structures that we mention here are most likely present in your institution, but might need a bit of tweaking for the Magnet journey. The quality improvement/performance improvement (QI/PI) structure is essential. One institution that we worked in had a PI structure that focused mainly on reimbursement outcomes (CMS core measures), and the PI Director reported to the Chief Medical Officer. It seemed that nursing PI was an afterthought, receiving little attention except the occasional harassment when numbers were poor. Remember the old saying, "You can't manage what you don't measure." It is true, and so with your PI structure comes consideration of your data collection structures. How do you get your data? Who collects it, and how do they collect it? Are you receiving data regularly on nurse-sensitive indicators? Is the collection methodology consistent with others with whom you benchmark? The National Database of Nursing Quality Indicators (NDNQI) has a somewhat strict methodology for the collection and submission of data. Without this, benchmarks would be useless; you would not know if the data you are using to compare to is the same as what you have collected. For example, pressure ulcer data is required as a 1-day prevalence study (American Nurses Association, 2009). If your institution decides to do the prevalence study over 1 week instead of a single day, you might be duplicating your counting or missing some that should have been counted. The data would be inaccurate, and because your data also influences the benchmark, you are actually making the benchmark less reliable for others. Data collection methodology is important.

Staying with the example of pressure ulcer prevalence, there is still some variation in data collection methodology. Some institutions have each nurse collect data on his or her patients, and the unit clerk compiles the unit's data, sending it off to the data entry person. Other institutions have a specific team of wound care nurses, intensively trained, who examine every patient to collect pressure ulcer prevalence data. Which is better? Does it make a difference? Most studies that have looked at this are case studies and not generalizable. It is somewhat logical that having the same nurses doing the same collection of data would help to maintain competence and consistency. Also, it is easier to maintain up-to-date training on pressure ulcer staging utilizing a small group than it is spread over all nurses in your institution.

Now the drawbacks. The cost of pulling a group of direct-care staff to assess each patient and collect data is more costly than having each nurse assess his or her own patients. Also, taking away the responsibility for assessing pressure ulcers from most direct-care staff may lessen their competence, something you definitely do not want to do. So, this is one of those situations where you will need to consider a cost/benefit analysis, as well as the culture of your institution. Any data collection structure needs to work in your institution and be integrated into related structures.

Yes, we know you are probably thinking of a structure we have missed. It is inevitable we will not get them all, not in this short space. Just remember the basic principles we have discussed when creating structures in your institution. Look to what similar institutions have done, and do not reinvent the wheel. Sound familiar?

CREATIVE SOLUTIONS

Creative Solution Title: *Implementing the Baby-Friendly Hospital Initiative*
Creative Solution Author: **Marie Bosco BSN, RN, IBCLC**
                                           Lactation Consultant
                                           Royal Oak Beaumont Hospital

Purpose: The goal of Royal Oak Beaumont Hospital is to implement the Ten Steps to Successful Breastfeeding as outlined by UNICEF/WHO Baby-Friendly Hospital Initiative and ultimately receive the designation of a Baby-Friendly Hospital. The purpose of this creative solution was to improve initiation of breastfeeding within an hour of birth (step 4 of the initiative) by addressing areas for improvements and barriers for staff and patients.

Legend

     Overall Rating: **ADVANCED BEGINNER**

     Financial: **$**

     Time:

     Personnel:

     Other Resources: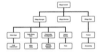

     Efficacy: **A**

     Transferability: **A**

     Malleability/Adaptability: **A**

     Ease of Implementation: **B**

Synopsis: A collaborative effort was enlisted to implement step 4 of the Baby-Friendly Hospital Initiative (BFHI) Ten Steps to Successful Breastfeeding. The purpose of this step was to help mothers initiate breastfeeding within an hour of birth. The goal was to have 80% of all healthy, vaginal deliveries offered skin-to-skin care within 30 minutes of delivery for at least 60 minutes, and offered breastfeeding assistance within the first hour. It was thought that Beaumont Hospital Royal Oak lacked the information, skills, and documentation needed to implement this step. So, a process change was initiated including staff education and changes in computer documentation.

Description of Organization: William Beaumont Hospital Royal Oak is an acute care hospital in Royal Oak, Michigan. It is one of three acute care hospitals in the Beaumont hospital system. Beaumont, Royal Oak, is a major academic medical center with fellowship, residency, and nursing education programs. The facility has Level 1 trauma status and has 990 beds, of which 904 are adult and pediatric, 18 are coronary care, and 68 are intensive care. It is a Magnet-designated hospital.

The Case Study: The goal of Royal Oak Beaumont Hospital was to implement the Ten Steps to Successful Breastfeeding as outlined by UNICEF/WHO Baby-Friendly Hospital Initiative and ultimately receive the designation of a Baby-Friendly Hospital. The Baby-Friendly Hospital Initiative (BFHI) is a global program sponsored by UNICEF and WHO to encourage and recognize hospitals that provide exceptional breastfeeding care. The BFHI promotes, protects, and supports breastfeeding through the Ten Steps to Successful Breastfeeding. BFHI assists healthcare facilities in providing breastfeeding mothers with information, confidence, and skills needed to successfully initiate and continue breastfeeding their babies. Healthcare facilities can provide support for both initiation and duration of breastfeeding immediately following birth by providing evidence-based care outlined in step 4: Help mothers initiate breastfeeding within an hour of birth. It was found that Beaumont Hospital Royal Oak lacked the information, skills, and documentation needed to implement this step. While breastfeeding was often initiated following delivery, much improvement would be needed to support this step as outlined by BFHI. The goal was 80% of all healthy vaginal deliveries would be offered skin-to-skin care within 30 minutes of delivery for at least 60 minutes, and offered breastfeeding assistance within this first hour. All mothers who have had a cesarean delivery will be given their babies to hold skin-to-skin within 30 minutes *after* they are able to respond to their babies for at least 60 minutes, and offered breastfeeding assistance with that first hour.

A collaborative group was developed to improve both skin-to-skin and breastfeeding initiation and thus the quality of maternal and newborn care. The group consisted of the director of Maternal Child Health, the nurse manager of the maternity unit, the QS Clinical Systems Coordinator, a staff RN (BFHI mentor), a Lactation Consultant, and the Manager of Anesthesia. The group discussed specific areas for improvements and their barriers. These areas included the need for updated breastfeeding education for staff, the need for recovery room initiation of breastfeeding for cesarean deliveries, the need for updated computer documentation regarding breastfeeding and initiation of use of computer documentation in the recovery room. A process change initiative began in September 2008 with a roll out date of July 1, 2009. The process began with Breastfeeding Support Services evaluating the breastfeeding initiation through chart review by Lactation Consultants. A newborn vital signs/feeding care plan was then developed for interim use in the Recovery Room. Documentation revisions were made and approved in the computer charting system. Education for staff regarding the new initiatives in place was provided via PowerPoint presentations distributed through e-mail and posted for viewing in the unit. Contacts were made to appropriate individuals needed to continue to promote the change process, and data continues to be monitored for compliance and improvements are instituted as needed. Problems with the current process were identified by the intervention group, and resolution plans were created and implemented. The official roll out of the new process began July 1, 2009 with goal of 90% compliance with skin-to-skin offering and breastfeeding initiation. In the first week, 82% compliance with breastfeeding documentation of vaginal deliveries and 19% compliance with all cesarean deliveries was found. During the next week, process improvements were implemented. A bonding nurse from NICU was assigned to assist with skin-to-skin contact, breastfeeding initiation, and documentation in the recovery room for 6 weeks. Charge nurses began to provide reminders of the importance of the initiative for all nurses during change of shift report. In August 2009, after the process change was implemented and periodic evaluations and improvements were continued, 86% of vaginal delivery mothers received breastfeeding assistance with appropriate documentation, and 70% of cesarean delivery mothers received breastfeeding assistance with appropriate documentation. This initiative is a perfect example of the people and processes needed to enhance nursing quality and improve patient outcomes and the successes possible if such people and processes are utilized appropriately.

Outcome Measures:

Formative/Compliance: Weekly evaluation of percent compliance with new process via documentation evaluation.

Summative/Outcome: Achievement of goal of 90% compliance after 1 year of implementation of process change.

Evidence Supporting this Creative Solution: Healthy People 2010 Breastfeeding Initiative, Baby-Friendly Hospital Initiative, The Ten Steps to Successful Breastfeeding, WHO, and UNICEF all support and encourage modalities to promote initiation of breastfeeding in hospitals. The American Academy of Pediatrics (AAP) also supports the Ten Steps to Successful Breastfeeding Initiative. Healthy People 2010 also supports initiation, exclusivity, and duration of breastfeeding as outlined: breastfeeding initiation (75% in early postpartum) and duration (50% and 25% at 6 and 12 months, respectively), and exclusivity (50% and 17% at 3 months and 6 months, respectively). It is well established through research that breastfeeding promotes the optimal health of mothers and their infants, with immediate and long-term benefits.

The need for people and process-centered efforts to improve care and outcomes in health care, as presented in this creative solution, is extensively discussed in a book by Smith and Flarey (1999). They highlight management principles of reengineering as they apply to health care and note that reengineering and process centered infrastructure has transformed healthcare organizations and allowed huge performance improvements.

Smith, P., & Flarey, D. L. (1999). *Process-centered health care organizations*. New York: Aspen Publishers, Inc.

Recipe for: *Implementing the Baby-Friendly Hospital Initiative*

Ingredients:

1 Director of Maternal Child Health

1 Nurse Manager of the maternity unit

1 computer documentation coordinator

1 staff RN (BFHI Mentor)

1 Lactation Consultant

1 Manager of Anesthesia

2 additional computers for the Recovery Room

PowerPoint program

Step-by-Step Instructions (see Figure 2-1 for Step-by-Step Instruction Timeline):

Step 1: Evaluate current breastfeeding initiation practices/processes via chart reviews.

Step 2: Develop a new care plan for newborn feeding for use in the Recovery Room.

Step 3: Develop a collaborative group comprised of individuals from multiple disciplines as needed for the initiative.

Step 4: Develop a group dedicated to improvement of skin-to-skin and breastfeeding initiation. Identify current problems with the process and create resolution plans.

Step 5: Make revisions to the computer documentation system and add additional computers as needed for documentation of new processes.

Step 6: Develop process plans and staff education, and disseminate in PowerPoint slides via e-mail and unit postings.

Step 7: Roll out new process.

Step 8: Evaluate compliance and outcome data post-process implementation. Plan and implement improvements as needed.

Step 9: Reevaluate for achievement of goal, and communicate results with all people involved so the process can be continually implemented, evaluated, and improved as needed.

Additional Outcomes to Consider Measuring:

Formative/Compliance: No additional measures.

Summative/Outcome: No additional measures.

Figure 2-1   Timeline for "Implementing the Baby-Friendly Hospital Initiative."

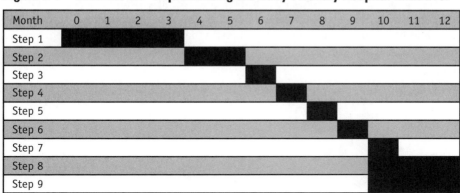

Insights from Original Implementation: A collaborative and supportive group can accomplish great things. The people involved in a process change are key. They must be invested in the change. Also, a process change takes time. You must be patient and change can and will happen.

For Further Guidance Contact:

Marie Bosco, BSN, RN, IBCLC
William Beaumont Hospitals Royal Oak
3601 W. Thirteen Mile Rd.
Royal Oak, MI 48073
mbosco@beaumonthospitals.com

Creative Solution Title: *Clinical Links*

Creative Solution Authors: Bette Schumacher, RN, CPN, MS
Clinical Nurse Specialist
Sanford USD Medical Center

Bonnie Becker, RN, BSN
Perinatal Data Center Coordinator
Sanford USD Medical Center

Patricia Dysthe, RN, BA
Clinical Care Coordinator
Sanford USD Medical Center

Sheri Fischer, RN, BSN
Nursing Unit Director
Sanford USD Medical Center

Purpose: The goal of this creative solution was to put information at the bedside nurses' fingertips in an easy to use format that was also printable, making clinical reference materials easy to locate, as well as use. A second goal was to have current and updated information that reflected today's fast-paced and changing practice in nursing and medicine.

Legend

Overall Rating: **PROFICIENT**

Financial:

Time:

Personnel:

Other Resources:

Efficacy: **A**

Transferability: **B**

Malleability/Adaptability: **A**

Ease of Implementation: **B**

Synopsis: A desktop accessible (online) reference menu was created for bedside nursing staff to have clinical information (Clinical Links) at their fingertips. Using Excel as a shell program to support the links, files are housed within the program. Several tabs were added, and color was used to make links appealing. Beginning with high-risk, low-frequency reference materials, online references provide bedside staff nurses with easily accessible information, all from one network location. Source files have grown and an indexing system has been added. Nurses use materials to support a variety of functions including: looking up information, performing weight-based calculations for medications, enabling just in time training, and calculating selected physiologic measures, to name a few. Prompt cards are available for selected nursing actions, such as central line dressing care, pain assessment, blood transfusion, moderate sedation monitoring, administration of high-risk medication, etc. A hyperlink to the related policy/procedure is imbedded so nurses always have the most recent issue of the policy/procedure. Information can be updated and instantly be available to the clinical staff. The Clinical Links concept has spread from the innovation unit (NICU) to multiple other units at the medical center.

Description of Organization: Sanford USD Medical Center is a Midwestern 545-bed tertiary care teaching hospital which is part of a large comprehensive integrated health system, Sanford Health-Merit Care System. The Medical Center serves an average of more than 50,000 inpatients annually. The Boekelheide NICU, a 58-bed Level IIIb Neonatal Intensive Care Unit, is located on the Sioux Falls, SD, campus at the Medical Center. Sanford USD Medical Center has been a Magnet organization since 2003.

The Case Study: The Clinical Links online reference tool was born from the dilemma faced by the Perinatal Data Center Coordinator at Sanford USD Medical Center of how to maintain communication and provide up-to-date information for more than 160 nurses in a busy NICU. The coordinator founded the idea after a discussion with the Practice Council chairperson regarding a means to keeping the nurses informed of ongoing and evolving practice changes. They looked at how other nursing units in the hospital made information accessible to staff. They found that online communication books and drug references were being used. They expanded on these ideas by utilizing Microsoft Excel as the basic vehicle for a one-stop menu to lead to all needed information. A trial access menu of references was developed, demonstrated, and tested. Feedback from the users always guided the development as the project evolved. The Clinical Nurse Specialist, bedside staff and unit Education and Practice Nursing Councils participated in this project. Any staff nurse request for information to be made available through clinical links was (and continues to be) considered. The nursing staff take ownership of their information as a result. Multidisciplinary contribution of resources was key in the development process. Multidisciplinary teams came on board and contributed clinical information. For example, the nutritionists developed their own nutritional page, the clinical pharmacist gave her expertise on the medication and IV pages. The initiative began in the NICU, but quickly expanded. The NICU Nurse Practitioners requested their own clinical reference page and then pediatric staff requested one for their unit. It continued to expand to other units by their request.

Outcome Measures:

Formative/Compliance: No formal compliance data generated, but frequency of nurse access of Clinical Links could be used. Staff reported accessing and using information from Clinical Links several times throughout their shifts.

Summative/Outcome: Positive feedback from staff and continual use and expansion of the program.

Evidence Supporting this Creative Solution: Support for the implementation and use of easily accessible computer information systems is evident in the current literature. Hohler (2004) found that handheld computers help nurses organize information and find the latest resources without having to leave their patients' bedsides. These resources help nurses do their jobs and can be used to enhance nursing practice. Domrose (2004) states that nursing students and new grads having quick, up-to-date reference materials to back up their decisions makes them feel more confident. Use of online information resources was studied in the Usage of Online

Information Resources by Nurses Project, which was designed to provide clinical nurses with accurate medical information at the point of care by introducing nurses to existing online library resources through instructional classes. It was discovered that clinical nurses will readily use these resources if they are formally introduced to them and taught how to access and use them (Wozar & Worona, 2003).

Domrose, C. (2004). *A new dimension*. Nursing Spectrum. Available at: http://www .nursingspectrum.com/StudentsCorner/StudentFeatures/ANewDimension.htm. Accessed March 7, 2010.

Hohler, S. E. (2004). A pocket full of knowledge: Enhancing nursing practice with handheld computers. *AORN Journal*. Available at: http://findarticles.com/p/articles/mi_m0FSL/ is_2_79/ai_113802519/. Accessed March 7, 2010.

Wozar, J. A., & Worona P. C. (2003). The use of online information resources by nurses. *Journal of the Medical Library Association, 91*(2), 216–221.

Recipe for: *Clinical Links*

Ingredients:

Computers accessible to bedside nurses

Excel computer program

IT personnel

Expert clinicians to create computer program content

Expert data manager

Unit Nursing Director

CNS

Nursing Practice Council

Step-by-Step Instructions (see Figure 2-2 for Step-by-Step Instruction Timeline):

Step 1: Discussed with Practice Council chairperson to brainstorm how to effectively communicate nursing practice issues and updates. Evaluated how other units are communicating to staff and explore how the computer could be of assistance.

Step 2: Set up a trial menu using Excel as the shell, to test a process of opening resources quickly. Received feedback and suggestions from the unit Practice Council members and CNS who reviewed the new program. Continue to revise the process until it was usable. Consulted with IT staff on the process when technical advice was needed. IT also provided desktop icon access and necessary security.

Step 3: Demonstrated use of Clinical Links at unit Professional Practice Meeting, and set the icon on the desktops for nurses to use. Continue to solicit feedback and add additional information to the menu as feedback was provided by CNS, multidisciplinary team, and Nursing Councils.

Step 4: Additions made such as an index cross-referenced by topic, so a resource could be looked up alphabetically, by title, or subject matter and a Bulletin Board page which chronologically details new information that has been incorporated, so staff easily find the latest information.

Step 5: Maintenance of Clinical Links including additions and linking of new information, updates to existing information, and periodic backups of the information. Estimated time varies from one to several hours per week, depending on content requests. Old references are dated and moved into a retired file folder.

Figure 2-2   Timeline for "Clinical Links."

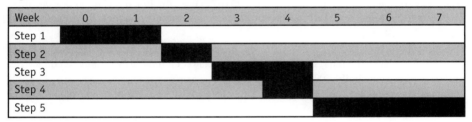

Additional Outcomes to Consider Measuring:

Formative/Compliance: No additional measures.

Summative/Outcome: Might survey nurses for increased job satisfaction and knowledge and comfort with daily nursing tasks after the implementation of Clinical Links. It may be possible to also look at patient outcomes before and after implementation of the system.

Insights from Original Implementation: Build the program for expansion. Give thought to how you want the clinical information organized in the menu first, before you add and link the reference sources. It is always fluid and never completed. Give thought to how you will update the resources (e.g., annual review and add a posting date to all references). It was learned that once the information is available and it is being used, going back to reorganize is quite a task.

For Further Guidance Contact:

Bette Schumacher, RN
Sanford USD Medical Center
Sanford Children's Hospital
Boekelheide NICU
1305 W 18th Street PO Box 5039
Sioux Falls, SD 57110-5039
schumabe@sanfordhealth.org

REFERENCES

American Nurses Association. (2009). *The national database*. Available at: http://www.nursingworld.org/MainMenuCategories/ThePracticeofProfessionalNursing/ PatientSafetyQuality/Research-Measurement/The-National-Database.aspx. Accessed December 19, 2009.

American Nurses Credentialing Center. (2008a). *Application manual Magnet Recognition Program*. Silver Spring, MD: Author.

American Nurses Credentialing Center. (2008b). *Search Magnet-recognized organizations*. Available at: http://www.nursecredentialing.org/MagnetOrg/searchmagnet .cfm. Accessed December 19, 2009.

American Nurses Credentialing Center. (2010). *Consultation for Magnet Recognition Program®*. Available at: http://www.nursecredentialing.org/Magnet/ResourceCenters/ Consulting.aspx. Accessed March 21, 2010.

ChangingMinds.org. (2009). *The psychology of change*. Available at: http://changingminds .org/disciplines/change_management/psychology_change/psychology_change.htm. Accessed December 19, 2009.

Donabedian, A. (1966). Evaluating the quality of medical care. *The Milbank Memorial Fund Quarterly, 44*(1), 166–203.

Drumm, C. (2005, Apr. 1). The Magnet journey. *Healthcare Traveler*. Retrieved October 19, 2009, from http://healthcaretraveler.modernmedicine.com/healthcaretraveler/The-Magnet-journey/ArticleStandard/Article/detail/154384.

Goal Setting Guide. (n.d.). *Smart goals*. Available at: http://www.goal-setting-guide.com/ smart-goals.html. Accessed December 19, 2009.

Havens, D. S., & Johnston, M. A. (2004). Achieving Magnet hospital recognition. *JONA, 34*(12), 579–588.

HealthStream® Research. (2009). Available at: http://www.healthstreamresearch.com/ Pages/Default.aspx. Accessed December 19, 2009.

Herzberg, F. I. (1968). One more time: How do you motivate employees? *Harvard Business Review, 46*(1), 53–62.

Hospital Consumer Assessment of Healthcare Providers and Systems. (2009). Fact Sheet. Available at: http://www.hcahpsonline.org/files/HCAHPS%20Fact%20Sheet,%20revised1, %203-31-09.pdf. Accessed December 19, 2009.

Kübler-Ross, E. (1969). *On death and dying*. New York: Simon & Schuster/Touchstone.

McNamara, C. (2008). *Basic guide to program evaluation*. Available at: http://managementhelp .org/evaluatn/fnl_eval.htm. Accessed December 19, 2009.

Pierson, P., Miller, J., & Moore, K. (2007). Engaging staff in the Magnet journey: The key is communication. *MedSurg Nursing*. Available at: http://findarticles.com/p/articles/mi_ m0FSS/is_1_16/ai_n18744577/. Accessed October 19, 2009.

Structure. (2006). In E. McKean (Ed.), *New Oxford American dictionary* (2nd ed.). New York: Oxford American Press.

University of Iowa. (2007). *Magnet champions*. Available at: http://www.uihealthcare.com/ depts/nursing/magnet/champions.html. Accessed March 21, 2010.

## CHAPTER 3

Project Development and Implementation

*"Trying to manage a project without project management
is like trying to play a football game without a game plan."*
—K. TATE (PAST BOARD MEMBER, PMI)

*"You can only elevate individual performance
by elevating that of the entire system."*
—W. EDWARDS DEMING

This chapter serves two purposes. The first, to further initiate you into the formal project management process, and the second, to provide a framework for implementing the creative solutions you will find within this volume. This chapter is by no means meant as a substitute for coursework or certification in project management. It is merely a brief overview, sprinkled with advice and experience to help make project implementation more structured and less chaotic for you. We recommend purchasing a book like *Absolute Beginner's Guide to Project Management*, 2nd Edition (Horine, 2009) or *The Everything Project Management Book*, 2nd Edition (Morris, 2008) for reference and further guidance. You will find that having a reference book easily available is a necessity. Also, having one main volume for reference instead of sporadically searching the Internet for information every time an issue arises will help you to develop a familiarity with and a confidence about the volume at your side. We hope this volume will also be at your side, extensively annotated, guiding you to project management and patient care excellence.

DEVELOPING THE CREATIVE SOLUTION

Each creative solution is actually a project to be managed. It is so tempting to say, "Why don't we just try it tomorrow?" Now that you have gotten this far in the volume, you probably know what we would say in return. If you do not plan and manage your project adequately, you probably will not have success. At least, you will be hard pressed to show that it was your project that made the difference. Why chance it? There is a right way to do it. What you need more than anything else is patience. As nurses, we are used to immediate feedback. We give a pain medication, and in 30 minutes we expect to see results. We have grown accustomed to operating in crisis mode constantly. Planning is seen as something we learned in school, but seems to be of little use when you are immersed in an eight patient assignment without assistance. Too many nurses we have met feel this way, and we need to nip it in the bud! Planning is the only way to get results short of serendipity. Although, as we have heard, it seems nothing ever happens according to plan. Maybe we need better planning skills, and a lot more patience. These anecdotes might or might not ring true to you, but we have experienced much apathy and resistance when it comes to planning and process approaches to implementing initiatives. It may just be the fast pace of health care, but you will need to slow it down when putting one of these creative solutions to use. So, we hope we have helped to set your expectations that things that make a difference will not happen overnight. Now, let us get to work.

WHAT IS PROJECT MANAGEMENT?

First we would like to provide you with a formal definition of project management. Project management is the application of knowledge, skills, tools, and techniques to a broad range of activities in order to meet the requirements of the particular project. A project is a temporary endeavor undertaken to achieve a particular aim, in this case, a creative solution. Project management knowledge and practices are best described in terms of their component processes. These processes can be placed into five process groups: initiating, planning, implementing, monitoring, and closing; along with nine knowledge areas: project integration management, project scope management, project time management, project cost management, project quality management, project human resource management, project communications management, project risk management, and project procurement management (Project Management Institute, Inc., 2009). These are not just skills to use, but a way of thinking about a project as a whole.

The Five Stages of Project Management

The following are the five basic stages of project management. We have dedicated some of these topics to their own chapters, such as Chapter 4: Motivation, Buy-In, and Enculturation; Chapter 5: Measuring Outcomes; etc. The following bulleted outline provides a sequence to the entire process. This outline is generic, therefore we have tried to provide more specifics throughout this volume. We think, however, it is valuable to see a step-by-step synopsis of the project management process.

1. Initiation
   - Define a Project: The proposed project has clear start and end points, a defined set of objectives, separate resources, and an organized plan to meet the objectives.

- Identify, Understand Roles, and Involve Stakeholders: Key players in the process, such as the sponsor, the project manager, stakeholders, team members, customers, and suppliers, all have distinct roles in the process. Identify those stakeholders who could have a significant effect on the project and involve them early. Consider how regularly they should be consulted. Form strong alliances with stakeholders who control the resources.
- Have Clear Goals: Goals and expectations must be identical for everyone involved. Scope must remain consistent to achieve what it sets out to accomplish.
- Gain Commitment: An eager, skilled, and committed team is needed. Provide training to team members, if necessary. You must gain commitment from superiors and stakeholders.
- Check Feasibility: Make sure there is a good chance the project will be successful. Before going ahead, assess if the project is appropriately timed, feasible for the institution, and worthwhile. Is the project in line with the mission/goals of the institution? Identify driving forces. Identify any resisting forces.

2. Planning
   - Define the Vision: Have a clear idea of what the project will achieve. Create a statement of project vision "What are we going to change and how?" Examine the idea and plan realistically.
   - Involve Stakeholders: Make sure you are aware of the goals of the stakeholders and plan with them in mind.
   - Set Objectives/Goals: List the specific objectives to achieve. Make sure they cover the areas of change that the project involves. Include targets for objectives. Goals/Objectives should be specific, measurable, attainable, realistic, and tangible (SMART).
   - Assess Constraints: Limit change to what is necessary. Limit resources as much as possible. Use existing processes if able. Assess time constraints.
   - List Activities: Break down the project into separate activities and determine on who each activity depends. Make sure the list is complete; go through the project step-by-step.
   - Committing Resources: Estimate who needs to be involved in each activity and how many work hours and days will be needed. Identify manpower and physical resource costs and obtain commitment to meet these costs.
   - Order Activities and Assign Responsibility: Put activities into a logical time sequence, estimate the duration of each activity, and create a schedule. Assign responsibility for each activity. Gain agreement from key people as to the dates assigned for each activity.
   - Validate the Plan: Discuss the final plan with stakeholders. Anticipate threats and prevent problems.

3. Implementing
   - Build a Team: Examine your role in the project. You are the leader of the team. Draw up a list of roles needed and candidates who can fill those roles. Choose those you need to complete the project. Consider the roles of each of the team members.
   - Communication Methods and Schedule: Keep written documentation of plans, meetings, and assignments. Choose how you and your team will communicate, and how often.
   - Lead and Resolve Conflict: Assess your leadership style. Use a style that best suits the tasks involved. Work through conflict as a mediator or decision maker.
   - Develop Teamwork: Encourage teamwork and remember team development process (forming, storming, norming, and performing).
   - Put Plan in Place: The team, in a coordinated effort, implements the plan.
   - Motivate and Maintain Momentum: Establish a logical process to make team decisions. Make SAFE decisions: the most Suitable, Acceptable to all stakeholders, Feasible to implement given the constraints, and Enduring to the end of the project and beyond.
   - Manage Information: Establish a schedule for collection of data and who will review it. Establish a method for collecting and organizing data.
   - Communicate, Communicate, Communicate: Share knowledge. Consider who needs what information in what format. Encourage two-way communication, and invite feedback.
4. Monitoring
   - Track and Evaluate Progress: Have an early warning system for problems. Compare schedules against budgets. Monitor supplies. Compare progress with plan. Revise plan/speed of project if necessary.
   - Evaluate Implementation Procedure: Assess how well the plan was actually implemented, and if compliance with the project/change is occurring. Troubleshoot problems.
   - Hold Review Meetings: Regularly hold review meetings to assess progress, brainstorm problems, and reinforce objectives.
   - Update the Plan: If necessary, update the plan with considerations from monitoring activities. Assess the impact of the change on the plan.
5. Closing
   - Deal with the Change Introduced: Understand the change process and how all stakeholders will be affected.
   - Assess Impact: Evaluate the results of the change made, both physically and psychologically.

o Plan to Integrate and Enculturate: If the change is successful, plan the process to integrate and enculturate. This might mean changing policies and procedures. An ongoing educational component may be necessary.
o Plan for Follow-Up: Plan to follow up periodically to evaluate if there is compliance with the change and the change is effective.
o Communicate Success—Write Progress Report: Write progress report with project team and disseminate to all stakeholders.
o Thank the Team and Close the Process: Hold a final meeting with team and sponsor to recap what has been accomplished and what has been learned (Lewis, 2007). Celebrate your achievement!

PLANNING, PLANNING, PLANNING . . . WITH OUTCOMES IN MIND

In this chapter, we will refer to your desire to implement a specific creative solution as managing a project, as they are one in the same. Some creative solutions may be so simple, that you need not go through all the steps of implementing a formal project, yet you will need to think about the implementation in the same way, to be able to evaluate the project and determine realistically which steps you may need and which are superfluous. Whichever the case, a good knowledge of how to manage a project and all that it encompasses, will be a valuable asset. The first step is, of course, need. What is the impetus for the project? We visited this topic in other chapters, but it is worth mentioning again. The impetus for the implementation of the project will help you shape your data collection, which will help you shape your action plan. The impetus may be regulatory, required by an accrediting agency. It may be for quality improvement, or it may be that resources will no longer support the current way. There are many reasons, just determine what the reasons are and use them to gain buy-in and determine through your data collection how you can show your implementation has made a difference, or heaven forbid, made things worse.

As you progress through the five stages of project management, you will want to read or reread certain sections of this volume that elaborate on specific topics and provide further insight. You will also want your reference project management book close by. This volume will provide you with specific tools you can use in each stage of the process. Listing all the project management tools available to assist you would probably take up this whole volume, so we will encourage you with your project management reference book and your enhanced searching skills to read Chapter 6: Implementing Evidence-Based Practice and Chapter 7: Involving Everyone in Research to search out tools to facilitate your efforts.

Whenever you are able, utilize electronic versions of tools. For example, in Chapter 5: Measuring Outcomes, we provide directions for creating a Gantt chart. The Gantt chart is easily created by hand, but is much more versatile if an electronic version is produced. This will allow you to make frequent updates and e-mail the new, updated schedule to all stakeholders involved. And let us warn you now, project management is all about visual tools and forms. Just remember, all of these forms are tools, not necessarily requirements. The purpose of a tool is to help you achieve your goal, not as penance for *volunteering* to lead a project. If the difficulty in using a tool outweighs the benefits derived from the tool, it is time to find a new tool. Consider the following software programs to support your project: word processing software, forms creators, business graphics and presentations, spreadsheets, databases, data analysis software, day planners and schedulers, and if budgeting is complex, you may want to include some type of accounting or budgeting software (Portny, 2007) . For those of you who were actually technology-fluent project managers in a past life, Microsoft project management software may be for you. Beware, this is not for the faint of heart; it is an intensive project managing program used by many professional project managers with complex and costly projects. For your purposes, we think this may be overkill.

PROCESS MAPPING

One tool we highly recommend is a process map. Although not a tool directly applicable to project management, it can be a great adjunct to many of your projects. A process map is the

> "[s]tructural analysis of a process flow . . . by distinguishing how work is actually done from how it should be done, and what functions a system should perform from how the system is built to perform those functions. In this technique, main activities, information flows, interconnections, and measures are depicted as a . . . graphic representation [which] allows an observer to 'walk-through' the whole process and see it in its entirety". (Process Mapping, n.d.)

Process mapping is merely the process of creating the process map. Basically what you are doing is creating a map of a process from start to finish. Creating a process map is a bit of brainstorming, a bit of self-awareness, and an exercise in mentally recreating a process probably performed countless times. You will typically not create the map on your own. Ideally, you would get a sampling of people together: those who currently use the process, those that know how the process should take place, those who know the requirements of the process, whether regulatory, for quality, or reimbursement, and someone who is familiar with process mapping and can facilitate the activity.

Uses of a Process Map

You can use process mapping for a number of functions. Here are a few:

- To clarify a process: Ask five different nurses how to administer medications to a patient and we bet you will get five different processes. Hopefully all will contain the essential five rights for administering medications and fall somewhere near how your institution's policy says it should be done, but that may not be the case. You may find that staff members vary drastically on their processes, and none resemble what the policy states. This is a red flag that either education is necessary or that, as it stands, the current process as defined in the policy is not practical. Either way, you have uncovered some valuable information about a practice that has the potential to put patients at risk. Process mapping is an excellent tool for seeing a process as it is actually done, without fear of retribution. What you are after is the truth, not a version of what should be happening.
- To describe and communicate a procedure: A process map can be utilized in conjunction with a policy. This provides a visual, step-by-step representation of the process that, for many, is easier to understand than a version in prose. This is especially true for more visual learners. The process map is an elementary way to portray an algorithm or a decision tree type process. At one institution, practically every nursing policy has a process map as an addendum. This helps new nurses learn institution-specific procedures more quickly and is used as an aid to educate nurses on new processes.
- To identify potential areas of variability: A process map, after it is completed, can be analyzed for areas where the process is unclear and left to individual interpretation. This could potentially result in risk for untoward events, depending on the specific process involved. Analyzing a process in this way can also illuminate areas where evidence-based best practices could be utilized to better the process, possibly resulting in safer patient care.
- To get everyone "on the same page": To fix or better a process, the first thing that needs to happen is that everyone agrees that the potential for enhancing the process exists. For this consensus, everyone needs to be "on the same page" as to where the process is currently and what is the ultimate goal for the process. Everyone needs to be "on the same page," otherwise the effort to change the process may be undermined by apathy and disbelief in the need to fix the process.

For process mapping to work, those involved must be honest. Participants need to be assured that you want to know how they really carry out the process in practice. This may not be how the process should be carried out, but it provides insight into what is going on currently, work-arounds and all. The process must not be punitive. If participants feel that it is, you will not get a true picture of what is really going on.

How to Map a Process and Create a Process Map

Step 1: Determine the boundaries. Determine where the process begins and where it ends. This will help define the scope of your map and provide everyone with distinct boundaries.

Step 2: List all of the steps involved in the process. Here you can be as broad or as detailed as you think appropriate. We advise first completing a broad process map. If you identify an area of concern, create another process map just for that area, defining your boundaries as just that segment of the overall process. For example, you may want to map the process of medication administration. After completion and analysis, you see an area of the process is poorly defined, for example, the steps to obtain medication from the pharmacy. Now, with stakeholder input, of course, map just that segment: the process of obtaining medication from the pharmacy. Using this stepwise approach will eliminate the unnecessary minutia from cluttering the overall process, providing a more macroscopic view of what is going on.

When creating the map, use a verb to start each task description. Tasks should be actions, and you will want to start each task for the process with a verb, usually an action verb. Write each task on a note card so you will be able to arrange the tasks easily.

Step 3: Sequence the steps. After you determine all the tasks necessary to complete the process within your defined boundaries, arrange the note cards so that the process flows from start to finish. Do not draw the arrows that show the sequence until later.

Step 4: Draw appropriate symbols. There are many different disciplines that make use of the process map. It is relatively new in health care, but old hat in engineering. The difference is not in the concept, but the level of complexity and the corresponding symbols used.

Remember, the process map is a communication device. You are communicating the process by the steps involved, by the decisions that need to be made, and by the boundaries of the process. To communicate effectively, everyone needs to understand the language. Different symbols mean different things, but typically they are standardized within a specific discipline. Engineers will utilize many symbols that are irrelevant to nursing. The symbols you will usually utilize are simple and there are relatively few. Here are the basics:

- o Ovals show the input to start the process and the output at the end of the process.

○ Boxes or rectangles show the specific tasks or activities performed in the process.

○ Arrows show the process' direction flow. Usually there is only one arrow out of a task/activity box. If there is more than one arrow, you may need a decision diamond.

○ Diamonds show the points in the process where yes/no questions are asked or a decision is required.

○ Triangles are used to denote a step where waiting is involved.

○ Every feedback loop should be closed (i.e., it should take you back to the input box, to the end of the process, or to a task where you continue the process until the end).

Step 5: Use a systems model approach. You want to use input based on people, technology, equipment, evidence-based best practices, and the economic and cultural environment within your institution. Your output should be your desired result of the process, which theoretically should get you the excellent outcomes you desire, assuming the process is evidence based and able to be translated to your environment.

Step 6: Check for completeness. Show the drafted chart to all stakeholders, asking their suggestions for other possible unaccounted for or for redundant steps. Alter the process until all agree that it is complete. Achieve consensus within the group that this is how the process is occurring. Make sure the process map is titled and dated, and also list the names of those involved in creating the map. This will be important as you use the map and possibly revise the process. Dating the map will help everyone distinguish the most recent version.

Step 7: Finalize the process map. Look at the process to determine if it is being performed the way it should be. Are people following the process as it is mapped? Revisit your reasons for creating the process map in the first place, and determine whether the map fulfills your goals. Utilize the completed map to address the purpose for its creation (Ahoy, 1992).

Remember, the main purpose of process mapping is to use diagramming to understand a process that is currently used, to communicate it to others, and to ask ourselves what is expected, appropriate, and best practice; in other words, what should we be doing to provide better patient care and satisfaction. The process map will help to identify what best practices are needed to be incorporated and find appropriate benchmarks for measuring how to arrive at better ways of performing. Figure 3-1 is an example of a simple process map showing the process for policy, product, and practice changes within the department of radiology in a community hospital.

Figure 3-1   Example of process map.

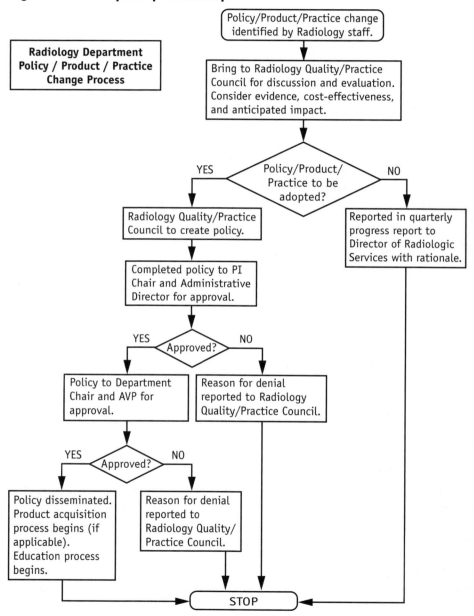

Pilot Study

In research,

a pilot study typically is conducted with a small number of research participants to determine the feasibility of conducting the study with a large number of people, including the utility of the selected research design, the adequacy of the approach used to recruit and retain research participants, the adequacy of the instruments used to measure study variables, and the procedures used to collect data, as well as to obtain an estimate of the size of the correlation between study variables or the amount of difference between experimental and control groups. (Fawcett & Garity, 2009, p. 130)

The pilot study can show flaws in the methodology of a proposed study so that it may be altered prior to the formal study proceeding. Many researchers utilize the pilot study for this purpose, while some undertake only a pilot study, looking for a sense of the viability of a study based on preliminary results. If the pilot does not show promising results, they frequently do not pursue the full study proposed.

Statistical Significance vs Clinical Significance

In project management/implementation, the concept of a pilot study is the same. It is done to try the methodology and see if it makes a difference. We need to make a definite distinction here between quality improvement and research. We discuss this more extensively in Chapter 6: Implementing Evidence-Based Practice. Here, we want to reinforce that in research, you are looking for a statistically significant difference. In quality improvement, it would be nice to show a statistically significant difference between a new intervention and the way it has been typically done. However, many times this is not necessary. Quality improvement projects are seen from a number of different aspects. It is not just asking if the care was better, but also asking how much the better care costs and whether or not the clinical benefits outweigh the increased costs. You may not actually be looking explicitly for statistical significance. You are probably more concerned with demonstrating clinical significance. Greenstein (2003) discusses the difficulty in defining clinical significance. He states the differences in definitions are because of "the specific clinical field being addressed, the size of the effect, the measurement used to evaluate a therapy and the clinical importance of the findings" (para. 15) and cites some of the various definitions found in the published literature.

LeFort (1993) has a definition of clinical significance that best matches what we believe will help you to understand the concept. He mentions that the term "clinical significance" reflects "the extent of change, whether the change makes a real difference to subject lives, how long the effects last, consumer acceptability, cost-effectiveness, and ease of implementation" (p. 58).

What constitutes a meaningful clinical result is usually subjective and should probably be defined by experts in a specific field. Keep this in mind when you design the implementation of your project, as you will need to demonstrate clinical significance to your institution's leadership. Determine the outcomes that will address the clinical significance of the intervention to your internal and external stakeholders. Ask yourself what differences will demonstrate that your intervention or project made a clinically significant difference. These are the outcomes on which you will need to collect data.

We recommend always doing a pilot study when feasible. At times, you will be carrying out a project with a specific deadline for completion. In such a case, you might need to forgo the pilot study and proceed with full implementation. Some believe that you do not need to be concerned with measuring outcomes and executing a systematic implementation if the project is required. Why worry about measuring all this stuff when we have to keep doing it, no matter what the results show? No. No. No. You need to treat all projects as if you are deciding whether or not it has clinical significance. Even a required initiative can be implemented in many different ways. If you discover your design is not producing the results you expect, tweak it or scrap it for an alternative method.

In the end, your pilot study will just be a scaled-down version of your proposed project. In the project management realm, managing a pilot study or pilot project is similar to managing the full project. The main difference is that you will not unnecessarily affect the entire institution if the methodology fails or if the project has poor outcomes. There are some tradeoffs, however. When you do a pilot study or project, keep in mind that what works for a few does not always work for many. Consider what implementation strategies were specific to the pilot population and then develop these to target your larger population.

It would be somewhat unusual to show clinical significance in a pilot study or program and not to show significance in a full rollout of the program. If this occurs, check your data for validity and reliability, and then stratify your data into subsets of your population that make sense. For example, you might pilot your new program on the medical acute unit with good results. You then roll it out to the hospital and find no difference in outcomes. Of course, you will make sure you have good compliance with the initiative. If you do, then look at your data by unit, noting on which units clinical significance was demonstrated. It may be that you find this initiative is not suitable for certain types of units. It may be that you need additional interventions to properly implement the initiative in certain units. This may mean changing other processes to accommodate your initiative. Whatever the case, looking at the data unit by unit will help you to diagnose the problem.

PROJECT LEADERSHIP

Yes, you're right. This chapter is titled Project Management. But the distinction between management and leadership is an important one, and leadership in any project is essential. Much of this volume is geared toward developing leadership capacity, confidence, and skill. Motivating, creating a vision, and facilitating are facets of leadership necessary for the Magnet journey and any quality initiative undertaken. Some business authors believe that there is a hierarchy; that it is preferable to be a leader, giving a short shrift to those who excel in managerial roles. We believe that both are necessary and valuable. A leader without a manager is no better than a manager without a leader. Rarely do you find an individual with the capacity to do both well and at the same time. Leadership and management overlap, there is no denying that, and each is incredibly time consuming, but each utilizes a different paradigm to view a situation.

Leadership approaches a situation from a global, change-oriented perspective. Management approaches a situation by dividing it into doable tasks and achievable goals. We see management as more compliance oriented and leadership as more outcome oriented. We are not trying to make judgments. Without compliance, outcomes will not be achieved, and without outcomes, all the compliance in the world is meaningless. So, where are we? We are looking to make sure that each project has both leadership and management (Portny, 2007). That is not to say one individual cannot act as both project manager and project leader. In fact, this is frequently what happens. It is important to have the awareness that both are valuable and both are necessary for the success of the Magnet journey and any quality initiative.

With vs For

I am working with the Chief Nursing Officer (CNO) to achieve Magnet designation for our institution.

I am working for the CNO to achieve Magnet designation for our institution.

What is the difference between these two sentences? Actually, there is a world of difference. The first implies camaraderie, equality, engagement, and internalized accountability. The second implies hierarchy, externalized accountability, control, and separateness. Which situation would you prefer? These sentences allude to the possible extreme opposite situations that can occur in an institution as a whole or in the implementation of a specific project. It is obvious that you would want to be a part of a situation where you perceive that you are working with, not merely for, the institution's or project's leadership. But as the leader, are you comfortable with that perception, and able to give up the need to control? Are you aware of what leadership style you use and how it is perceived? Can you modify your style to fit the needs of others and still achieve your goals?

On starting a newly created job in a new institution, I sat down with my boss to discuss the vision for the position, the expectations, and the tasks and responsibilities. I was told, "I'm a very hands-off manager unless you show me I can't be." Wow. I was certainly speechless. In that moment, I knew I was working for, not with. It set the stage for what has definitely been a trying relationship. Our advice, do not do this. Instead of telling someone what type of manager you are, ask them with what type of manager they work best. Ask your employee to tell you about his or her best manager and what made him or her so good. A superior manager alters his or her style to fit the needs of the employees being managed. This is the type of manager you want to be. No two employees can be managed in exactly the same way, not if you want to get the most productivity and engagement. You need to individualize. We think this advice will serve you well.

Delegation

Nurses are familiar with the topic of delegation from nursing school. It is sort of drilled into you what you can, should, and should not delegate, and who you can delegate to. The American Nurses Association (ANA) defines delegation as "[t]he transfer of responsibility for the performance of a task from one individual to another while retaining accountability for the outcome" (2005, p. 4). The ANA's *Principles for Delegation* (2005) lists five rights of delegation: right task, right circumstance, right person, right directions and communication, and right supervision and evaluation (p. 7). Here they are referring more to patient care activities, geared more toward licensure and the activities a registered nurse, a licensed practical nurse, and unlicensed personnel can professionally and legally perform. You cannot delegate medication administration to unlicensed assistive personnel. It is not acceptable either professionally or legally. This is obvious. What we are talking about here is delegation in the project management realm, the things a project manager can assign to others to carry out. The five rights above can be carried beyond direct-care nursing into the realm of project management. The principles of delegation are really the same as we learned in nursing school.

Unfortunately, the project manager cannot do everything, nor should he or she be expected to. The project manager should first and foremost manage the project in its entirety. This means coordinating activities, assuring accountability, holding to the established timeline and budget, communicating to all involved, and the many other activities that fall under the project management umbrella. But again, the project manager cannot do it all. The manager needs to look for things to delegate. The issue here is really guilt. It is the guilt nurses feel from not being able to do it all themselves. We have got one thing to say to you: Get over it. Realize that a successful project is a team effort. You need to be able to let go of total control, and focus on managing. Delegate whenever you can.

How Should You Delegate?

Here are some principles to help you delegate successfully:

- Clearly articulate the desired outcome to whomever you are delegating. Begin with the end in mind and specify the desired outcome.
- Clearly identify constraints and boundaries, the lines of authority, responsibility, and accountability. How much independence does the person delegated to have? Make clear when the individual should wait to be told what to do or ask what to do, when he or she can recommend what should be done, and when he or she can act independently. Be sure to specify when the results of his or her actions should be reported and to whom. Also, where possible, you want to include your team in the delegation process. Empower them to decide what tasks they can take on and when.
- Always match the amount of responsibility you give an individual with the amount of authority he or she has. There are things you can delegate to a director that are inappropriate for a direct-care nurse. Understand that you can delegate some responsibility, but you have the ultimate accountability for the project. The buck stops with you!
- You should delegate to the people at the most appropriate organizational level. The people who are closest to the work are best suited for some tasks because they have the most intimate knowledge of the processes and challenges of everyday patient care. This might also help to increase workplace efficiency, and might help to develop the self-motivation that builds leaders.
- You will need to provide the people you delegate to adequate support and resources. Be available to answer questions, and make sure the timeline for activities is adhered to through regular and consistent communication and monitoring. Agree on a schedule of times when you will review the progress of the task you have delegated.
- As the project manager, your focus should be on results. Concentrate more on what is accomplished rather than specifying exactly how the task should be done. Your way might not be the only way or even the best way to achieve results. Do provide advice on finding the best way to accomplish the task, and stress evidence-based best practices. Suggest contacting other institutions to see how they have carried out the task and note their successes. Allow the person to have some control over his or her own methods and processes. This will help to facilitate trust and critical thinking.
- Be aware of "upward delegation," where the person you have delegated to shift responsibility for the task back to you when there is a problem. Help him or her to find the solution, do not simply provide an answer (Mind Tools, 2009).

The project leader needs to build motivation and commitment through communication, discussing how success will impact patient care, financial rewards, future opportunities, professional development, and other desirable outcomes. Recognition is essential in delegation. Discuss the importance of the completed task to the overall project and inform supervisors of the person's contribution. Recognize contributing individuals as publicly as possible to both reward the person and possibly recruit others who see the difference participation can make to the overall success of a project.

Who is accountable for what by when . . . Communicate!

Possibly the most important thing you can do in managing your project is to communicate effectively, timely, and accurately. This attention to communication will assist you in keeping those involved informed and accountable. A Gantt chart in electronic format can be updated frequently and e-mailed to display due dates and any added or deleted activities. Just make sure you have a way to denote when the chart was updated, so that those receiving the chart will know which is the most recent. If you use other tools for communication such as a monthly newsletter, include an updated chart in each. This way, recipients will know the most recent chart is in the current monthly newsletter.

Training and Resources for Those Involved

One of the most common pitfalls we have found in project management is that those involved do not have the knowledge, skills, or resources to understand instructions, complete tasks, or receive and comprehend communications. We are not saying that they are not good at what they do, whether direct patient care or management. But we are saying that there are just some skills you do not learn in nursing school. For example, you send out an updated Gantt chart to all stakeholders, yet many might not be familiar with a Gantt chart and do not know how to read it. You send out a chart with interim project compliance and outcome data, but some do not have the software installed on their computers to open the file. Or, you have delegated a task for data collection to someone without access to the necessary data. These are all scenarios that can and most likely will happen at some point. Our goal here is to simply bring awareness to you, and for you to make sure those involved have what they need to see the project through.

The key to assuring that what is necessary is available is through assessment. The knowledge, skills, and resources necessary will be different for different groups of people, as discussed in Chapter 2: Structures, Processes, and People for Nursing Quality. Before you assign, disseminate, or communicate anything, think about your audience and assess whether they have the resources and abilities to perform, understand, and utilize what you are sending. If you think there might be an issue with something, show it or send it to a couple of people that represent the group you are trying to reach, and ask their opinions. If delegating to an individual, present the task and ask whether he or she has done something like this before. Ask them also to summarize back to you what you have asked them to do, to assure the instructions are understood. If there is a gap between what you are sending and what you want the receiver to do or to understand, either provide the necessary education and resources, simplify the task or message, or delegate to an individual better suited for the task (Cook, 2005).

ACTION PLANNING

Whenever you implement an initiative or intervention, you will want to compose an action plan. Action planning forms can be used as tools to help organize and standardize the way implementation planning is carried out in your institution. These forms should include your goal, which should be broken down into measurable and time-specific objectives, the tasks necessary to meet each objective, and who is responsible for each task by what date. The action plan is actually a step-by-step breakdown of tasks necessary to achieve your goal. Creating an action plan is a precursor to creating your Gantt chart. The Gantt chart visually displays the activities and the timeline your action plan dictates.

An action plan is one of those essential tools of project management. We suggest perusing various action planning forms to see if one fits your needs. If not, create your own composite from the elements of the retrieved forms that work for the types of projects you do and the needs of your institution. We created a form for one institution that contained sections to remind users to consider both compliance and outcome data (see end of chapter). This may work for your institution, or it may be too prescriptive. It is your choice.

Steps for Writing an Action Plan

Here are the basic steps for writing an action plan:

- Determine your overall goal. Typically, the goal will have some impetus, some reason why you want to spend the resources, time, and money. For example, it may be a noted significant decrease in patient satisfaction. Thus, your goal would be to increase patient satisfaction. Usually the data that specified the opportunity for improvement (baseline data) is the same data that will show if you meet your overall goal.
- Determine the evidence-based interventions you will implement to reach your goal. Your objectives must be measurable and have a definite time for completion. The acronym SMART is frequently used for goals, and may be

also extended to objectives: Specific, Measurable, Attainable, Realistic, and Timely. Specific goals and objectives have a better chance of success than general ones. To set specific goals, answer the following six questions:

Who: Who is involved?
What: What do I want to accomplish?
Where: Identify a location.
When: Establish a time frame.
Which: Identify requirements and constraints.
Why: Specific reasons, purpose or benefits of accomplishing the goal.
(Top Achievement, n.d., para. 1)

Example: Specific: A general goal might be to increase patient satisfaction. A specific goal would state, "Increase patient satisfaction through initiating daily rounding, service recovery within 24 hours of an incident, and daily patient discharge phone calls by December of this year." Measurable: You want to establish concrete criteria for measuring progress toward the attainment of your goal. Seeing success through measuring your progress can help you stay on track with your project and keep to your timeline. Each achievement produces the positive reinforcement that motivates you to continue your efforts to reach your ultimate goal. Measurable objectives and goals will typically use some data collection and analysis to determine achievement. For example, you can measure the amount of days within a certain amount of time that you do daily rounding on patients; rounding 25 out of the 30 days demonstrates 83% daily rounding. Attainable: Make your objectives and goals achievable within the frame of resources available and institutional culture. Plan your steps wisely and establish a time frame that allows you to complete those steps. You may be surprised at how, through incremental attainable objectives, goals become achievable and within reach. Be flexible with your timeline. Frequently, events occur with little or no notice, and may delay your objectives and goals. Do not get discouraged, just adjust your timeline accordingly. Realistic: You must be willing and able to work toward a set goal. A goal can be both visionary and realistic; let your team help decide how imaginative your goal should be. Every objective should represent substantial progress toward your goal. A goal that is visionary, but is something that your team truly believes in will be easier to reach than a goal eliciting indifference. One way to know if your goal is realistic is to determine if you have accomplished anything similar in the past. If not, do not let this deter you. Do you know others that have achieved the same goal? How did they do it? Timely: A goal should be grounded within a specific time frame. This will create a sense of urgency. There are some that can only get something accomplished if it has a deadline attached.

For each objective necessary to meet your goal, write each step and how long that step will take (Figure 3-2). Determine who is the best person to carry out that task and delegate. You will see that there are some steps that have precursors that cannot be completed before a previous task is finished. And, there are some steps that can occur simultaneously. You will be able to visualize this better when you create a Gantt chart for the objectives.

Note on the action plan who is responsible for each specific task and by when. Determine the data you will need to ensure each objective is completed successfully. Consider if the objective requires both compliance and outcome data to demonstrate effectiveness, or if it is merely a task that needs a level of compliance to help meet the goal.

Monitor the implementation of your plan through the data as well as if the time-specific milestones are met. Review the plan regularly, and update the plan as frequently as necessary. Again, we advise you to create a Gantt chart from the action plan and revise the Gantt chart whenever a revision is made to the action plan timeline (Time-Management-Guide.com, 2002).

DATA COLLECTION AND ANALYSIS

We bet you thought, "Thank goodness we're done with data!" Well, not quite. We want to revisit some of the concepts previously discussed and talk about a few more that we think will be helpful in managing your Magnet journey and quality improvement projects. First, if you are trying to improve something, it just makes sense that there must have been some data that showed that there was an opportunity for improvement. That data will be your baseline data. You can use your baseline (preintervention) data to compare with your postintervention data to see if you have made a difference. If you have baseline data, make sure you collect the same data for your postintervention comparison. You want to compare apples and apples, not apples and pomegranates.

Scrutinize the validity and reliability of your data. This means evaluating your data collection process and those collecting your data. Is your data complete? Are those that are collecting the data trained properly in the process? Who compiles the data, and how do they do it? Are the same people consistently collecting the data or are they different each time? If possible, it is nearly always preferable to collect data electronically. This helps to eliminate the possible human error inherent in a paper and pencil data collection process.

Trending the Data

One data concept we did not discuss is trending. Many times, you will want to see that a specific intervention has a distinct impact on the outcome you are trying to improve. In reality, there may be many interventions and initiatives occurring simultaneously in your institution affecting the same outcome measure.

Figure 3-2   Example of action planning worksheet.

Action Planning Worksheet

Prepared By: _____

Date: _____

Opportunity For Improvement/Goal

Objectives/Interventions for This Goal:

What outcomes do you wish to achieve? (Objectives)	By when? (Target Dates)	How will you measure success? (Measures)

Actions/Steps to Achieve These Objectives:

What must be done? (Action)	By whom? (Responsibilty)	Starting? (Start Date)	Completed? (Due Date)	Comments: (Contingencies, resources, etc.)

	What are you going to measure?	When are you going to measure?	How are you going to measure?	Who is going to measure?
Overall Compliance				
Overall Outcome				

Do you stop all other initiatives and implement only one at a time? Well, in a perfect world you would, however, in the real world, you do the best you can to determine a single intervention's effect. One way to look at the impact an intervention is having is by trending the outcome measure the intervention is meant to improve. Trending data can be beneficial when trying to better an outcome and also trying to maintain gains made from successful initiatives. It also might help to show cyclical variations in your outcome data, possibly because of a seasonal effect. It can help you to know when to react to changes in the outcome data, and when to continue to monitor. The best format to utilize for trending, in our opinion, is a control chart. If you are using a more simplified run chart, we suggest including at least 13 months of data (assuming it is collected monthly) to note an annual trend and to enable comparisons to the same month of the previous year. Ultimately, you want to be able to show that your initiative made a positive difference in the unrealized outcome, and that this difference is cost-effective. Plan what data you will need to collect and how you will go about collecting it as you create your action plan. Consider both compliance and outcome data, and data to communicate the progress of the initiative (Cook, 2005).

One last word on the data front: Be careful of interventions designed to benefit one outcome but worsens another. We have experienced a situation where a hospital utilized mattress overlays to protect patients at risk for nosocomial pressure ulcers. The overlays worked beautifully for preventing pressure ulcers, however the overlays were so thick, the patient was raised nearly to the level of the side rails. Patients began falling off the bed just from reaching for their personal items. There was no barrier preventing them from rolling. This was noticed when mining the fall incidence data. Our advice is do not solely look at the outcome metric under scrutiny. Peruse all the related outcomes and be aware if there is some reciprocal effect on another metric. This is really just an appeal for you to be aware.

CREATIVE SOLUTIONS

Creative Solution Title: *Topics in Evidence-Based Nursing Practice Conference Series*

Creative Solution Author: Daniel J. Singleton, RN, BSN
Nursing Performance Improvement Coordinator
Aria Health, Philadelphia, PA

Purpose: The vision of the Topics in Evidence-Based Nursing Practice Conference Series is to offer nurses from the Tri-County area the resources to begin to think differently. Offering them the time, resources, and environment to effectively bridge the gap between evidence-based concepts and evidence-based practice in a variety of nursing venues.

Legend

Overall Rating: **COMPETENT**

Financial: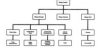

Time:

Personnel: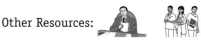

Other Resources: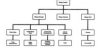

Efficacy: **A**

Transferability: **A**

Malleability/Adaptability: **A**

Ease of Implementation: **C**

Synopsis: Through comprehensive literature reviews of evidence-based nursing trends for policy and practice review, the Evidence-Based Practice (EBP) council at Aria Health identified learning gaps and educational opportunities for advancing and implementing the utilization of evidence-based practices in a variety of nursing-sensitive venues. The Topics In Evidence-Based Nursing Practice (EBNP) Conference series is an annual conference, focusing on EBNP implementation strategies and EBNP education. The Topics In Evidence Based Nursing Practice Conference consists of both professional presentations, by local and nationally renounced presenters, as well as educational workshops tending to the needs of acute care providers, nursing educators working in clinical and academic settings, and nurse administrators seeking to adopt EBNP practices.

Description of Organization: Aria Health is a multiple hospital system with 485 beds. They are a teaching hospital system. Aria Health consists of three inpatient facilities and two outpatient sites. They are located in Northeast Philadelphia, PA, and Lower Bucks County, PA. Aria Health is not currently Magnet designated.

The Case Study: Nurses of the Evidence-Based Practice Council and the Resource and Professional Development Council at Aria Health had the drive and passion to deliver evidence-based practice concepts to a broader audience that main staged the multiple evidenced-based initiatives and policy developments within Aria Health. After an initial proposal by the Magnet Director to organize a conference series, the two councils coordinated a system-wide initiative to plan, organize, and implement an EBP conference series that incorporated nursing from the Tri-County area. Although this initiative is an excellent example of how to educate, dissemi-nate, and encourage the use of EBP in nursing, it also serves as a strong depiction of effective project management. The organization of an educational conference such as this that includes multiple presenters, participants from several counties, and a large syllabus requires a team effort and project management techniques and skill. The project team charged with the organization of the EBP conference was comprised of multiple individuals with varying talents, such as registered nurses, nurse administrators, unit clerks, and clinical nurse assistants. The project was sup-ported by the Chief Nursing Officer (CNO) and nursing directors. To carry out the project, the project coordinators created subcommittees and delegated to them the management of resources, public relations, and speaker selection. They contracted audio/visual technicians, a Web designer/programmer, and national and local speakers to present topics. Funding was needed to support this undertaking as the cost was found to be greater than the health system could support. The project manager then needed to orchestrate a grassroots effort with members of the EBP council to develop grant proposals, which earned the team approximately half of the funds needed to complete the project. The outcome was a 2-day conference attended by nurses throughout the region surrounding Aria Health.

Outcome Measures:

Formative/Compliance: Periodic risk analysis.

Summative/Outcome: Overwhelming positive response to the conference was apparent in the exceptional postconference survey results. A survey scaling system of 1 (poor) to 5 (excellent) was utilized to evaluate the effectiveness of each speaker and the overall conference.

Evidence Supporting this Creative Solution: Schlichter and Thomas (2009) dis-cuss the importance of effective project management in health care, especially in the current economy. It is necessary to strategically plan healthcare activities to assure that all stakeholders are satisfied and that spending is minimized (HIMSS Project Management Task Force, 2008b). Hospitals are being challenged to do more with less in an environment that demands innovation and effective performance. Using project management methodology will allow for improved project outcomes and avoidance of common causes of project failure (HIMSS Project Management Task Force, 2008a). This creative solution combines a means for providing infor-mation and education on EBP, which is necessary for effective performance in health care with project management strategies to allow for mass dissemination of the information in a cost-effective and time-efficient manner.

HIMSS Project Management Task Force. (2008a). *How to deliver successful projects.* Available at: http://www.himss.org/content/files/WhyHaveProjectManagementMethodology .pdf?src=enews20080109. Accessed December 29, 2009.

HIMSS Project Management Task Force. (2008b). *Why have a project management methodology in healthcare.* Available at: http://www.himss.org/content/files/WhyHaveProjectManagementMethodology.pdf?src=enews20080109. Accessed December 29, 2009.

Schlichter, J., & Thomas, D. (2009). Healthcare project management in the new economy. *PM World Today, 11*(8), 1–8.

Recipe for: *Topics in Evidence-Based Nursing Practice Conference Series*

Ingredients:

Project manager

Administrative support (CNO/Directors)

Project team members

Subcommittee leaders

Venue for conference

Room

Meals

Budget/funding

Health system sponsorship

Grant proposal/award

Program presenters

Syllabus/course content

Handouts

PowerPoint/slides

Binders

Pens

Audio/visual equipment/technicians

Advertisement/marketing materials

Direct mailers

E-mails

Flyers/posters

Step-by-Step Instructions (see Figure 3-3 for Step-by-Step Instruction Timeline):

Step 1: Conduct literature reviews to identify gaps in learning and needed educational opportunities for effective implementation of evidence-based practice.

Step 2: Create initial proposal for the conference to address educational needs within the institution.

Step 3: Obtain administrative support and approval from CNO/nursing directors.

Step 4: Appoint project manager and recruit personnel for the project planning team and subcommittee members.

Step 5: Create a budget including costs related to conference venue, materials, personnel time, and honorariums and assess financial resources within the hospital. Recruit someone with grant writing knowledge to write a grant proposal to gain additional financial support.

Step 6: Design the conference syllabus and recruit presenters. Assure presenters know presentation requirements and due date for slides and handouts to be submitted for inclusion in the conference binder.

Step 7: Choose and schedule the venue. Request inclusion of meals, refreshments, and audio/visual equipment.

Step 8: Develop a marketing plan. Design and distribute mailers, posters, and e-mails to advertise conference.

Step 9: Complete conference binder and organize slides for presentations. Create sign-in sheet and certificates of completion for attendees and a post-conference evaluation form.

Figure 3-3   Timeline for "Topics in Evidence Based Nursing Practice Conference Series."

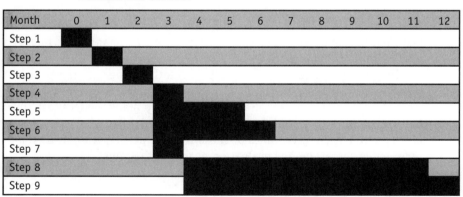

Additional Outcomes to Consider Measuring:

Formative/Compliance: There are many compliance measures in the management of a project, some of which include adherence to the timeline planned for the project, attendance of project team participants at scheduled meetings, timely response from presenters/speakers, return of their content to be presented, and ability to keep costs within budget.

Summative/Outcome: Evaluation of overall adherence to budget and planning schedule. Comparison of preconference and postconference tests for attendees to evaluate the effect of the conference material.

Insights from Original Implementation:

- An undertaking of this magnitude was difficult given the limited resources. With dedication and perseverance, the team was able to conduct a conference that was comparable to others with more endowed budgets. The need for extensive financial backing of the institution was balanced with the acquisition of grant funding and personal sacrifice.
- It is all about presentation. As with fine dining, it is the appearance more than anything else that drives the overall experience. The utilization of professional sound and visual technicians enhanced the overall experience. Even when the content was lacking in depth and breath the visual and audio delivery helped drive the experience.
- Establish a timeline for the project and maintain track of the tasks at hand. With a changing of the guard midway through the development phase, there was potential for areas of the project to be mismanaged. A rapid focus plan-do-study-act (PDSA) was conducted to reestablish control and accountability for various aspects of the project.
- Avoid the "Ready, Aim, Fire" approach, in other words action without planning, for project implementation.
- Plan time for planning. The most important phase of any project is the planning phase. Often teams spend little to no time planning, which is a predictor of a failed initiative.
- Conduct a risk analysis early and often. Another aspect of the planning phase is the risk analysis. Planning for variables prepares the team for possible threats to the project. Having contingency plans reduces lost time. This can be directly proportional to lost revenue.
- Clearly define each of the roles of those who are participating in the planning, implementation, and evaluation phases of the project.

For Further Guidance Contact:

Daniel J. Singleton, RN, BSN
Nursing Performance Improvement Coordinator
Aria Health
Knights and Red Lion Rds.
Philadelphia, PA. 19114
dsingleton@ariahealth.org

Creative Solution Title: *Implementation of a Computerized Medication Administration System Utilizing Bar Code Technology*

Creative Solution Authors: Ruben D. Fernandez, PhD(c), MA, RN
Vice President, Patient Care Services
Palisades Medical Center, North Bergen, NJ

Lorna Schneider, MSN, RN, APN, BC, CS, CCRN, CCNS
Clinical Coordinator
Palisades Medical Center, North Bergen, NJ

Fay Spragley, DNP, RNC, APRN, BC, CCRN
Clinical Coordinator / Nurse Practitioner
Palisades Medical Center, North Bergen, NJ

Purpose: The overarching goal was to ascertain quantifiable data that will provide the organization with information to benchmark against best practice. This would assist us in our goal toward improving the organizational culture of safety. This was our departmental/organizational response to the Institute of Medicine's initiative for creating safer delivery systems as illustrated in the publication: "To Err is Human: Building a Safer Healthcare System" (1999), and the Institute for Healthcare Improvement's 100,000 Lives Campaign (2004). Palisades Medical Center's (PMC) nursing department had suspected an overall underreporting as well as unidentified number of medication errors, as identified in the literature. The nursing department therefore wanted to create a nonpunitive environment where medication errors would be identified, causes analyzed, and at the same time, promote an organizational culture of safety that led to better patient care outcomes.

Legend

Overall Rating: **COMPETENT**

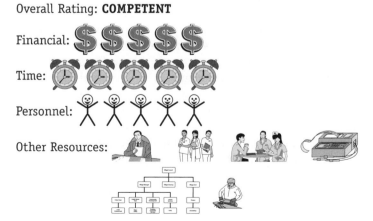

Financial:

Time:

Personnel:

Other Resources:

Efficacy: **A**

Transferability: **C**

Malleability/Adaptability: **B**

Ease of Implementation: **D**

Synopsis: PMC nursing department undertook the development of a project to implement a computerized medication administration system. Siemens's Medication Administration Check (MAK) was the technology used. It was initiated by the nursing management team and championed by the nursing department, but the project was completed with a multidisciplinary framework. The project was developed to provide safer medication administration for patients and to improve patient outcomes. The MAK system allowed the organization to quantify medication error data. This was initiated and implemented within a nonpunitive environment, which encouraged the support of the system and a culture of safety. It brought technology to the bedside and moved the hospital toward an environment of information technology.

Description of Organization: PMC is a hospital in North Bergen, NJ. The hospital has approximately 202 beds and serves approximately 350,000 people in Southern Bergen and Hudson counties. It has been a member of the New York Presbyterian Hospital network since 1999, and is affiliated with the Columbia University College of Physicians & Surgeons.

With comprehensive medical services, a quick-response emergency department, which includes a heliport, and a centralized location overlooking Manhattan, PMC serves as a major healthcare resource for Hudson and Bergen counties in New Jersey. Over the years, the hospital has been consistently improved and renovated and modern technology added to meet the changing needs of the patients.

More importantly, the medical center has reached beyond hospital's walls to offer the most innovative healthcare services. The board-certified physicians, skilled nurses, and devoted staff assure that each patient receives the very best medical care, administered with a personal touch. The Palisades Mission: To enhance the health status of the diverse communities we serve and deliver patient care in a safe and nurturing environment consistent with the highest standards of excellence, quality, and efficiency, and with strict adherence to ethical practices. The Palisades Vision: To be the healthcare provider of choice in northern Hudson and southeastern Bergen counties. PMC is not Magnet designated.

The Case Study: In 2005, PMC recognized the need to implement an electronic medication administration system that included bar code technology. During a strategic planning retreat, the nursing management team identified this project as a priority to move the hospital into a culture of safety, as well as to promote compliance with The Joint Commission's National Patient Safety Goals (2005).

The department of nursing led the project by identifying the need and consequently garnered support from all levels of the organization.

Although championed by the nursing department, there were many stakeholders involved in this project. It was a multidisciplinary effort inclusive of: medical staff, pharmacy, information technology, respiratory therapy, education, engineering, and finance.

The choice of system to implement, Siemens's Medication Administration Check (MAK), was based upon current contracts that the vendor held within the hospital and the vendor's ability to meet the organization's needs. A committee was formed that was delegated the task of implementing the system. This included learning the system, tailoring it to the organization's needs, shadowing it along with the current system, policy development, and education of staff and administration. This project was a major change in the culture of the institution, as well as the practice and performance of every nurse and therefore needed to be carefully planned and managed to achieve the desired outcomes.

The MAK system uses bar code technology to assure that five rights of medication administration are achieved. Prior to administration, the medication must be scanned, then, the patient identification band scanned. The system checks for the right drug, right dose, right time, and right route. By scanning the patient identification band, the right patient is assured. The clinician then electronically charts that the medication was administered.

During the shadowing phase of this system, multiple medication errors were found that would have gone unnoticed. These errors included orders that were not transcribed, incorrectly transcribed orders, illegibly transcribed orders, orders unknown to pharmacy, orders profiled wrong by pharmacy, and orders that were not recopied, or recopied incorrectly. These medication variances were unknown to the nursing practitioners and pharmacists at the time of discovery. This system brought medication error data to the next level, and ultimately brought the organization closer to a culture of safety. We were able to see exactly what the nurse had in his or her hand, at what time, and which patients the medications were being administered to. This information was deemed crucial in making medication error data meaningful in promoting safe medication practices. Intrinsic to the system is the ability to highlight potential errors that might be related to look-alike, sound-alike medications, as well as to provide us with the ability to investigate and trend possible medication errors. This information adds to the growing body of knowledge about medication errors and assists us in avoiding future errors.

Furthermore, the identification of near misses leads to analysis of practice behaviors and ultimately the delivery of safe and efficient patient care. The system as unfolded at PMC is a critical component of our patient safety program and is a conduit for our culture of safety initiatives. PMC was the first hospital in

Hudson County and among the first ones in the state of New Jersey to implement this state of the art technology.

Outcome Measures:

Formative/Compliance: MAK reports enabled identification of incorrect patients, incorrect medication scanned, medication omissions, pharmacy interventions, and overrides of the system, among others.

Summative/Outcome: Performance improvement data, inclusive of National Patient Safety Goal data; successful The Joint Commission Survey and compliance with other regulatory bodies accreditation standards; patient satisfaction data related to medication administration; chart reviews; and staff interviews.

Evidence Supporting this Creative Solution:

Medication errors unfortunately occur frequently in and out of the hospital. These errors account for one out of 131 outpatient deaths and one out of 854 inpatient deaths (Institute of Medicine, 1999). They are costly and are the cause of preventable morbidity and mortality. Crane and Crane (2006) describe a method of solving this widespread problem with a systems approach consisting of a failure mode effects analysis (FMEA) combined with technology such as the MAK system used in this creative solution. Avoiding medication errors using IT solutions is at the top of healthcare providers' priorities, according to a study released by the Health Information Management Systems Society, surpassing even HIPAA-related concerns (Kenedy, 2003). Since 2000, the Food and Drug Administration (FDA) has received more than 95,000 reports of medication errors. In 2004 the FDA mandated bar coding of medications so that when used with a bar code scanner and computerized patient information systems, it can help ensure that the right dose of the right drug is given to the right patient at the right time. The implementation of a computerized medication administration system such as MAK supports National Patient Safety Goals (The Joint Commision, 2005) and the 5 million lives campaign goals. It is the future of medicine.

Kenedy, K. (2003). FDA's Medication Bar-Code Proposal Raises Awareness. CRN

Crane, J., & Crane, F. (2006). Preventing medication errors in hospitals through a systems approach and technological innovation: A prescription for 2010. *Hospital Topics, 84*(4), 3–8.

Institute of Healthcare Improvement. (2006). *5 million lives campaign.* Available at: http://www.ihi.org/IHI/Programs/Campaign/. Accessed March 8, 2010.

Institute of Medicine. (1999). *To err is human: Building a safer health system.* Washington, DC: National Academy Press.

Johnson, K. (2004). Keeping patients safe: An analysis of organizational culture and caregiver training. *Journal of Healthcare Management, 49*(3), 171–179.

Leape, L., & Berwick, D. (2005). Five years after *To Err is Human,* what have we learned? *Journal of the American Medical Association, 293*(19), 2384–2390.

McRoberts, S. (2005). The use of bar code technology in medication administration. *Clinical Nurse Specialist, 19,* 55–56.

Ruchlin, H., Dubbs, N., & Callahan, M. (2004). The role of leadership in instilling a culture of safety: Lessons from the literature. *Journal of Healthcare Management, 49,* 47–58.

The Joint Commission. (2005). 2010 National patient safety goals. Available at: http://www .jointcommission.org/patientsafety/nationalpatientsafetygoals/. Accessed March 8, 2010.

Recipe for: *Implementation of a Computerized Medication Administration System Utilizing Bar Code Technology*

Ingredients:

Project coordinators

Senior management and Board of Trustees

Nursing department (bedside nurses, nursing instructors, case managers)

Respiratory therapists

Physicians

Pharmacists

Education Department

Information Technology Department

MAK committee and super users

Siemens Consultants

Siemens MAK program

Lionville medication carts

Infologix medication carts

Bar code bracelets

Bar code scanners

Computers

Batteries

Step-by-Step Instructions (see Figure 3-4 for Step-by-Step Instruction Timeline):

Phase I – Planning and Shadowing

Step 1: Organize and carry out a strategic planning retreat.

Step 2: Preview the system: MAK leadership education and training.

Step 3: Schedule preparations, testing, and shadowing.

Step 4: Formulate team and super users.

Step 5: Schedule Siemens nurse visits and site visits.

Step 6: Develop educational and training materials.

Step 7: Formulate policy and procedures, downtime protocols, and implementation guidelines.

Phase II – Pilot on a medical/surgical unit.

Step 8: Educate and train staff on pilot unit.

Step 9: Pilot MAK system on unit.

Step 10: Set up medical carts.

Step 11: Collect data and analyze reports and monitoring.

Step 12: Monitor and implement continuous improvement.

Step 13: Troubleshoot and revise policies and procedures.

Step 14: Report to executive administration and Board of Trustees.

Phase III – Implementation in all inpatient areas.

Step 15: Educate and train additional super users.

Step 16: Educate and train staff on all inpatient areas.

Step 17: Develop schedule to go live.

Step 18: Collect data and analyze.

Step 19: Monitor and implement continuous improvement.

Step 20: Report to executive administration and Board of Trustees.

Phase IV – Implementation in outpatient areas

Step 21: Educate and train staff on all outpatient areas.

Step 22: Develop schedule to go live.

Step 23: Collect data and analyze.

Step 24: Monitor and implement continuous improvement.

Step 25: Report to executive administration and Board of Trustees.

Additional Outcomes to Consider Measuring:

Formative/Compliance: No additional measures.

Summative/Outcome: No additional measures.

Insights from Original Implementation: Prior to implementing this creative solution, the following must be assessed:

- All levels of the organization must be committed.
- The budget must be specific to the project.
- Training resources should be included in budget allocation.
- The culture of the organization must be ready and willing.

Figure 3-4   Timeline for "Implementation of a Computerized Medication Administration System Utilizing Bar Code Technology."

	2005	2006				2007				2008				2009	
Activities	4Q	1Q	2Q	3Q	4Q	1Q	2Q	3Q	4Q	1Q	2Q	3Q	4Q	1Q	2Q
Phase I - Planning and Shadowing															
Step 1	■														
Step 2		■	■	■	■										
Step 3			■	■	■										
Step 4			■	■	■										
Step 5			■	■	■										
Step 6				■	■	■	■								
Step 7				■	■	■	■								
Phase II - Pilot on a Med/Surg Unit															
Step 8								■							
Step 9									■						
Step 10								■							
Step 11									■	■	■	■	■	■	■
Step 12									■	■	■	■	■	■	■
Step 13									■	■	■	■	■	■	■
Step 14									■				■		
Phase III - Implementation in All Inpatients Areas															
Step 15									■	■					
Step 16										■					
Step 17										■					
Step 18											■	■	■	■	■
Step 19											■	■	■	■	■
Step 20										■			■		
Phase IV - Implementation in Outpatient Areas															
Step 21													■		
Step 22												■	■		
Step 23														■	■
Step 24														■	■
Step 25															■

- Must have a multidisciplinary approach and commitment.
- Must designate champions.
- Must have the buy-in of the staff involved; suggested to use the Council of Nursing Practice as a conduit of change, and the use of staff nurse champions.

The following was learned after implementation:

- There is a very large time commitment involved.
- It is a long-term process and all involved must have a good understanding of that.
- You must have a realistic budget.
- You need a dedicated champion for the project.
- A nursing informatics expert would have facilitated the process.
- A need for flexibility is required.
- Change is a process.

For Further Guidance Contact:

Ruben D. Fernandez, PhD(c), MA, RN
Lorna Schneider, MSN, RN, APN, BC, CS, CCRN, CCNS
Fay Spragley, DNP, RNC, APRN, BC, CCRN
7600 River Road
North Bergen, NJ 07047
rfernandez@palisadesmedical.org
lschneider@palisadesmedical.org
fspragley@palisadesmedical.org

REFERENCES

Ahoy, C. (1999). *Process mapping*. Available at: http://www.fpm.iastate.edu/worldclass/process_mapping.asp. Accessed December 1, 2009.

American Nurses Association. (2005). *Principles for delegation*. Available at: http://www.nursingworld.org/MainMenuCategories/ThePracticeofProfessionalNursing/workplace/PrinciplesofDelegation.aspx. Accessed December 2, 2009.

Cook, C. R. (2005). *Just enough project management*. New York: McGraw-Hill.

Fawcett, J., & Garity, J. (2009). *Evaluating research for evidence-based nursing practice*. Philadelphia: F. A. Davis Company.

Greenstein, G. (2003). Clinical versus statistical significance as they relate to the efficacy of periodontal therapy. *Journal of American Dental Associates, 134*(5), 583–591.

Horine, G. M. (2009). *Absolute beginner's guide to project management* (2nd ed.). Indianapolis, IN: Que Publishing.

LeFort, S. M. (1993). The statistical versus clinical significance debate. *Journal of Nursing Scholarship, 25*(1), 57–62.

Lewis, J. P. (2007). *Fundamentals of project management* (3rd ed.). New York: Amacom.

Mind Tools. (2009). *Successful delegation*. Available at: http://www.mindtools.com/pages/article/newLDR_98.htm. Accessed December 1, 2009.

Morris, R. A. (2008). *The everything project management book* (2nd ed.). Avon, MA: Adams Media.

Portny, S. E. (2007). *Project management for dummies* (2nd ed.). Indianapolis, IN: Wiley Publishing, Inc.

Process Mapping. (n.d.) In *BusinessDictionary.com*. Available at: http://www.businessdictionary.com/definition/process-mapping.html. Accessed November 30, 2009.

Project Management Institute, Inc. (2009). *About project management*. Available at: http://www.pmi.org/AboutUs/Pages/About-PM.aspx. Accessed November 27, 2009.

Time-Management-Guide.com. (2002). *How to write an action plan*. Available at: http://www.time-management-guide.com/plan.html. Accessed December 4, 2009.

Top Achievement. (n.d.). Creating SMART goals. Available at: http://www.topachievement.com/smart.html. Accessed December 4, 2009.

## CHAPTER 4

Motivation, Buy-In, and Enculturation

"In motivating people, you've got to engage their minds and their hearts.
I motivate people, I hope, by example, and perhaps by excitement, by having
productive ideas to make others feel involved."

—RUPERT MURDOCH

"Conduct is more convincing than language."

—JOHN WOOLMAN

MOTIVATION

There is one question we hear over and over again. How do you get people motivated and on board? Those posing the question are usually looking for a magic bullet answer, something that will immediately get everyone to buy-in and desperately want to be a part of the initiative they are undertaking. However, it can actually be dangerous for this kind of immediate acceptance and blind following. Take, for example, any of the highly publicized cult cases, where it is possible to see where blind following can lead. In health care, blind following can lead to negative outcomes such as poor financial straits, staff apathy, or poor patient care. Blind following is actually the antithesis to the Magnet philosophy, stifling the voice of others who may believe a peer's logic is faulty and his or her initiative, detrimental. These voices are necessary so that whatever you decide to implement will have the best chance for positive outcomes.

Of course, when immersed in a sea of negativity, it is hard to fathom the necessity. True, not every voice is a constructive voice. And this is where you can have your greatest affect. Instead of trying to convince everyone that your way is best and that everyone should believe what you tell them, encourage others to speak their minds, but do so constructively. It has been said that the opposite of love is not hate. Hate has passion and emotion. Instead, the opposite of love is indifference or apathy. Indifference lacks passion and emotion, and implies that the subject of the indifference is meaningless and void of enough importance to even stir some modicum of emotional response. We believe blind following leads to apathy and indifference. You do not want this in your institution.

So, your goal now becomes one of turning negativity into constructivism. There are volumes of advice written to guide you. The FISH! Philosophy (Charthouse Learning, 2009), for example, is a program designed to change attitudes and instill passion to encourage staff to work together constructively to better the working environment. Building relationships and teamwork is the core of your initiative and will most likely be a part of whatever you implement. Besides building relationships and enhancing teamwork, you should consistently and collaboratively set expectations and standards that both facilitate and require constructive approaches in all situations. This may already be the culture in your institution. If it is, consider yourself lucky. If not, you will need to change the culture; no small feat. And how do you change a culture? By bringing on board one person at a time. This will be our theme here and is another of our mantras. Try it when a nurse leader comes to you and asks why everyone will not get on board: One person at a time. Say it with us.

The Message

So, what is the message you will give when you are on the Magnet journey? The message is quality patient outcomes and patient and staff satisfaction. There will be those who will challenge your message. You will need to not only believe the message, but also know why you believe it. The Magnet framework is an evidence-based framework. That means it was constructed on a foundation of research. In the 1980s, there was a pretty severe nursing shortage. Hospitals could not hire fast enough, offering huge sign-on and retention bonuses to staff units as best they could. Nurses were leaving hospitals in droves, many times looking for the most attractive bonuses and benefits packages. What some astute researchers noticed was that there were some institutions that appeared to be insulated from the nursing shortage, not just retaining their staff, but also attracting new staff. What was happening at these hospitals that made staff nurses want to stay and new nurses want to join? What researchers found were certain common attributes that created an environment sought after by nurses and facilitated nurse retention. These attributes were categorized and became what we know as the 14 Forces of Magnetism (American Nurses Credentialing Center, 2009a). Research on the characteristics of hospitals that were able to retain and recruit nurses demonstrated that these hospitals had an environment characterized by the 14 Forces. (American Nurses Credentialing Center, 2010).

The Magnet framework has changed. The 14 Forces are still present, and research continues to demonstrate their importance in nurse retention and recruitment. Recent research is focusing on the relationship of the 14 Forces to patient outcomes, and patient and staff satisfaction (American Nurses Credentialing Center, 2009b). The framework has been redesigned into five model components to better reflect the importance of the overarching attributes necessary to create a Magnet environment. The five model components are: (1) Transformational Leadership; (2) Structural

Empowerment; (3) Exemplary Professional Practice; (4) New Knowledge, Innovation, and Improvement; (5) and Empirical Outcomes, all functioning in an environment of global issues in nursing and health care (American Nurses Credentialing Center, 2008). Each of the 14 Forces is subsumed under one of the 5 model components. As research has progressed and the healthcare environment has changed, the focus on patient outcomes, nursing research, and care innovation is appropriate. First-time Magnet applicants are judged more on structure and process. Hospitals seeking redesignation are judged more heavily on outcomes and innovation (American Nurses Credentialing Center, 2008). It is rightfully assumed that their structures and processes are Magnet worthy, now they need to grow further and demonstrate superior outcomes and care innovation. You are now armed with the most potent weapon in your arsenal, tangible evidence-based positive outcomes.

Another potent weapon is a probenefit cost/benefit analysis. That is to say, you will want to demonstrate that the financial benefits of the Magnet journey outweigh the financial costs. This is not as straightforward as it appears. Both costs and benefits are frequently buried within standard operating costs and standard performance improvement interventions. Can the reduction in the patient fall rate be attributed to the Magnet journey or to the ongoing efforts to better the evidence-based fall prevention program? Can you separate the Magnet journey out of the total hospital environment? The challenge of what can be attributed to the Magnet journey and how to value some of the intangible benefits creates a distinct air of subjectivity to the cost/benefit analysis. Not every board of directors will consider nursing research valuable, yet it does cost money. How do you quantify professionalism, attitude, and camaraderie? Can you demonstrate clearly that the Magnet journey results in better patient outcomes? That is exactly what current research is attempting to do. The ANCC reprinted a volume of the Journal of Nursing Administration (JONA), which contains articles looking at the relationships between Magnet designation and patient-related outcomes (Aiken, Clarke, Sloane, Lake, & Cheney, 2009; Aiken, Havens, Sloane, & Douglas, 2009; Armstrong, Laschinger, & Wong, 2009; Drenkard, 2009; Stone & Gershon, 2009; Stone et al., 2009; Ulrich, Buerhaus, Donelan, Norman, & Dittus, 2009). Familiarizing yourself with this literature may help you build your case for the Magnet journey.

Who Gets the Message?

As we have said previously, your message needs to be tailored to your audience. Your audience should be stratified, and you would do well to have a ready message for each stratified group. When you speak to one of these groups about the Magnet journey, you will need to be prepared. The groups may vary, but we have found that there are some typical staff groups. The "I'm excited, tell me more about it" group is probably the most enjoyable group to address. They genuinely want to know about the journey and its benefits. They are typically champions for new initiatives and excited by change and progression. The message for this group consists of the amazing benefits the Magnet journey can bring, which is better patient care and a better working environment. You will need to convey a sense of excitement and motivate this group to buy-in and join the journey. You can mostly use generalizations about the benefits, and not mention fiscal considerations or time commitment at this point.

Then there is the "What's it going to do for me?" group. These people are a bit more difficult to sway and a bit more cynical. This is not a negative, so long as their cynicism does not result in premature dismissal. This group is typically less team oriented and more individualistic. The challenge here is twofold: to get them on board with the journey and to develop their teamwork. These are the people who might say, "I just do my shift and go home." Unfortunately, they have not realized that nursing has changed. It is no longer just about providing direct patient care. It is also about getting involved in initiatives to continuously better patient care, about recognizing opportunities for improvement in the work environment and working to realize these opportunities, and about increasing and constantly updating your knowledge and skills to keep abreast of the most effective evidence-based practices. The hard part is getting this group to get on board. Be patient. Culture change occurs through one person at a time. The message for this group is similar to the message for the first group, but be prepared to diffuse some negativity. They may try to take you down the road of addressing issues that are purely personal. Remember to bring the conversation back to the group.

It is okay to not have all the answers. Introducing the journey as something that, while some have much success and we can learn from their successes, can be a varied experience since every institution has a unique combination of structure and culture. The journey is not a step-by-step replication of other's experiences, but a unique expedition. While others can provide the route, the journey is truly one's own. You may want to address some issues with those who have had success. Just preface or end it with "That's not to say we have to do it this way."

In this group, stress flexibility and the variation permitted to arrive at the Magnet journey goals. This can alleviate some of the fear of change this group typically displays. Realize that some people are more rational, while others are more emotional. If someone is caught up in an emotionally charged issue, do not feed into the situation. You need to first reduce the emotionalism by starving it of any substance. Change the topic and move on. Losing one member of a group is better than losing the entire group.

The next group you might encounter is the "Whatever it is just leave me out of it" group. Do not spend a great deal of time on this group initially. They will usually do what they have to do, and will not necessarily work against the initiatives for the journey. You may not achieve total acceptance from this group, but you may recruit a few if they see some results from the efforts.

There is and will always be the "Nothing you can say will make me believe" group, in other words, the negative group. You will need to buffer the negativity of this group. Actually, this group tends to be just a few isolated individuals. Like a virus, however, they can spread negativity and infect others. Use the principle of isolation to keep them out of any group they could possibly negatively influence and do damage to the journey. Also, do not put these individuals together in any group where they could feed off each other. Eventually, these individuals will either join the more moderate "Whatever it is just leave me out of it" group or leave your institution. Either way, progress will have been made.

Probably the largest group will be is the "I'll just wait and see" group. Members include those individuals who are ambivalent and not really invested in the journey, but have no alternative agenda. They will take a wait-and-see approach; the jury is out until they see some evidence of progress from the journey. These are the ones you want to court. You do not want to overwhelm them, but rather, you will want to provide them with a steady stream of achievements from your Magnet journey initiatives. Work to get these people involved. They may be a bit shy in accepting a leadership role, but they can usually be convinced to play a supportive role in specific initiatives. As they see more and more progress, you will see more and more acceptance.

The nursing leadership groups can be classified into three types. You will have the excited group, the apathetic group, and the advancement-focused group. The first group are your champions, the second are your challenges, and the last are your most frustrating. Here's where your chameleon leadership ability is most important. For the first group, the excited group, you will need to be a transformational leader, motivating and empowering. For the second group, the apathetic group, you will need to be transactional, making sure you get what you need regardless of their feelings. You have to keep in mind that these nurse managers are your portals to the staff. If they are working against you, it will be telling in the staff's attendance at councils and work groups. So keep them accountable to senior leadership with a written account of their staff's attendance and their assistance with initiatives. For the last group, the advancement-focused group, you will have to involve senior nursing leadership in helping to keep them accountable for their role in Magnet journey initiatives.

We do not want to come off as overly negative or cynical, but our view of people is shaped by our experience, and this is what we have experienced. Your experience may be more or less challenging. Remember your resources and your methods to keep people accountable. Use education as much as possible to inform everyone and to help change the attitudes of those who are not enthusiastic or on board. Have semiannual or quarterly reviews highlighting how much has been accomplished and the benefits to the work environment and patient care.

Possibly the most frequent question you will encounter is "Why do we need to change?" This comes from the apathetic individuals. There is nothing inherently wrong with this question, but it assumes that your goal is to maintain the status quo and to just keep things going. However, the Magnet journey believes in constant striving for improvement. Maintaining the status quo is not good enough. Constant change is the norm and is necessary to make use of the constantly changing technologies and techniques to better patient care. This new paradigm also appropriately addresses the information explosion in the Internet-driven push to get information to everyone as quickly as possible. It seems that we still have not fully adapted many of our structures and processes to work within this new paradigm, and unfortunately many of us in health care have neither accepted nor prepared ourselves with the skills necessary to accommodate this change.

Refuting Negativity

Refuting negativity may be one of the most trying yet necessary actions you can do to keep moving on the Magnet journey. When you consider how to refute negativity, consider both the message and the messenger. It may be much easier to refute the message than to discredit the messenger. There are some people who others believe due to their personality, education, position within the hierarchy of the institution, or to the group with whom they associate. So it is not just about what is said, but who is saying it. If the negativity is coming from the CEO, you might as well stop the journey now. The support of senior hospital and senior nursing leadership is critical. But remember, not every leader has a title. Your institution has many informal leaders whose voices can sway many opinions.

One of the best strategies for refuting negativity is to have the factual, rational, and evidence-based rationale for the journey and the associated initiatives and interventions. A second strategy is to be aware of where the negativity is coming from, what the content of the negative message is, what formal or informal influence the messenger has, and who he or she is influencing. In other words, think of refuting negativity in a strategic way. Do not simply address it as you come across it, but prune it before it grows and flourishes. Sometimes isolating the source works. It can help to pull the messenger into the initiative prominently, having him or her own it; this then converts the negativity into endorsement. In the same vein, refuting negativity also depends on the characteristics of the messenger providing the positive message. If you are this individual, think about how you are perceived by others and how this may affect the message you deliver. You may want to partner with someone else to help achieve acceptance, or you may be the one everyone in your institution trusts. Sometimes just by being the "right" messenger, the message is more easily received.

On a grander scale, you could seek out an individual to speak about the Magnet journey from a recently designated Magnet facility. This could be an excellent way of informing and motivating key persons in your institution. An individual who has experienced the journey (and lived to tell the tale) and has no motivation other than helping other institutions is a powerful portrayal of beneficence and selflessness in the desire to better patient care and the work environment for everyone. Also, it sometimes seems staff are swayed by those from outside the institution more than those internal. You may have experienced the situation where someone knowledgeable in your institution has an idea to solve a contentious problem. Instead of trying the suggestion, a consultant is hired who suggests an identical idea. Suddenly the recommendation is taken seriously. We will call this the "insider bias," where insiders are seen as biased by nature of their position within an organization, and therefore unable to perform an accurate assessment.

Champions

In Chapter 2, we discussed some of the champions you will need for the Magnet journey. Find your champions and cherish them. You will most likely need at least one champion per unit for the journey. You will also need leadership champions. It is important to have champions from disciplines other than nursing as these will be your ambassadors for the Magnet journey. Here we would like to discuss a bit more about how to choose champions and how to reinforce their roles in the journey. For champions from other disciplines, you will need individuals who are influential in their departments, who can get things done, and who have a structure for communicating the information and initiatives undertaken. It is best to have volunteers that believe in the journey and the many benefits it can bring. Using individuals who have no real desire to contribute can be counterproductive. This is where your leadership abilities will be tried. Give the champions control. Let them decide how best to communicate with their units or departments. Let them choose which initiatives they wish to lead. Use their talents to accomplish your goals. If you need posters made to educate staff on the Magnet model, recruit champions who are creative and would enjoy the work. Provide the time for them to work and the materials they need. Provide food and you will be showing your appreciation.

You can guide your champions to have a specific focus when beginning the journey, such as where your gap analysis shows weakness. An institution we visited challenged their champions to develop a community outreach program, and provided them with the guidance and resources necessary so they could assess the community's needs, establish relationships with other community organizations, and plan interventions to help meet the community's needs. The institution allowed the champions to be creative, and gave them both the authority to decide on specific interventions (with guidance) and the responsibility to carry out the initiative. Many successful interventions were completed, such as food drives for local food banks, adopt-a-family programs for the holidays, education programs and screenings at malls and senior centers, a school supplies drive in coordination with local religious charities, and talks that focused on careers in nursing at local schools. They definitely made a difference in the community.

It is key to make initiatives for champions positive and fun. Look at what perks you can provide to the group for their hard work and dedication. Remember that this group is typically composed of volunteers, so be sure to keep them active, happy, and motivated. Frederick Herzberg, mentioned in Chapter 2, is a psychologist who researched job satisfaction and developed the motivation-hygiene theory (1968).This model has been a powerful influence on administrators. Although there is criticism of the theory, it does still provide insight into how employee motivation may be achieved.

His model distinguishes between motivators, which are needed to motivate individuals, and hygiene factors, which are needed to ensure employees are not dissatisfied. Hygiene factors do not provide the employee with positive satisfaction, but if absent, will lead to dissatisfaction. Hygiene factors are things like job security, salary, fringe benefits, and status; factors that are extrinsic to the work itself. Motivators include challenging work, recognition, and responsibility; factors that provide positive satisfaction from the work itself and facilitate the growth of the employee. What the model does, in our opinion, is to instill an awareness of the need to go beyond the carrot and stick approach to motivating employees. There are a number of motivation theories, models, and programs available for use and guidance. Look at some of these programs and the goals you want to achieve. Find one that is compatible with your goals and your institution's culture.

Stages of Change

You might be a bit frustrated because you have tried and tried to introduce new initiatives and you just cannot seem to get the staff to change their old ways of doing things. How many times have you heard the phrase, "Well that's how we've always done it," or "That's the [hospital name] way," implying that there is no other way it can be done. First, we advise you to be patient. Second, you should understand that, like the stages of grief we are all so familiar with (Kübler-Ross, 1969), there are stages of change individuals go through when letting go of one behavior and adopting another. There are a few theories and models that describe the various stages of change or transition. We will describe a few of the theories and models here, but if they do not seem applicable to your situation, just know that there are others that may help guide you to success.

The stages of change theory highlights the pattern of behaviors and feelings individuals and groups experience as they proceed through the process of change. This progression is based on research by Elisabeth Kübler-Ross (1969). The stages apply to change, good or bad. The sequence of emotions and behaviors begins sequentially with shock, feelings of denial, and anger. The individual is on a downward trend with respect to well-being and the emotional state. The individual begins bargaining to find a way out ("If this can be stopped, I'll do something to compensate") and then feels depressed when realizing the change is inevitable. This typically encompasses the lowest emotional point of the change/transition process. As time progresses, the individual becomes resigned to the fact that the change will occur or is occurring and may become ambivalent or apathetic. Eventually, the individual becomes more open to the change, and will finally accept the situation. The process is thought to end as the individual becomes encouraged by and involved in the change (Figure 4-1).

The time it takes to progress through this sequence of emotions is different for every individual and every situation. Now you can see why it can take so long for individuals to accept change and demonstrate new behaviors. You have no doubt seen individuals who seem resistant to change, no matter what that change might be. These individuals might take longer to progress through the sequence than others who are more amenable to change at the onset. Those who are more committed to the original process, possibly those who have done it that way for a majority of their career, may experience greater fluctuations in emotional well-being during the change process and may take longer to progress through the stages. What does

Figure 4-1   Psychological/Emotional stages of change.

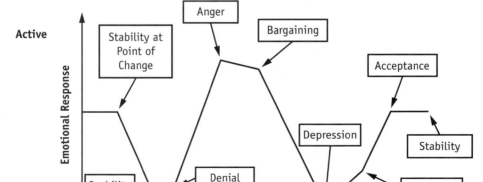

this mean to you? It means that you need to consider those most affected by the change and support them more intensely than those less concerned. This process is based on emotional response; while there are behavioral implications without a doubt, support needs to focus on the emotional state of the individuals undergoing change. Of course, if the change requires learning new skills and knowledge, much of the emotional turmoil can come from a fear of learning or ability to perform. You will need to ensure adequate educational time for learning the new process or procedure, and take into consideration that the individual who once was considered an expert in the process will be losing part of his or her identity, as they are now a novice to the new process. Definitely a confidence buster!

There are a number of other theories that also purport to describe the change process. Some are focused at the individual level, some at the group level, and many at the organizational level. Familiarizing yourself with a number of these will help you plan your rollout of the initiative and take into consideration the individual, group, and organizational skills and emotions involved in the change process. Volumes have been written that describe organizations' and individual's experiences with the change process. Many of these are anecdotal case studies, written by someone intimately involved, which can be good for advice. Because of all the many factors involved that can affect the change process, case studies should not be used as a strict prescription for success. Instead, think of these theories and case studies as guides, helping you to plan implementation and address possible issues. The more you know and understand, the better you can anticipate, prepare, and troubleshoot, and enhance your probability for success. Change happens differently for everyone, and, as we have observed, for some, not at all.

The Transtheoretical Stages of Change Model

James Prochaska and Carlo DiClemente developed a model for behavioral change called the Transtheoretical Stages of Change (Prochaska & DiClemente, 1983). This model is geared toward health promotion and individual behavior change, and states that there are distinct stages an individual passes through on his or her way to successful behavior change. This model, compared to the stages of change theory discussed previously, is more focused on behavior change with the corresponding emotional state playing a more minor role. The stage progression is, however, subjective, and defined by the individual undergoing the change. The stages are as follows:

- *Precontemplation* is when an individual has not yet acknowledged that there is a problem behavior in need of changing.
- *Contemplation* is when an individual knows a problem behavior exists, but is not ready or sure he or she wants to change.

- *Preparation/determination* is the stage where the individual is getting ready to change.
- The *Action/willpower* stage commences when the behavior is beginning to change and the individual proceeds throughout the behavior change.
- In the *Maintenance* stage, the individual maintains the behavior change, but may enter the next stage.
- The *Relapse* stage is where he or she returns to the old behavior instead of continuing with the new and is considered to be a normal part of behavior change.

The hope is that if an individual falls into the relapse stage, he or she will restart the process again at the preparation, action, or maintenance stage, continuing the resolution to change the behavior.

Of course, behavior change is never this neat. In the course of a single day, an individual might pass through several of the stages, while some will stay in one stage longer than others. That is why this model is typically seen as moving on a cyclical or spiraling timeline as opposed to a linear one. The variability and subjectivity in each individual makes it truly arduous to support a change in the behavior of many individuals simultaneously. Fortunately, Social Learning Theory (Bandura, 1977) demonstrates how an individual's behavior can also be shaped or reinforced by their learning environment. The theory stresses the main factors that affect behavior change: environmental influences, personal factors, and attributes of the specific behavior. Each of these factors may be affected by or may affect the other factors. Environmental influences can be everything from how the physical structure of the environment facilitates behavior change to how coworkers adhere to and engage in the desired behavior.

It sounds like common sense, but if you are changing a process and want individuals to eliminate the old process and change to a new process, remove the factors that are connected to the old process. You will be using the environment to facilitate the new process and change behavior. For example, to change behavior to order a different type of mattress for pressure ulcer prevention than the one that is typically ordered can be difficult. Take the old choice away: Eliminate it from the ordering form or as a choice on the computer order entry. This will force individuals to order the new mattress.

At the heart of Social Learning Theory are the concepts of self-efficacy and value. An individual must believe that he or she has the capability to perform the changed behavior and must value the outcome of the behavior change. It is easy to contemplate strategies you might use to support the behavior change based on these concepts. First, you will want to provide good instruction and feedback to individuals with respect to the behavior change. Positive reinforcement is essential. Also, you will need to convince individuals that the change will be beneficial both to the organization as a whole (if appropriate) and to each of them individually. Typically, we have found that addressing the question, "What's in it for me?" is essential in facilitating the behavior change and obtaining acceptance. Social Learning Theory provides a valuable awareness into how you can support the behavior needed. So far we have seen how learning and change theories and models can work synergistically to advance your change agenda.

Organizational Change Theories

Organizational change theories are in abundance, and every bookstore's business section is teeming with books touting the benefits of using the author's "proven" theory. The only problem is, the theory is typically proven in only one venue. Better to look for a theory or model with a more comprehensive base of evidence supporting its use. Here is an example of one you might choose.

In his book *Leading Change* (Kotter, 1996), a Harvard Business school professor, proposed an eight-step process for organizational change. In this model, the first step is to create an urgency for the change to obtain acceptance from management and staff alike. There are a number of ways this can be done. Of course, accurate data is best for convincing. If the impetus for your initiative is an opportunity for improvement, convey this by showing the current data and how it is not meeting the benchmark or goal. Go even further and show, if possible, how much, in dollars, satisfaction and reputation this deficiency may be causing. Kotter states that for an organizational change to be successful, at least 75% of a company's management needs to be on board.

The second step is to form a powerful coalition of influential people whose influence comes from various sources, such as position in the company, expertise, company politics, financial acumen, and status as a formal or informal leader.

In step three, you create a vision for change so that everyone will understand the specifics of what you want to achieve. This is best accomplished when you have a concrete strategy to achieve your articulated vision.

And in step four, you communicate your vision frequently and with fervor, integrating it into everything you do. You will need to not only communicate the vision, but also demonstrate the behavior you want from others. Be a role model for the change. There is nothing quite as hypocritical as someone attempting to change another's behavior when he or she cannot change their own. It is like a nurse who smokes, but who also gives smoking cessation education. How much would you believe this person? You would probably believe them very little, and for good reason.

In step five, you need to look for and remove any obstacles which may inhibit the change process. Look specifically for those who are resisting change and determine their barriers, whether process, products, or personal, and take action to eliminate the barriers as soon as possible. Reward those who are appropriately making the necessary change, and find out what might have helped them make the change. It might just help others.

For step six, you will want to create some short-term successes. Break up a long-term goal into a series of short-term targets for which success can be demonstrated periodically. Each of these smaller successes can be used to further motivate the staff and to demonstrate leadership that your plan is working. Make the first couple of targets "sure things" that are nearly impossible to blunder. And, of course, continue to acknowledge those that help you meet your targets.

Now that you have some short-term successes, you will want to build on these to develop and establish the change, step seven. Build on what changes went right and learn from those that may have faltered. You will be learning which techniques work in your institution with its unique organizational personality and culture. Of course this culture may change, but for now this knowledge may be a powerful ally in strategizing to further the change process. After each success, reflect on what went right. After each mistake, reflect on what you could have done differently. Continue looking for new, fresh, and innovative ideas. Stagnation is a dirty word!

In the last step, step eight, you will need to enculturate the change. The change should become part of your organization's behavior. To help this happen, you will need to put the change into policy, procedure, and performance. Put the change into hospital policy, making it standard procedure. To reinforce and hold staff accountable, the change needs to be integrated into performance evaluations. Linking money with metrics is a mantra in the business community. Even if you are not quite as direct, the change must still be linked to some evaluative process that is valued by the employee. We have found that in a number of institutions, performance evaluations are nothing more than a formality, linked to neither salary nor promotion. To enculturate any change and assure accountability, the performance of the behavior change must be measured and evaluated, and this evaluation must be linked to an incentive valued by the employee under scrutiny. If not, the process is generally meaningless.

So we have gone through Kotter's eight steps and thrown in a bit of advice of our own. You might choose to use a different model or theory for organizational change. Just do not forget the basics: support, encourage, plan, incentivize, learn, evaluate, hold accountable, enculturate, and by all means, keep changing!

Teamwork

There are possibly as many books and articles written about teamwork and team building as there are about organizational change. Peruse a few volumes and you will see commonalities. Everyone has a bias on what is the most important aspect of team building, but as a general rule, you can hardly go wrong no matter which you choose. Of course, you want to make sure the authors have credibility (credentials, experience). Many of these volumes will give you a number of distinct rules for team building. *Why Teams Win: 9 Keys to Success in Business, Sport, and Beyond* (Miller, 2009); *6 Habits of Highly Effective Teams* (Kohn & O'Connell, 2007); and *Twelve Tips for Teambuilding: How to Build Successful Work Teams* (Heathfield, 2009) are just a few options.

Learning about team building is a matter of noting the relevant concepts. Heathfield (2009) makes an important distinction between building an overall sense of teamwork and constructing an effective team. They are truly two distinct goals, yet many times the goals get intertwined and interventions miss the mark. Creating an overall sense of teamwork is geared toward engagement and cama-raderie. Building an effective team is more concrete and objective. Instead of developing general abilities, you are constructing a purposeful, focused work team, capable of fulfilling a mission and purpose that can be measured objectively.

Creating an overall sense of teamwork will be discussed a bit later. Here we want to focus on constructing an effective team. And as you have probably noticed by now, we are big advocates for planning. The better you plan your team, the better your results will be. The time spent on planning is nothing compared to the time spent trying to rectify problems from a lack of planning. Good planning, no matter how good, will always miss something. Therefore, in your planning, it is good to plan for an unexpected situation. How do you do this? Provide for extra time and resources within your overall team building plan, as most situations that arise consume time and resources. You will be glad you did.

Creating a Team

As for creating a team, you should first be aware that there are some typical stages that teams proceed through as they develop. Bruce Tuckman, an educational researcher, in his classic article *Developmental Sequence in Small Groups* (1965), termed the stages: *forming, storming, norming, performing,* and *adjourning*. The first stage, *forming*, occurs when the team is formed and when members' roles are defined. Next comes the *storming* phase where conflict becomes an issue as members are determining loci of control, reacting to individual's personalities and diverse points of view. Eventually the group progresses to the *norming* stage, when the team finds ways of compromising and are beginning to operate more as a unit instead of a bunch of individuals. The *performing* stage is when the team is working at maximum productivity to obtain its goal and fulfill its purpose. After the goal is met and the purpose fulfilled, the *adjourning* stage follows and the team disbands.

Now this sounds like a nice easy progression, but you probably already know it is not. Some teams never make it beyond the early stages and just fall apart. The key to a successful group lies in its leadership. In *Teambuilding That Gets Results,* Diamond and Diamond (2007) provide some actions necessary for each specific stage of the team's development. In the *forming* stage, you will want to establish ground rules, clarify the mission and purpose to the team, set goals, evaluate resources, and create the individual roles group members will play. Be careful to watch for personality discord and disputes among members as to what the team's vision should be. Members may become defensive as they deal with control issues among one another.

In the *storming* stage, you will want to encourage communication (both participating and listening), create an open environment where members are not afraid to voice their opinions, develop individual and team goals, and support and facilitate compromise so decisions can be made and the team can move forward. In this stage, be wary of cliques and power struggles where anger and frustration dominate. Things may move slowly at this stage, but with good leadership, compromise will be achieved and team cohesiveness enhanced.

The *norming* stage is the calm after the storm. Take advantage of the emotional tranquility and proceed to work as a team toward the goals, stressing both team and individual strengths. In this stage, watch for "groupthink," where members censor themselves for the good of maintaining a milieu of calmness, possibly inhibiting innovative ideas and silencing unpopular opinions. The team may also become complacent and operate on autopilot, stifling innovation and slowing progression. Emphasize the importance of and facilitate critical debate. Keep on target.

The *performance* stage is when you can sail to success, taking advantage of individual and team strength and maintaining an environment of open communication. Watch for the regression to earlier stages when under pressure. A change in leadership is commonly an impetus for regression. You and your team need a bit of flexibility as the workplace dynamics change during the group's tenure. Diamond and Diamond (2007) also describe the *adjourning* stage as "deforming and mourning." Here, teams that are formed for a specific purpose disband and may continue to meet infrequently to monitor the results achieved. For this type of team, closure is needed by summarizing the team's purpose, goals, and achievements, and disseminating the information to the appropriate stakeholders. Then the only thing left is a goodbye and a celebration acknowledging member's contributions and the team's success.

But what if the team is not disbanded; if the team is an ongoing task force charged with continuous monitoring and improvement in a specific nurse-sensitive indicator such as nosocomial pressure ulcer prevalence. Members never collectively reach the *adjourning* stage. The challenge in this type of team is preventing attrition from complacency and apathy. There is a greater opportunity for a group like this to revert back to earlier groups stages. The leader of the group needs to keep things fresh, but focused. Facilitate the establishment of continued goals, frequently reviewing the successes achieved and the opportunities that exist. Recruit new members at intervals and possibly limit the expected term of members. Of course, you cannot have a mass turnover, but a staggered, gradual influx and exit may bring new life to a stagnant team.

Team Building

In *6 habits of Highly Effective Teams*, Kohn and O'Connell (2007) discuss how to define teams and team effectiveness, and how those teams that were deemed effective demonstrated specific characteristics. They have congealed these characteristics into six habits, each discussed in depth in their book. They found that effective teams strengthen their emotional capacity to improve the internal and external team relationships, specifically the team member's relationships to each other, the team member's and team leader's relationship to the team as a whole, and the team's relationship to external groups and stakeholders. They provide models to frame and define this "strengthening of emotional capacity" as well as practical advice to help others achieve this habit within their own team.

The second habit is to expand the team's self-awareness, mainly through the development of a mission statement, a vision, and a list of unanimously agreed upon values. This can and should be formalized in a team charter, a document that sets the foundation for the group by explicitly defining the group's purpose, organization, and operations.

The third habit discusses team ground rules to ensure members practice empathy and respectfulness within the team and hopefully outside the team as well. Ground rules may also be included in the team charter and should be unanimously approved with specified repercussions for violations.

The fourth habit is about establishing and regulating the team's norms. Each team will have different norms, those implicit and explicit rules of behavior with which the team operates. These norms are dependent upon many factors that need to be collectively considered and managed by the team's leadership such as socialization, individualization, team purpose, and environment, to name a few. Good and active facilitation can lessen the chaos, enhancing team cohesion.

The fifth habit is lateral thinking, where a team can begin to align members' thinking patterns instead of using the paradigm of conflict and challenge to discuss new ideas. Lastly, effective teams entrust team members with roles appropriate to their specific competencies and comfort. This, the authors state, helps to establish mutual trust among team members, a sure sign that the team is cohesive and operational.

Although we believe that Kohn and O'Connell volume provides valuable insight into teams and team building, again we advise you to peruse the business section of your local bookstore and familiarize yourself with the various volumes on team building to find a guide that works for you and your institution's culture.

BUY-IN

By now you know you will need stakeholder input and support, and you have planned how you will present the rationale for your project, whether it be the Magnet journey or a simple practice change. Of course, the larger the project, the more individuals it typically affects. So your plan will need to consider education and communication strategies for all stakeholders involved. Remember, communication is two-way: You need their input as well as their acknowledgment and approval. We have discussed in other chapters the need to tailor the level of stakeholder involvement to your needs and their needs. If there are meetings that are purely informational, you could possibly send them the information via e-mail instead of taking up their time and requiring their attendance. One of the most powerful efforts that will help you obtain buy-in is consideration of others' time, abilities, and resources. But do not be modest and hide it. Make it blatant to the other individuals involved. You may begin an e-mail with, "In an effort to be considerate of your time, I am sending you the information that will be presented at the meeting. You are more than welcome to attend, but the group understands and appreciates the value of your time. If you have any questions about the information, just contact me." Here you want them to perceive that you are doing them a favor. This then obligates them to you. Think of it as strategic consideration.

Involve stakeholders as much as you need to, but at a minimum, establish a regular time and venue for communication to maintain an awareness of your initiative and to perpetuate buy-in. As we stated in previous sections, keep individuals accountable for their part in your initiative. Forming symbiotic partnerships with other individuals or departments may help to further your agenda and facilitate buy-in. Partnerships between nursing and hospital leadership are crucial for success in the Magnet journey. Think of the roles others can play in your initiative and how they may benefit from it. This incentive may act as a motivator for engagement. You can also form partnerships with external agents, whether they are other institutions that have successfully traveled the Magnet journey or consultants that give credibility to your cause.

Incentives vs Motivators

Previously, we discussed Herzberg's motivation-hygiene theory (1968) and stated that what most see as an important incentive (such as money) is not necessarily a motivator. We would like to make the distinction between an incentive and a motivator a bit clearer so you can keep it in consideration as you plan how to motivate others on the Magnet journey or whatever your initiative might be. Incentives are mainly for short-term behavior change. They can be effective and we think everyone can agree on that. Do you need a nurse to cover an open shift? Provide a financial bonus (an incentive), and you will probably find someone who will do it. But short-term behavior change does not necessarily correspond to long-term behavior change, engagement, or motivation. Incentives are better at direct cause and effect behavior and are more contractual.

Motivators are things that foster engagement and facilitate an internal process that becomes mostly self-generating. We see incentives as more external and motivators as more internal. Are incentives ever motivators? They can be. You can consider whatever motivates someone as an incentive for their behavior, but the motivator also implies an engagement and internalization not implied by an incentive. It is sometimes a fine line of distinction, but an important one to consider.

Now there is nothing wrong with incentives. On the contrary, we believe incentives are necessary and should be an integral part of planning. Incentives are not just tangible. One of the most powerful incentives is recognition. Recognition of an individual's contribution to an initiative goes a long way. There are a number of companies providing advice on increasing staff satisfaction. A standard intervention is recognition. A handwritten letter from a senior leader goes a long way in acknowledging and perpetuating an individual's contribution to the institution. Financial incentives work well to achieve immediate behavior change, much better than punitive measures. A rule of thumb is, if you have the opportunity to use either a positive incentive or a punitive measure, try the positive intervention first.

If that does not work, the second option might be a bit more punitive. But do not start by extreme punitive measures. Instead, start with a conversation outlining your expectations and the consequences of not meeting these expectations. The first step is truly creating and communicating expectations. Frequently we might think, "They know what they're supposed to do, they just don't want to do it." But, do they really know or do you just think they know? You cannot hold someone accountable for an expectation that he or she is not aware of. Spell it out so you are both on the same page, along with the behaviors you are looking for and by when. Make sure they are competent to perform the expected behaviors. Follow up in the stated time providing positive or corrective feedback.

You may not hear it verbalized directly, but you will probably find it implicit in conversations and actions: It is the "What's in it for me?" thinking and it is pervasive. Even the most selfless, team-focused individual gets something out of whatever they are engaged in. So the selfish issue needs to be addressed whenever something new is implemented or behavior needs to be changed. It is a huge part of obtaining buy-in and provides individuals with a distinct connection to the initiative or behavior change. This is where incentives come into play. The sometimes difficult part is individualizing these incentives. It is difficult because you need to know what acts as an incentive for each person, and you may not know each of them well enough to deduce this. In fact, for large-scale initiatives, you may not know them at all. So what do you do? You could brainstorm with managers and determine a number of incentives that will motivate most of the individuals you are targeting. You could also look at what worked in the past. What incentives did most staff respond to? Another approach is a bit more scientific. Survey your staff. Ask them what they would like to see as an incentive or, even better, what motivates them. It may be as simple as saving them time or frustration in their workday. It may be the opportunity to learn a new skill or better their current skill level. What you will get is an idea of your staff's expectations. If you can use these results and offer these incentives, you have also made the incentive and implementation process participative. This in itself will help achieve buy-in.

The Selling Point

Your initiative should also have a universal selling point. What we mean by this is that the selling point should result in something that is undeniably better, even if this better result is not something everyone cares about. This selling point should be understood as beneficial to as many of your staff as possible. A prime example is the implementation of a bar-coded medication administration process and technology. Some may find that the process takes more time, some may find it frustrating during the implementation process, but few can argue with the main selling point, which is patient safety. With a selling point that is beyond reproach, individuals are forced to acknowledge that, no matter what the drawbacks are, there is a result that cannot be trivialized, a result that outweighs the burdens the initiative's implementation may bring.

Achieving buy-in is all about the psychology of selling. Someone once asked us, "How do you get nurses to buy-in?" There are many factors involved, but the most important is having a great salesperson, someone who can sell the initiative and incite excitement about what the initiative can do, for both the individual and for the greater good. In most cases, this is better patient care. Selling is all about convincing. Convincing entails establishing credibility, a credible rationale for the initiative, and credible reasons why individuals should believe the initiative will achieve what you say it will achieve, a result better than what is currently happening. Health care is like traveling up a down escalator; stand still and you are actually regressing, moving farther behind. Every organization is rushing forward with change. You need to be quicker. You need to be running up the escalator just to keep competitive. It is difficult to convey this global view to direct caregivers. That is why you need to be a great salesperson: part expert, part motivational speaker. Remember you are selling, but you are selling substance. It is all about the universal selling point. Believe in it and others will also.

Many volumes written on implementation will advise you to have an arsenal of responses in your repertoire to be able to respond to a variety of questions, concerns, and challenges. Again, the better your planning, the better your result. Be able to describe a world after the implementation of your initiative that will be better because of your initiative. Of course you might embellish a little, or let idealism carry you away, but your vision should incorporate your universal selling point and portray a world better than what it is now. We are not implying that you are going to change the world with your initiative (although you may) but probably just your own piece of it. Live and breathe your vision during the implementation process. You of all people should exemplify total buy-in.

ENCULTURATION

Work-Arounds

For us, enculturation is habit. It is what is usual, the standard process or procedure. It is total change and implementation, eliminating the way it was done previously into extinction. It actually becomes part of the culture, hence the word en-*culture*-ation. Let us forewarn you though; this is not easily achieved. It takes patience, persistence, responsibility, and accountability. It takes multiple methods of facilitating compliance and some astute strategic planning. Not everyone responds to a single strategy. Strategies need not be complex and hugely time consuming. Some are actually quite simple and common sense. For example, as we have stated previously, if you want individuals to change to a new process you need to not only use education and accountability, but also eliminate the physical things that support the outdated process, such as paperwork, forms, and whatever else could allow individuals to revert back to the old process. Establish incentives for using the new process or procedure. One of the crucial things to keep in mind during the implementation of any new initiative that requires a change in behavior is work-arounds. A work-around is a process where individuals work around a process, usually because the process is too time-consuming or not practical. Usually, these work-arounds are established after the implementation phase, more likely when scrutiny is lax and the new process or procedure is seen as cumbersome. Be on the lookout for these work-arounds. They are possibly the largest threat to enculturation. If not recognized and eliminated, the work-arounds themselves will become enculturated.

Typically, work-arounds are seen as negative, going against the established procedure and taking unauthorized license in deciding what process should be followed. Staff utilizing work-arounds are seen as rogue employees, unable to conform to established rules and regulations. However, there are some positive aspects to work-arounds that we would like to discuss. For example, work-arounds may demonstrate creativity and critical thinking. They may also provide insight into a better way of doing things. Before chastising those using work-arounds, look at the reason for the work-arounds. Is it because staff are unable to get what they need in a timely fashion? Is it because there are not enough staff? Is it because the process does not achieve the outcomes it should? Our advice is to be aware of work-arounds, and then try to address their purpose in the newly established process. This may mean eliminating barriers to performing the established process, or modifying the established process so that work-arounds become unnecessary. Until you find and eliminate work-arounds, enculturation of your newly established process will not be achieved.

Enculturation in Your Implementation Plan

Enculturation should be addressed in your implementation plan. What we have found is that many believe implementation and change are complete as soon as a good outcome is demonstrated. This could not be further from the truth. You will need time, energy, and resources to achieve your enculturation strategy. Just as you strategized and created an implementation plan, you will also need to strategize and create an enculturation plan, a post implementation plan designed to focus on compliance with the initiative and continued monitoring of outcome measures. Depending on the initiative and your institution, enculturation could take a year or more. Your enculturation plan should encompass:

- Methods to continue integration
- Measuring compliance and intervening when necessary
- Analysis of data at regular intervals
- Rooting out work-arounds and possibly modifying processes
- Standards for accountability
- Defined authority and responsibility for the initiative, whether it is you or another individual
- Communication relating the status of the initiative to appropriate individuals, departments, and leadership

Incentivize and Celebrate

The last thing we would like to recommend is that you need to incentivize and celebrate success in your implementation and enculturation plan. During the implementation phase, incentives should be more of a celebratory nature and somewhat larger in scope then during the enculturation phase. After, you may continue to celebrate milestone outcomes to reinforce the initiative, but incentives can be more subtle and provided when positive outcomes are communicated. For example, by simply acknowledging that these outcomes would not have been possible without the compliance to the specific process or procedure. Making that constant connection between the initiative, compliance, and positive outcome is an incentive and an association that may actually help increase ongoing compliance.

The message we want to get across in this chapter is that you need to be realistic and not become apathetic in your quest to garner support and engagement with the Magnet journey. To some extent, you have to take things for what they are and not what you want them to be. Not everyone is as excited, committed, and engaged as you are. It is inevitable that some will doubt, some will scrutinize, and some will refuse to be part of the journey. By dealing with and strategically planning for these responses, you will be better prepared and more pragmatic. Do not discard people because they do not see it your way. Have a true democratic dialogue with them and find out what makes them feel the way they do. Set aside your own views and truly engage with others. It is all about building relationships. Enjoy the relationships and enjoy the journey.

CREATIVE SOLUTIONS

Creative Solution Title: *The Product and Intervention Fair*

Creative Solution Authors: Joanna Galletta, BA(c)
Magnet Program Assistant/Administrative Assistant/
Nursing Project Coordinator
South Jersey Healthcare, Vineland, NJ

Patricia Sanchez, RN, BSN
Nurse Manager, Medical Acute Unit
South Jersey Healthcare, Vineland, NJ

Purpose: The goal of this project is to engage and empower staff, to establish staff ownership of and enculturate the falls prevention initiative, ultimately helping to decrease inpatient falls. We want to involve the bedside nurse in the decision making process and encourage them to create interventions for their patient population. We also want to individualize care for our patients, providing equipment and interventions specific to their needs.

Legend

Overall Rating: **NOVICE–ADVANCED BEGINNER**

Financial:

Time:

Personnel:

Other Resources: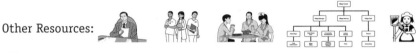

Efficacy: **A**

Transferability: **A**

Malleability/Adaptability: **A**

Ease of Implementation: **B**

Synopsis: The Product and Intervention Fair was designed to facilitate staff engagement, buy-in, and ownership of patient safety initiatives. It was also hoped that this would help individualize care for patients, utilizing products and interventions specific to their needs. Utilizing the shared governance structure and a Materials Management/Purchasing liaison, vendors were contacted to bring samples of their patient safety products to the fair, so that unit-based practice council (UBPC) chairs could view them, possibly choosing to adopt them in their unit based on their unit specialty, population, product efficacy, and culture. Evidence-based patient safety interventions that could be effective on specific units were found through literature searches and written up in a specification sheet format. Fair participants were encouraged to also peruse these interventions and choose ones that they may want to adopt in their unit. After leadership and UBPC approval, products were tested and interventions were implemented.

Description of Organization: South Jersey Healthcare (SJH) is a Magnet-designated, multiple-hospital system. The health system encompasses two full service in patient hospitals consisting of approximately 350 inpatient beds, comprehensive health centers, and outpatient and specialized services such as a Bariatric Center of Excellence, Wound Care Center, Sleep Center, and Balance Center. In 2008, SJH performed over 18,700 surgeries and the emergency department visits topped 97,400. The health system also serves as a clinical site for nursing students from a number of local colleges and maintains a professional relationship with Cumberland County College, which is adjacent to the Regional Medical Center (RMC) campus.

The Case Study: Our goal was to encourage staff and facilitate them taking part in the process of providing consistent products throughout the organization that were evidence-based and best practice for the bedside nurse to implement, and to provide safe and quality care to our patients. This initiative was lead by the Fall Prevention Task Force and shared governance council chairs. SJH has a robust shared governance structure, which was seen as essential to the success of this initiative. The members of the Coordinating Council, Quality Council, Nurse Executive Council, and staff nurses participated in this initiative.

The idea for this initiative came from the Falls Prevention Task Force Team. Staff nurses who attended the Quality Council meetings were troubled that the fall prevention program was not working to its full potential and suggested a fall prevention task force be formed. From their suggestion a committee was formed that developed evidence-based and innovative initiatives and monitored the efficacy of the patient falls prevention program.

The idea was brought first to leadership and management for support and then to the shared governance councils for support and buy-in. Some of those involved were: the Chief Nursing Officer, Vice Presidents of Patient Care Services, Quality Director, Finance Manager, Care Center Directors, Unit Managers, and the Materials Management Manager.

The Product and Intervention Fair was a vigorously promoted event that brought together three vendors from different companies to display their falls prevention wares for the members of the Coordinating Council, one of the councils in the SJH shared governance system. The membership of this council consists of the chairs of each unit's UBPC. The chair of each UBPC was charged with perusing the vendor's assortments of fall prevention aids to determine what would be most cost-effective for their unit, considering the unit's population and culture. They also perused evidence-based patient fall prevention interventions. These were formatted into specification sheets to mimic the commonly seen product specification sheets, and were gathered from the fall prevention literature by the Director of Quality and the Manager of the Medical Acute Unit, both members of the Falls Prevention Task Force at SJH. This was an interdisciplinary initiative that incorporated staff from the Materials Management Department to contact the vendors and facilitate the product acquisition and trial process.

The Product and Intervention Fair lasted 2 hours and was promoted vigorously to management and staff. The event was publicized as an important way to individualize falls prevention initiatives and products to specific patient populations, and also offered participants a continental breakfast. After choosing unit-specific products and initiatives, the UBPC chairs brought their suggestions back to their unit manager and outcomes manager for evaluation of cost appropriateness and effectiveness. Products and interventions were finalized by each UBPC chair and submitted on unit summary sheets to the administrative mentor of the Coordinating and Quality Councils for compilation.

The staff nurses were anxious to trial the new products and interventions that they selected for their patient populations and specialty units. Several unit chairs volunteered their unit to be the trial unit and were selected to test the new products before implementation to the entire system. Once the items were validated, they were implemented to the appropriate units; however, items can be utilized by any and all areas within the organization when appropriate. Each Unit Manager maintains their own budget in which they would be able to purchase products as needed throughout the fiscal year. During the process, staff nurses demonstrated the stewardship values of the organization.

Outcome Measures:

Formative/Compliance: For evaluation we measured staff attendance at the fair, number of products and interventions considered, number of unit summary sheets submitted for consideration, anecdotal satisfaction of the vendors, anecdotal satisfaction of the council member participants, and the costs for this initiative.

Summative/Outcome: For evaluation we measured the number of units testing new products and interventions, the number of products and interventions tested, the number of products and interventions adopted, the cost of the products and interventions, and the patient fall rate.

Evidence Supporting this Creative Solution: Product fairs are a common part of professional conferences where vendors display products appropriate to the conference's purpose and focus. This creative solution is an extension of that process. No literature could be found on the efficacy of using a product or intervention fair in this way, leading us to believe that this is a truly novel and creative way to engage staff, to facilitate staff ownership of an initiative, and to individualize patient care.

Recipe for: *The Product and Intervention Fair*

Ingredients:

CNO, leadership, and management support

Materials management/purchasing liaison

Staff buy-in

Shared governance structure

Time allowance for staff with salary

Vendors and their product safety wares

Product specification sheets and intervention specification sheets

Unit summary sheets

Venue to accommodate fair

Person to plan and coordinate the event

Food

Step-by-Step Instructions (see Figure 4-2 for Step-by-Step Instruction Timeline):

Step 1: Obtain support from CNO, leadership, management, and staff.

Step 2: Involve Materials Management/Purchasing liaison in event planning, product acquisitions, and product trials.

Step 3: Plan the date and time to coincide with a scheduled shared governance meeting to facilitate attendance.

Step 4: Contact vendors, discuss the event, and invite them to attend with samples of their company's patient safety products. Ask the vendors to bring a supply of patient specification sheets for each product. Finalize the time and date.

Step 5: Vigorously publicize the event to staff and all stakeholders.

Step 6: Search the patient safety research and quality literature to find patient safety interventions that may be appropriate for the various unit specialties and populations within your institution. Create and duplicate intervention specification sheets.

Step 7: Hold the event. Instruct council participants to bring their chosen product and intervention specification sheets back to their unit leadership and UBPC for discussion. When they decide what the unit wants to trial, write each on the unit summary sheet (provided), and submit it to the event coordinator or administrative council mentor by the next council meeting.

Step 8: Collect the sheets at the next council meeting and summarize the unit's interventions and products, noting which units have chosen identical products for trial. Share this with the Materials Management liaison to obtain these products for trial. Collect and summarize formative outcome measures.

Step 9: In partnership with the UBPCs and unit leadership, facilitate the adoption of chosen interventions.

Step 10: Begin product trials for specific units.

Step 11: Evaluate products and determine their cost-effectiveness. Adopt products as desired. Products may be unit-specific, but if desired, can be made available to any staff who thinks patients may benefit.

Step 12: Incorporate the final products and interventions into the unit-based patient safety guidelines. At SJH, these guidelines are accessible at each nurse's station so that any nonregular staff will know what is expected.

Additional Outcomes to Consider Measuring:

Formative/Compliance: Formal survey to determine satisfaction of the vendors, satisfaction of the council member participants, and satisfaction of leadership or

Figure 4-2   Timeline for "The Product and Intervention Fair."

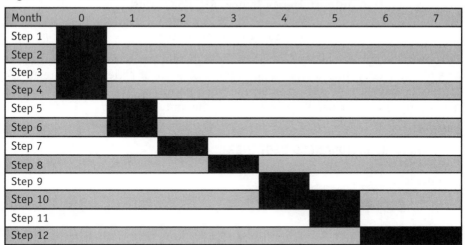

management with the initiative. Measure compliance with the use of products and interventions on a unit level.

Summative/Outcome: Possibly look at the correlation of the unit-based products and interventions adopted along with the unit's patient fall rate.

Insights from Original Implementation:

- A robust shared governance structure is necessary to truly involve and engage staff, and to develop staff ownership of the initiative.
- An interdisciplinary team approach is helpful with buy-in from leadership, finance, nursing, and Materials Management/Purchasing.
- Commitment of the staff and leadership is essential.
- There was some discussion of making this an annual event, where vendors would display their newest patient safety products to Coordinating Council members so we at SJH can keep abreast of the latest innovations in patient safety products and provide the best patient care possible.

For Further Guidance Contact:

Joanna Galletta, BA(c)
gallettaj@sjhs.com

Patricia A. Sanchez, RN, BSN
sanchezp@sjhs.com

Creative Solution Title: *Change of Shift Huddle*

Creative Solution Author: **Megan Bynoe, RN, BSN, CCRN**
Assistant Nurse Manager
CentraState Health System

Purpose: The purpose of the Change of Shift Huddle was to make all staff members of a telemetry unit in an acute care hospital aware of patients who are at risk for falling and alert all staff to intervene when necessary. The overall goal was to help decrease the number of patient falls on the unit.

Legend

Overall Rating: **ADVANCED BEGINNER**

Financial:

Time:

Personnel:

Other Resources:

Efficacy: **A**

Transferability: **A**

Malleability/Adaptability: **A**

Ease of Implementation: **A**

Synopsis: The Change of Shift Huddle is an intervention utilized to decrease the number of patient falls on a hospital unit. All incoming staff meet at a designated station and receive a brief report that takes approximately 5 minutes on all patients. The emphasis in the report is on mental status, history of previous falls, effects medications may be having, equipment in use on certain patients, and other information individualized to specific patients. The Change of Shift Huddle makes everyone aware of every patient on the unit. In that way, if any staff member observes a patient at risk of falling attempting to get out of bed without assistance, even if the staff member is not assigned to that patient, they will be aware that they have to intervene. The Change of Shift Huddle allows the nursing staff to make changes and manage crises before they occur, and make individualized patient care adjustments to facilitate patient safety. Many other interventions are used to help decrease the number of falls on the unit, but the personal interest shown by all staff in the Change of Shift Huddle is the most effective solution thus far.

Description of Organization: CentraState Health System is a not-for-profit, single hospital system with 271 beds and is a member of the Robert Wood Johnson University Health System. It is a teaching hospital with Family Residents and Geriatric Fellows from UMDNJ Medical School. CentraState Medical Center was Magnet designated in 2006 and is currently in the process of renewal.

The Case Study: A telemetry unit in an acute care hospital faced the great challenge of frequent falls. A large percentage of the patient population on the unit range between the ages of 65 and 100+ years old, and many are confused or demented. A change in their environment, the use of multiple medications, and the utilization of unfamiliar equipment are some of the things that contribute to falls. Unfortunately, some falls result in serious injury to patients.

The Falls Prevention Committee for the hospital was in search of a simple and inexpensive idea to prevent and reduce the number of falls that could be easily implemented. The Falls Prevention Committee requested the hospital librarian to conduct a literature search for articles describing falls prevention interventions. Several articles, which included evidence-based research information, were found and reviewed by Falls Prevention Committee members (ECRI, 2006).

An article by Stewart and Johnson (2007) describing huddles to improve office efficiency was chosen as a model after which a falls prevention intervention could be created. The Change of Shift Huddle was developed. The goal of the Change of Shift Huddle was to make all staff members aware of the patients who are at risk for falling and alert everyone to intervene when necessary. Many patients have an overly positive perception of their ability to ambulate without assistance, increasing their risk of falling. They see others at risk, but are reluctant to see themselves at risk for falling, and therefore, they neglect to see the need to practice preventive behavior. The job of caretakers is to help prevent patients from falling, and particularly, to help prevent serious injuries.

The article on the huddle was distributed to nursing staff for review. The nursing staff members were allowed 2 weeks to review the article and comment. Brief 10-minute discussions at different times with nursing staff members for feedback followed the review. Change of Shift Huddle was initiated on the unit with the night staff. After 6 months of using the Change of Shift Huddle, falls data was reviewed and the fall rate did decrease. The Change of Shift Huddle was then extended to include other shifts. The nurse manager of the unit kept the staff continually informed by providing a brief monthly report of the number of falls on the unit.

Outcome Measures:

Formative/Compliance: Monthly review of patient fall rates with unit staff.

Summative/Outcome: Monthly, quarterly, and annual falls reports are generated, which show the number of inpatient falls and the number of falls with injury by the Risk Management department. The Falls Prevention Committee calculates the rate of falls per 1000 patient days and uses this rate to compare with similar published rates. Hospital falls data are also submitted to NDNQI through which they can compare themselves to other similar institutions. After 6 months of the Change of Shift Huddle intervention, the number of falls decreased as shown in the chart below (Figure 4-3).

Figure 4-3   Patient falls.

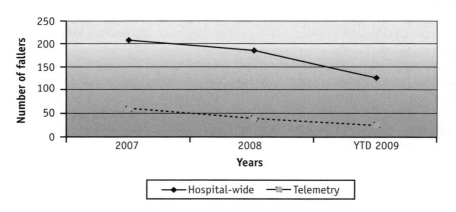

Evidence Supporting this Creative Solution: The idea of the Change of Shift Huddle came from an article written by Elizabeth E. Stewart, PhD and Barbara C. Johnson, PhD in Family Practice (2007). The term "huddle" was taken from the game of football when players came together to decide on their strategy for playing and winning the game. This article refers to the use of huddles to improve office efficiency, but this idea was adapted to the prevention of falls. However, the Change of Shift Huddle could be used to address many other problems, particularly when problems involve communication (Hendrich, 2006; Kimball, 2002).

ECRI. (2006). Focus on falls: prevention strategies that work. *The Risk Management Reporter*, *25*(6), 1–7.

Hendrich, A. (2006). Inpatient falls: Lessons from the field. *Patient Safety & Quality Healthcare*, *3*, 26–30.

Kimball, S. (2002). Breaking the fall factor. *Nursing Management*, *33*(9), 22–25.

Stewart, E. E., & Johnson, B. C. (2007). Huddles: Improve office efficiency in mere minutes. *Family Practice*, *14*(6), 27–29.

Most articles on Fall Prevention focus on the identification of patients at risk for falls, tools used for assessing risk, planning care for patients at risk, and identifying the costs involved when patients sustain serious injuries. Certainly, these are all aspects that need to be addressed. However, the simplicity and enhanced communication of the Change of Shift Huddle seemed to be the least expensive and most effective if done consistently.

Recipe for: *Change of Shift Huddle*

Ingredients:

Nursing and ancillary staff on designated unit/shift

Step-by-Step Instructions (see Figure 4-4 for Step-by-Step Instruction Timeline):

Step 1: Distribute the article on the huddle to nursing staff for review.

Step 2: Schedule brief 10-minute discussions with nursing staff members for feedback following the review.

Step 3: At the beginning of each shift, after the nurse-to-nurse report, gather all staff on the floor for that shift for the Change of Shift Huddle.

Step 4: In the Huddle, review each patient on the unit in a brief 5-minute report, focusing on patient mental status, history of previous falls, possible effects of medications, equipment in use for specific patients, and any other individualized patient information.

Step 5: Nurse manager conducts brief monthly reviews with staff to report the number of falls to keep staff informed about the Change of Shift Huddle results.

Figure 4-4   Timeline for "Change of Shift Huddle."

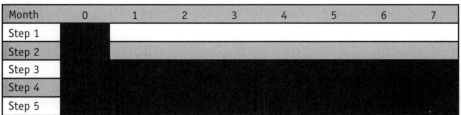

Month	0	1	2	3	4	5	6	7
Step 1								
Step 2								
Step 3								
Step 4								
Step 5								

Additional Outcomes to Consider Measuring:

Formative/Compliance: Attendance of all staff on each in the huddle and the frequency that the huddle is done. Is it done consistently on every shift?

Summative/Outcome: Survey staff to evaluate if they feel the huddle has improved communication of patient needs and risks and improved their ability to care for patients.

Insights from Original Implementation: This Change of Shift Huddle solution is simple, does not incur additional financial costs, and requires no additional training or skill. However, it must be done consistently. Keep the Change of Shift Huddle report short. Once accustomed to receiving this report, the staff would ask additional questions if it was not given in the report. We have received nothing but positive feedback on the Change of Shift Huddle from the staff.

For Further Guidance Contact:

Megan Bynoe, RN, BSN, CCRN
Assistant Nurse Manager
CentraState Healthcare System
901 West Main Street
Freehold, NJ 07728
mbynoe@centrastate.com

REFERENCES

Aiken, L. H., Clarke, S. P., Sloane, D. M., Lake, E. T., & Cheney, T. (2009). Effects of hospital care environment on patient mortality and nurse outcomes. *Journal of Nursing Administration, 39*(7/8), S45–S51.

Aiken, L. H., Havens, D. S., & Sloane, D. M. (2009). The Magnet nursing services recognition program: A comparison of two groups of Magnet hospitals. *Journal of Nursing Administration, 39*(7/8), S5–S14.

American Nurses Credentialing Center. (2008). *Application manual Magnet recognition program®*. Silver Spring, MD: Author.

American Nurses Credentialing Center. (2009a). *History of the Magnet program*. Available at: http://www.nursecredentialing.org/Magnet/ProgramOverview/HistoryoftheMagnetProgram.aspx. Accessed December 20, 2009.

American Nurses Credentialing Center. (2009b). *Magnet research references*. Available at: http://www.nursecredentialing.org/Magnet/ResourceCenters/MagnetReferences.aspx. Accessed December 20, 2009.

American Nurses Credentialing Center. (2010). *Forces of magnetism*. Available at: http://www.nursecredentialing.org/Magnet/ProgramOverview/ForcesofMagnetism.aspx. Accessed March 29, 2010.

Armstrong, K., Laschinger, H., & Wong, C. (2009). Workplace empowerment and Magnet hospital characteristics as predictors of patient safety climate. *Journal of Nursing Administration, 39*(7/8), S17–S24.

Bandura, A. (1977). *Social learning theory*. New York: General Learning Press.

Charthouse Learning (2009). *Welcome to the official home of the FISH! philosophy*. Available at: http://www.charthouse.com/content.aspx?name=home2. Accessed December 19, 2009.

Diamond, L. E., & and Diamond, H. (2007). *Teambuilding that gets results.* Naperville, IL: Sourcebooks, Inc.

Drenkard, K. (2009). The Magnet imperative. *Journal of Nursing Administration, 39*(7/8), S1–S2.

Heathfield, S. M. (2009). *Twelve tips for teambuilding: How to build successful work teams.* About.com. Available at: http://humanresources.about.com/od/involvementteams/a/twelve_tip_team.htm. Accessed December 20, 2009.

Herzberg, F. I. (1968). One more time: How do you motivate employees? *Harvard Business Review 46*(1), 53–62.

Kohn, S. E. & O'Connell, V. D. (2007). *6 habits of highly effective teams.* Franklin Lakes, NJ: Career Press.

Kotter, J. P. (1996). *Leading change.* Boston: Harvard Business Press.

Kübler-Ross, E. (1969). *On death and dying.* New York: Macmillan.

Maxwell, J. C. (2008). *Teamwork 101: What every leader needs to know.* Nashville, TN: Thomas Nelson.

Miller, S. L. (2009). *Why teams win: 9 keys to success in business, sport, and beyond.* Mississauga, Ontario: John Wiley & Sons Canada Ltd.

Prochaska, J. O., & DiClemente, C. C. (1983). Stages and processes of self-change of smoking: toward an integrative model of change. *Journal of Consulting and Clinical Psychology, 51*(3), 390–395.

Prochaska, J. O., Norcross, J. C., & DiClemente, C. C. (1994). *Changing for good: A revolutionary six-stage program for overcoming bad habits and moving your life positively forward.* New York: Harper Collins Publisher.

Stone, P. W., & Gershon, R. R. M. (2009). Nurse work environments and occupational safety in intensive care units. *Journal of Nursing Administration, 39*(7/8), S27–S34.

Stone, P. W., Larson, E. L., Mooney-Kane, C., Smolowitz, J., Lin, S. X., & Dick, A. W. (2009). Organizational climate and intensive care unit nurses' intention to leave. *Journal of Nursing Administration, 39*(7/8), S37–S42.

Tuckman, B. W. (1965). Developmental sequence in small groups. *Psychological Bulletin, 63*(6), 384–399.

Ulrich, B. T., Buerhaus, P. I., Donelan, K., Norman, L., & Dittus, R. (2009). Magnet status and registered nurse views of the work environment and nursing as a career. *Journal of Nursing Administration, 39*(7/8), S54–S62.

## CHAPTER 5

Measuring and Communicating Outcomes

"If you can't measure it, you can't manage it."

—ANONYMOUS

"You cannot improve one thing by 1000% but you can improve 1000 little things by 1%."

—JAN CARLZON

"Evaluate what you want—because what gets measured, gets produced."

—JAMES A. BELASCO

Outcomes are essential. Face it, without outcomes, all of your efforts are for nothing. Interventions may be well intentioned and make you feel good, but without measurable positive outcomes, they may have no additional benefit. We sometimes get so caught up in how we are doing something, that we forget why we are doing it. We believe that if we do the intervention correctly as prescribed, we will definitely get a good outcome. Unfortunately, this is not the case. You need to measure and communicate outcomes, whether good or poor, to either continue the intervention because it is making a difference or to stop the intervention because it is not demonstrating the desired results. This chapter will discuss some of the issues to consider when measuring and communicating outcomes.

OUTCOME DATA VS COMPLIANCE DATA

We will not repeat ourselves here, but instead refer you to Chapter 6: Implementing Evidence-Based Practice. The distinction between outcome data and compliance data is an important one, not just for the knowledge of those involved in measuring, but it is also a way of thinking about the type of intervention you are implementing. Compliance with policies, protocols, and interventions is necessary if you want to achieve the goal or purpose of your policy. Many times our focus is so narrowly concentrated on compliance issues that we get caught up in these issues, possibly to the detriment of our efforts. To make a difference in patient care outcomes, you need to measure compliance, but your focus should be on the outcomes. It sounds obvious, but basically compliance is what you do, outcomes are what occur to your patients. The distinction can get muddled through the language we use.

When we talk about patient compliance, are we talking about an outcome? Sure, it might be an outcome for example, if you have an initiative to increase patient compliance with the use of the call bell for assistance. So then what is the outcome of the initiative? It is an increase in patient compliance. But also think, ultimately, why am I doing the intervention? Why do I want patients to use the call bell more? Maybe it is to prevent them from trying to ambulate on their own and possibly falling. So, ultimately, your overall outcome measure of this initiative is the patient fall rate. This might be your outcome focus for this initiative. If you can show that your efforts have decreased the fall rate, you know your work has made a difference by bettering patient care.

PARTS OF A CHART

Have you ever received a chart or graph from the Performance Improvement (PI) Department or the Infection Control Department that you could not understand? You receive the same chart every month, and every month you look at it and either file it away or post it on the unit's PI board for all to see. Sure everyone sees it, but does anyone actually understand what it means? You basically know what it is, or what it is supposed to be, but it does not present the data so that you can use it. Things are missing, or just wrong. Maybe the sides of the chart have no labels or dates are missing. There are no units with the numbers or there are so many lines in the chart that you cannot tell which data is yours. Or maybe you are just given a number for the month. Is it good or bad? Who knows?

Charts and graphs vary in type. There are bar charts (vertical bars), line graphs, graphs of data points, charts with horizontal bars, graphs that look like a spider web; the list goes on and on. So how do you know which should be used? Usually the decision as to what type of chart or graph to use has to do with the type of data you have and the message you are trying to convey.

An effective chart or graph should be able to convey a number of things. For it to be an effective chart or graph, it must include the components necessary to convey the information you are trying to send out. The chart must be complete. Although charts and graphs differ in appearance and purpose, there are some standard parts of a chart you should know and look for when interpreting a chart or graph (Smith, 2008). We will admit now that the parts we see as universal, others will see as specific to distinct types of charts. We are not stating gospel, merely a guide for you to go by.

Figure 5-1   Example of an effective graph.

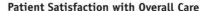

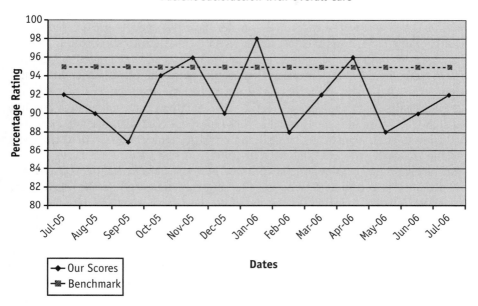

Patient Satisfaction with Overall Care

The chart in Figure 5-1 is relatively complete. The chart has both axes defined, the title tells you what data you are looking at. It not only tells you how you are doing for the month, but it also trends the data. Typically, the best chart to use for monthly data is a 13-month chart. In this way you can visualize the trend over a full year and compare the current month with the same month in the previous year. If you have quarterly data, use a 5-quarter chart for the same reasons. The chart in Figure 5-1 also contains the benchmark value, which allows you to compare how you are doing to how others are doing. It is important to know where the benchmark is from and why you are using that value as your benchmark. The legend should define what each set of data points represent.

The units of data also need to be provided. In this chart we can see that we are dealing with percentages. That needs to be explicit, whether each value has a percentage sign or it is collectively labeled as in this chart; it is crucial to know what units you are measuring. And of course, the benchmark data must have the same units, comparing apples with apples. The scale of the chart is also something to consider when you are creating a chart. If the y-axis scale (the vertical scale) was 0 to 100, the trend would be less obvious and the data would look more uniform. You would not notice as much variability because the scale would be larger, resulting in less discrimination. This is sometimes how people use charts to their advantage to make data look better than it actually is.

Much of the overall interpretation of a chart has to do with perception. Do not let the layout of the chart fool you. We have seen people use a trend line in charts, a line that shows the best linear trend estimation, to show that a program is indeed demonstrating an effect, lessening or increasing the targeted metric. This linear trend line is more perception than significance. The trend may be little more than a seasonal fluctuation. Be careful not to believe what you first perceive; dig deeper. Realize that the person creating the chart may have an agenda, possibly to show their data in a positive light. Those inexperienced with reading charts will fall prey to their agenda. Be cynical and critically look at the parts of the chart noting the scale, the benchmark, your value, and the trend. Furthermore, when you receive data, it is beneficial to know how the data was collected and how its accuracy is determined. Who is collecting this data, and do they have some expertise in collecting this type of data? Do they know what the data means, or are they just following a strict definition provided by a regulatory agency? Is it collected manually or is it automated in some way? We once saw a situation where nurse-sensitive pressure ulcer data was collected by medical coders who followed the strict regulatory agency's definition of what is considered a hospital-acquired pressure ulcer. The problem was that the definition did not include the recognition of nursing documentation, only physician documentation. Clearly they were classifying pressure ulcers as hospital-acquired when the nursing documentation proved they were present on admission. Knowing that this rate of hospital-acquired pressure ulcers was inflated, managers did not believe the data and did not take it seriously. In the end, the data collection and presentation was worthless.

We firmly believe data collection, presentation, and dissemination should always add value, whether as a base of knowledge or an impetus for action. If not, it is an act of futility, costing the institution money with no real benefit. For us, a complete chart or graph, appropriately used, is a thing of beauty. Its beauty is obvious in its ability to convey meaning, data, trending, the sender's agenda, and comparisons and standing within the comparison group and perception, all within a simple visual display.

THE CHART AS LANGUAGE/NUMBERS AS LANGUAGE

What many do not realize is that numbers are like words. They, like words, are placed to create meaning and get across some piece of information. If you think of numbers as language, you begin to understand that missing parts can cause a message to be incomprehensible to the receiver. *Please some bread and John lunch.* Does this sentence make sense to you? What is missing? Oh, we forgot the verbs.

Please buy some bread and make John lunch. Now it is understandable. The syntax is complete and you can decipher the sentence's meaning. You can also infer the intent of the sender. It appears that the sender is delegating an errand to a familiar person, possibly a wife speaking to her husband or vice versa, and asking that he or she make, possibly for their son John, lunch. Sure there are other interpretations, but what we are trying to show is that proper grammar leads to more than understanding; it leads to inference. This is the same for the language of numbers. With numbers, the chart becomes the syntax. Without a complete chart, the message is not interpretable and the only inference is that the sender is incompetent. To reinforce the idea that numbers are a form of language, and to blur the lines between the two a bit more, we propose a formulaic definition of communication:

$$\text{Communication} = (\text{Sender} + \text{Receiver}) \times \text{A Common Language}$$

The economy of writing the explanation this way emphasizes the power of syntax in numbers; one can convey a lot of meaning and information in a very compact and visual way. It is estimated that 65% of the population are visual learners (Riding & Rayner, 2000). So, there is a good chance that a visual display will help to convey what you intend.

What are You Trying to Say?

If numbers are a form of language and the chart is its syntax, then some of the same rules apply for sending out a chart full of data to managers and staff. I am sure you have heard the phrase "think before you speak." Hopefully this phrase was not recently directed to you, but we are pretty certain it is a parental standard and a mantra of grade school teachers. What we are cautioning here is that there is a lot of inference that goes along with language. Some of the inferences we make are possibly more valid in a face-to-face communication situation. This may be due to a bit of triangulation. When we communicate face-to-face, we are actually receiving two modes of communication simultaneously, verbal and nonverbal. They both work synergistically to give us not only the direct communication, but also provide us with interpretable gestures that help us to make inferences about the verbal message we receive and actually extend its meaning. Have you ever had a face-to-face communication with someone whose verbal communication relayed one message, but his or her nonverbal communication relayed another? You probably were not quite sure how to interpret what their ultimate meaning was. It is like a mother telling her child, "Come give mommy a hug," but her arms are folded across her chest and she is looking rather distracted. This is what we call a mixed message, and it happens quite frequently. Face-to-face verbal communication is, we believe, easier to interpret than written communication, where there is no verbal inflection or intonation, nor is there the nonverbal communication that reinforces or refutes the message.

We typically interpret face-to-face verbal messages using our deciphering skills of hearing, listening, relating, and inferring. But when it comes to written communication, we are definitely handicapped. Without the intonation, inflection, and nonverbal communication of face-to-face verbal communication, we need to rely on other cues for inference. So what does all this have to do with data and charts? Well, before you send out data and charts, you need to consider that, as a communication, your message is subject to misinterpretation. You need to consider first what you are trying to say, and then, after composing the chart (communication), consider if it says what you intended and reflect on how it could possibly be misinterpreted. What indirect messages are you sending along with the chart? Failure to address these issues can cause your chart to be just another paper, filed away. What a waste of time and effort! Frequently we see that when we receive charts and data, the sender failed to share the chart with a colleague prior to sending it. Having a colleague read over your data is the equivalent of having someone read your school paper before you turn it in to the teacher. You should always have another set of eyes that you trust take a look at the chart and data before it is distributed to your audience. Tell that person the purpose of the chart and what the data represents. Let him or her ask questions and see if you can modify your chart to account for his or her questions to clarify your message. Then you can send it out, confident that the message you are sending is the same message that is going to be received.

Stating that you are fluent in a language means that you can read, write, and speak the language, and understand the colloquialisms and the irregularities inherent in the language. You may not know every slang phrase or the latest local buzzwords, but you have a command of the language that goes beyond mere translation. You can decipher the implied meanings from the intonations and inflections in the spoken language. It is the same with the language of data and charts. If you are fluent in this language, you can decipher the implied meaning, but maybe there is not an implied meaning, or possibly the implied meaning was not intended. What we are trying to say here is that you need to make sure the receivers of your data or chart communication are fluent in the language of data and charts. If not, they may need some language lessons. Sending a message in English is worthless if the receiver speaks only Spanish. The same is true with sending data and charts. That is why before you send data in any format, you need to assess your audience for their level of understanding and comfort with that format. If they are not fluent, education is necessary. You might also simplify your presentation, the same as when you speak with someone who only has a superficial command of the second language. You will probably use words that are simpler and less colloquial. It is all about tailoring the message to your audience to assure your message is received as it is intended. What we have seen work well in environments where there is only a superficial knowledge of data or chart language is first simplification, then education, and gradual complexity. First, you simplify your message (data/chart) as much as possible. This may mean adding a narrative explanation to the chart at the beginning. Concurrently, you or others fluent in data/chart language are educating the receivers of the data/charts on how to interpret the information, analogous to a language course for nonnative speakers. As the receivers become more savvy and knowledgeable, the narrative can be eliminated, and the charts can become more complex without the fear that the audience will not understand. Frequently the mismatch between sender and receiver with respect to data/chart dissemination goes either unnoticed, or worse, is accepted without resolution. This makes the process worthless and frustrating.

As the sender of data, it is important to make sure the data has integrity, that it is believable. Those not fluent in data interpretation might see data as black and white, either good or bad. They do not yet see the integrity of data as a continuum, much like the hierarchy of evidence discussed in Chapter 6: Implementing Evidence-Based Practice. This all good or all bad extremism is common when there is immaturity in knowledge of a certain subject. Children go through this extremism phase, and unfortunately, some adults are stuck there. Data integrity is all about shades of grey, but until your audience has the knowledge and maturity in data analysis and interpretation, you as the sender need to make a special effort to provide the most accurate data possible.

And prepare to be challenged, especially by those individuals with opportunities for improvement. The now famous (or infamous) book *How to Lie With Statistics* (Huff, 1954) sums up what many believe, that you can make the data say anything you want. This line of reasoning may lead the receiver to blame the sender for data that shows poor performance. That is why it is essential that the data be as clean and accurate as possible and that the sender not take the challenge personally. We have seen firsthand how difficult this can be. Once, in a meeting with unit managers, the Performance Improvement (PI) coordinator began reviewing the performance metrics (nurse-sensitive indicators) of all the units. When she got to this particular unit, the manager, who was incidentally a novice at data analysis and interpretation, challenged the catheter-associated urinary tract infection (CAUTI) rate, stating that there was no way it could be that high. Unfortunately, even though the PI coordinator knew the data and tried to explain that the rate depended on the number of catheter days as well as the number of infections, she could not speak to the integrity of the data, having received it from the infection control department and being unaware of how and by whom it was collected. The manager then began attacking the PI coordinator, implying that she had no idea what she was doing and that the data was meaningless. This erupted into an all out battle until finally the meeting facilitator called an end to the meeting, without resolution. This episode tainted all further data sent by the PI coordinator for everyone who attended this meeting. That is why it is so important to address data integrity to the best of your ability, assuming you are the one sending the data.

RUN CHARTS, PARETO CHARTS, AND GANTT CHARTS

There are different types of charts for different purposes. Some of these charts are tools to help you communicate and some are tools to determine if a problem exists, to help decision making, and to help you organize. So it is essential that you use the correct chart or graph for the appropriate purpose. We will review three different types of charts that are utilized for specific purposes.

The Run Chart

A run chart is a chart that communicates data, showing trending over time and how a process is operating. There are various types of run charts, depending on what you are using the data for. A more formalized run chart is a control chart, which has horizontal lines defining the upper and lower limits of the process under scrutiny (George, 2003). For example, say you are making widgets, and the process has a limit to the amount it can make. Over this amount, there may be issues with the quality of the widgets. The process also has a lower limit. Below this, there is possibly something wrong in the process. You can also think of the process strictly as a machine that makes the widgets: too fast and it may be missing a step, too slow and maybe something is wearing out. Either way, you need to investigate the process or else you will have a poor quality or quantity of widgets. Now think of this in relation to nursing processes. It is a bit more difficult, but consider patient satisfaction as a process, something you are creating. It is not as tangible as a widget, but much more valuable. So your run chart displays the monthly patient satisfaction data, maybe the scores from the Hospital Consumer Assessment of Healthcare Providers and Systems (HCAHPS) survey and the Centers for Medicare and Medicaid (CMS) patient satisfaction survey that is publically reported and will eventually affect the way hospitals are paid by CMS. These scores are plotted and basically show how your patient satisfaction process is working. You might not think you have a distinct process, and maybe you do not. But think of the process as all the things you do to promote and deliver care that satisfies patients. Some statistical calculations could give you the standard deviation for the data. The standard deviation is basically a measure of how your data varies naturally within your process.

Rarely does patient satisfaction data stay exactly the same. There are so many variables affecting the data that a bit of variance is expected. It is not necessarily bad, but rather, is just part of the process. Sometimes institutions react to what they think is a drop in patient satisfaction scores that is truly just the variability inherent in their process. They immediately think their process is broken when it is not. If it is within the upper and lower limits you prescribe, then you know the process is working. The limits are somewhat subjective, depending on how varying you think your process is, and how much variability you can tolerate. It is typically based on a number of standard deviations from the mean.

There is one other line that is part of a run chart: the mean or median. The mean or median of the data is displayed as a horizontal line in the chart. This line can provide some important information without having to compute statistics. If a number of data points are consistently on one side of the mean (or median) line, there is statistically a shift or an improvement or deterioration in the process. You might have initiated a new patient satisfaction program and in keeping track of the data, you notice increases for a number of consecutive months after the initiative was implemented. What the run chart is showing you is that your new program is making a difference, causing higher patient satisfaction scores, something we would all like to see. If it keeps up, you would calculate and graph a new mean (or median) line on the chart and new upper and lower limits to control the new process and hopefully continue the improvements made in patient satisfaction scores. So, from a control chart you are able to tell if a process is operating properly, and if you have made a statistically significant difference in the process (good or bad). That is a lot of information from one chart, which is why it has become a popular method of displaying and disseminating data. It is part of the Six Sigma Program arsenal of tools. Unfortunately, most nurses are probably not able to read and understand a run chart in this depth. With some education however, the run chart could become the standard method of presenting and disseminating data for your institution.

Figure 5-2 displays a run chart that is likely the type you will use. The upper and lower limits are intentionally missing, but the mean or median line is present. It is difficult to say if anyone really needs upper and lower control limits for nursing processes. You may feel they are helpful. We believe their value does not outweigh the time and effort needed to teach what they are used for. We believe in the KISS (keep it simple stupid) principle. With that said, a run chart with the mean or median line plotted is sufficient. You might also want to plot the national benchmark on this chart for reference. Having the benchmark plotted provides more value than the upper and lower limits, and decreases the confusion when everything is plotted. And you do not necessarily need to use a computer chart. You can create a run chart by hand, however, it is a little tedious and is definitely not recommended if this is to be used institution-wide.

Steps to Make a Run Chart

- Assemble everything you need (graph paper, pencil, ruler, eraser, data).
- Draw x and y axes on the paper.
- Determine the range of values and the range on the y-axis. Label the y-axis.
- Determine time period for measurement. Label the x-axis.
- Plot the data points (Date [x], Score [y]).
- Connect the data points.
- Calculate the median or mean.

Figure 5-2 Example of a run chart.

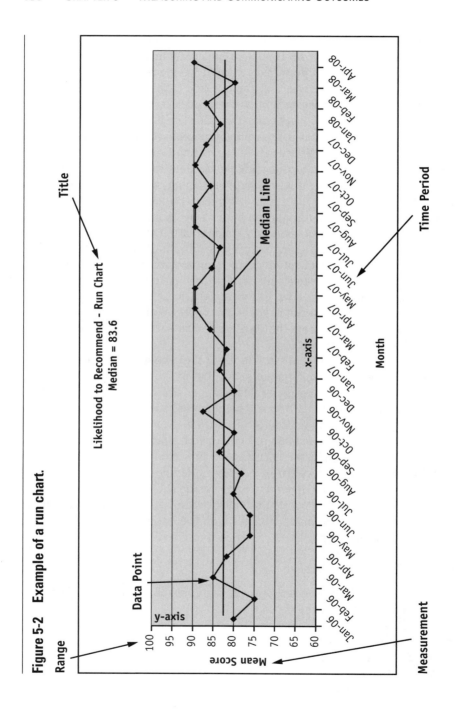

- Draw a horizontal line at the median or mean on the chart.
- Title the chart and put in source of the data.
- Label who created the chart and the date created/modified.

Hopefully you will create your chart electronically. We used Excel 2007, but there are programs that will create run charts automatically from the data you enter. If you are not comfortable with Excel, other programs might be beneficial. Even if you are creating run charts electronically, we suggest using the preceding algorithm to educate the audience of your run charts. We have presented educational sessions to staff nurses and nursing administrators, providing them with data and having them create a run chart using the algorithm provided. We believe it is a good way to utilize a hands-on approach to learning the parts of a run chart.

Should you use the mean or the median? We have looked at a number of sources, and determined the following guidelines based on both statistical and practical considerations.

- Use the **mean** for 10 or less data points.
- Use the **median** for 11 or more data points.
- If you are using the mean, when you get to 11 data points, switch to using the median.

The Pareto Chart

A Pareto chart is designed to look at the many causes of a specific problem and help you determine which causes, if rectified, would most take care of the problem. In other words, which causes should you spend time and resources addressing. The Pareto chart is based on the 80/20 principle, which posits, with respect to the situation, that 80% of the problem is caused by 20% of the causes. This rule is not exact, nor is it meant to be. It is meant to describe the phenomena seen in many situations: that there is a small portion of causes that account for a large amount of the variance. It is then logical, that if you fix the small portion of causes, you will have addressed much of the variance. The Pareto chart is a tool that you can use to look at your data and determine the things you might want to target with interventions to address these causes. As an example, we will consider catheter-associated urinary tract infections (CAUTI). Of course your goal is to have no CAUTIs, but some believe that is not achievable. Even so, let us say your rate is above the national benchmark. You delve into the causes and determine the percent of CAUTIs that each cause is responsible for. See Table 5-1 for an example of what this might look like in chart format.

Now it is not that difficult to determine from this chart, which causes to go after to make the biggest impact, but a Pareto chart makes this realization easier and helps to communicate this to others. If you have not used, sent, or received a

Table 5-1 CAUTI Causes Example Table

Cause	Percentage of CAUTI caused
Nonsterile insertion	6
In place too long	32
Poor catheter maintenance	26
Catheter too small	5
Catheter system sterility broken	7
Patient manipulating catheter	2
Catheter defective	1
Patient with undiagnosed UTI prior to catheter insertion	21

Pareto chart before, it takes a bit of education on how to interpret the data. Once educated, it is a valuable tool for improving processes and communicating data. The Pareto chart in Figure 5-3 is based on the previous CAUTI data.

Interpreting this chart is relatively straightforward. The bars represent the percentage of the CAUTIs caused by each distinct cause. The line adds these percentages to provide a cumulative percentage of CAUTIs caused by all the causes so far. So going by the 80/20 rule, we are looking for the causes that comprise roughly 80% of the CAUTIs. We can easily see from the Pareto chart in Figure 5-3 that three causes (in place too long, poor catheter maintenance, and patient with undiagnosed UTI prior) account for 79% of the CAUTIs. These are the causes you want to target. Forget the others for now. After these three main causes are resolved, collect further data on CAUTI causes and create another Pareto chart. You will most likely have lowered your CAUTI rate considerably and will find different reasons for the majority of CAUTIs. Use the 80/20 rule again and determine the CAUTI causes that account for about 80% of the CAUTIs. These are the next to be addressed. This cycle can go on continuously until, dare we say, you have no CAUTIs. While this sounds fairly simple, it is not. The most difficult part is addressing the causes of CAUTIs, of course. The Pareto chart does not tell you how to do this, it just tells you which problems, when resolved, will give you the most success for your effort. That in itself, we believe, is valuable information that can systematically guide your improvement efforts.

The Gantt Chart

Your run chart showed you there was a problem, or an opportunity for improvement. You delved deeper into the data and determined the causes of your problem.

Figure 5-3   Pareto chart example.

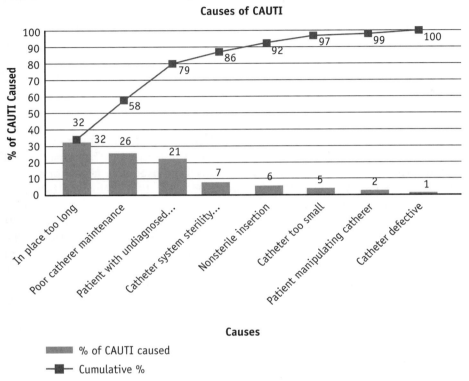

Causes of CAUTI

The Pareto chart helped you determine which causes you should address to make the largest impact. Now you have to address these causes. Of course you use the evidence-based practice process to find the best interventions to address these problems (see Chapter 6: Implementing Evidence-Based Practice). You have found the perfect intervention, one that is feasible and is transferrable to your population and your institution. So you go about developing an action plan to implement the intervention. Here is where the Gantt chart comes into play, to help you visually organize the activities necessary to implement your intervention. The Gantt chart is basically a timeline of events and actions necessary to reach your goal. The goal here is the implementation of a specific intervention, but it could be used for any project that requires multiple dependent and independent activities over a period of time. The Gantt chart is designed to visually display the activity timeline, but it also visually displays which activities could be done simultaneously, and which activities are dependent on an activity occurring prior to its initiation.

For example, if your intervention is to produce an educational pamphlet to address a patient need, before you can print and copy the pamphlet, you need to assemble and edit the contents. The activity of assembling and editing contents must come before printing. The Gantt chart would visually show this dependence. However, while you are assembling and editing the content, you could contact the printer and set up the general layout. So these activities could occur simultaneously. The Gantt chart would display this visually and help keep you on track to complete your activities and ultimately achieve your goal of implementing your intervention.

It is a great project management tool. But remember, as a tool it is there to help you. When a tool becomes an activity that is not adding value to you or to your process, it is no longer a tool, but rather a burden. It is then time to find another tool. The definition of a tool is "anything used as a means of accomplishing a task or purpose" ("Tool," n.d.). Once the tool becomes a task that must be done and is not used as a means to accomplish a task or purpose, it ceases to be a tool and becomes an activity done just for the sake of doing it. We see this happen often, mostly in the use of process improvement methods. The DMAIC (define, measure, analyze, improve, and control) methodology for process improvement and control can be a tool to help achieve your goals for a specific indicator. But when it just becomes a requirement that you have to write up a DMAIC process as a penalty for having a poor result or because of an untoward outcome, the DMAIC write up becomes a penalty, not a tool for improvement. That is when it is time to reevaluate the efficacy of your tool. Tools are meant to assist, not to become a way to penalize those who have had a poor outcome. Think of it as a hammer. A hammer helps you to place a nail in the wall. If the nail is already in the wall and you have to use the hammer as a requirement, then your pounding is meaningless. The nail is already there; using the hammer is just going through the motions and is a waste of time and effort.

Creating a Gantt chart is easy. You can do it electronically or you can use paper and pencil, whatever you prefer and whatever makes most sense. If you think the timeline will be tentative and might need to be updated frequently, you would be better off creating your Gantt chart electronically. This also allows you to e-mail updates to all the members in your group working on the project. Printing the updated Gantt chart and posting it will take little time. However, if you are more comfortable doing so, using a pencil and paper will work fine. Just think about how you will disperse updates. We utilize a Gantt chart in the creative solutions that accompany each chapter. Figure 5-4 shows the Gantt chart from the creative solution, "Don't Let Research Scare You!" in Chapter 7.

As you can see, the Gantt chart shows when each step should occur. It shows what has to be done, and when it is due. Steps 1 through 4 can be done simultaneously, while steps 5 through 7 need to be done afterward. Step 1 will take

1 month or less, while step 7 occurs over 3 months. The number of steps and the timeline should be determined by the entire group working on the project. Of course, nothing is written in stone, and you may need to adjust the chart if the number of steps or if the time necessary to complete the steps changes. We used Step 1, 2, and so forth, to denote which step of the process we are referring to. This is fine as long as everyone has the definition of what each step is. You may want to list the specific steps so that if any are added or eliminated, those receiving an updated chart do not get confused. You also must title and date the chart, when it was created or revised. In this way, when you or a recipient of the chart retrieves it, they can be assured that they have the most updated version. A Gantt chart is a great organization tool. Look at it frequently to make sure your project is on time and on target. The Gantt chart works best when it is paired with a corresponding action plan. The action plan is developed first, and then the Gantt chart is created. The action plan will guide the Gantt chart, providing the necessary steps and time frames necessary to complete the project. When you update your action plan, do not forget to update your Gantt chart.

Figure 5-4   Gantt chart example.

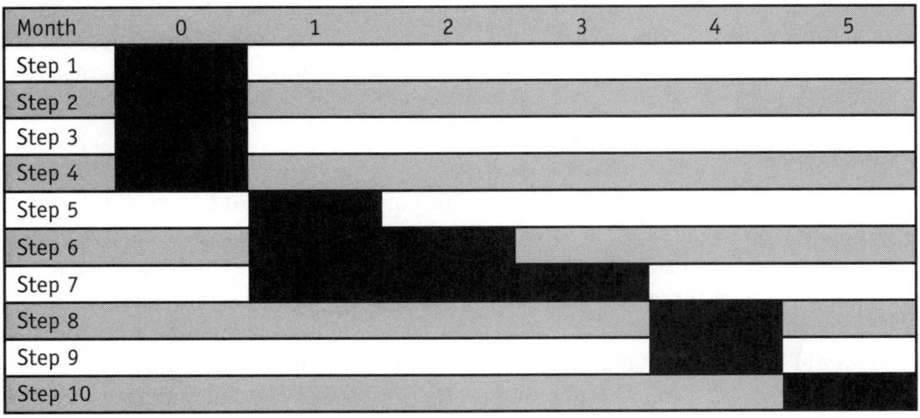

Month	0	1	2	3	4	5
Step 1						
Step 2						
Step 3						
Step 4						
Step 5						
Step 6						
Step 7						
Step 8						
Step 9						
Step 10						

Databases, Report Cards, and Dashboards

Databases

Databases are ongoing collections of data. Keeping a database is easy and allows you to go back and see trends in the data that might show things that are important when determining priorities. Of course, it is always better when someone already has a database established with the data you need. You might need to add to it or pull from it what you need, but if you are starting a brand new initiative looking at a brand new indicator, you might not have the data or database necessary to use, so you need to create a database. A program such as Excel is probably the best in which to create your database. Besides allowing you to sort and manipulate your data, it permits you to create charts from your data, which can help you communicate trends and show the progression of the initiatives addressing the indicator over time. Run charts, described earlier, are created from databases containing data on specific indicators. If you have not created a database before, we suggest familiarizing yourself with some of the databases already in use in your institution, specifically in the Performance Improvement (PI) department. PI people are experts in databases, possibly not in their creation, but definitely in their content. They can guide you on what data you should include and what you can leave out. Do not replicate what someone else already has. If PI already has a database of indicators by unit, there is no need for you to maintain your own. If you are not computer savvy and have never used Excel before, we suggest taking a noncredit course at the local community college. If you are computer savvy, but just not familiar with Excel, Microsoft offers online tutorials that will guide you through some basic Excel functions at http://office.microsoft.com/en-us/training/FX100565001033.aspx. For the self-learners, there are many instructional books on Excel's functions covering everything from creating charts to data analysis. Just look in your bookstore's computer section. You will be amazed at what you find.

Report Cards

What is the easiest and fastest way to communicate data to staff? We have found that report cards are a format that seems universally accepted and understood. We were all in school at one time and remember, some fondly and some not so fondly, what a report card is. We understand its purpose, and what it should tell us about how we are doing. The report card can be as simple or complex as you would like, but remember who the receiver of the report card is and their capacity to understand the document. Again, the KISS principle applies here. What we have found is that when people create these report cards, they try to include every indicator possible. This is a huge mistake. Data overload equals data apathy. If there is too much, staff will not be able to remember it all and to take it all in. Studies have been done on the short-term memory of people. It is said that people can hold up to seven items in their short-term memory. That is why a telephone number (without the area code) is the perfect length, seven digits. The point is, do not overload. No one can remember and focus on 20 indicators at once. So be strategic in creating your report card. Determine how many indicators you want your staff to focus on at one time. At one of the author's institutions, he developed a PI report card. With the input of staff and nursing leadership, it was decided that the report card should focus on four indicators, pulled from the strategic goals of the nursing department. Not everyone agreed that these were the most important indicators, just that improvement of these indicators fulfilled the strategic goals of the nursing department and the strategic goals of the institution as a whole. They had the most "bang for the buck" and were universal across the institution. Strategic value, universality across the institution, cost-effectiveness, nursing control, and data availability and integrity are all things to consider when choosing your indicators. In another institution, their report cards were structured to be unit-specific, deciding that tailoring the needs to the specific unit outweighed the benefits of universality. This institution employed outcomes managers, advanced practice nurses responsible for evaluating their unit's data and determining what indicators are in most need of attention. They acted as the data analysts for their units and, with the leadership team, helped to strategically develop action plans to address opportunities for improvement in the unit's indicators.

You can decide which indicators to use on your report cards based on your own criteria. If you decide to use unit-specific indicators, more often than not, these indicators will remain on the report card for 4 to 6 months, until the opportunity for improvement is realized and the improved results are stable. Then you can look for other indicators with opportunities for improvement. We are asked the question, "How long does it take to make a change in an indicator and know that the change will be maintained?" It is a great question with no simple answer. The fact is, you need to continue monitoring an indicator for a period of time after you have made a significant improvement. This is due to the Hawthorne Effect. The Hawthorne Effect is a phenomenon that asserts whatever is scrutinized will improve, strictly because it is the focus of attention. So if you are targeting an indicator with a specific intervention, expect improvement on that indicator strictly because you are focusing on that indicator. Once the indicator is no longer the focus of attention, expect compliance with the intervention to decrease. This is typical and should be anticipated and planned for. See the Creative Solution at the end of this chapter entitled, *The Unit-Based Report Card,* for an example of a report card that one of the authors created. This report card conveys an incredible amount of information to those who can read it. And that is the key: assuring everyone (your audience) can read the report card. The top section shows simply this month's number and last month's number for comparison. It also provides the benchmark/goal. So, to know how you are doing as a report card is supposed to tell, it takes very little time and data analysis ability. The red, yellow, and green code makes interpretation even that much quicker. You can easily see which indicators have the greatest opportunity for improvement, thus where you might want to focus your efforts. The charts are possibly the most important part of the report card. For each indicator, a chart shows 13 months of data, allowing you to compare this month of this year with the same month last year. The charts also show trending of the data, or possibly an indicator that is not controlled. We made the decision to use incidents as our data instead of a rate. As discussed previously, rates can be difficult to interpret for the data interpretation novice. What rates typically do is take into account the number of patient days, making comparisons more valid (i.e., comparing apples with apples). For example, if you have twice the number of patient days this month as you had last month, you would expect twice the number of patient falls or CAUTIs. Simply stating that there were three CAUTIs this month and two last month does not tell the whole story. In this instance, to account for the absence of patient days or catheter days in the incident data, we have charted the number of catheter days as separate data. This way, you can determine if your incidents are increasing with increasing patient days, or if there is no correlation. Looking at data trends can provide some important insights into interpreting the data and the expectations for the data. For instance, you might look at the trending for pneumonia data and find patterns that repeat each year. These fluctuations might be due to seasonal disease patterns and are not under internal control. The trends might also show you what to expect in the future to better prepare your resources, being proactive instead of reactive. Without noticing these trends, one might think an increase or decrease in an indicator might mean they need to take action. This is not always the case. It might also leave you scrambling to obtain resources, which you may have been able to prepare in advance.

Trending data is a powerful tool to better understand how an indicator reacts over time. Of course, to trend the data, you need to measure the data with an acceptable frequency. In measuring an indicator once a year, it might take you a decade to notice a trend. Also, you will not have the ability to notice seasonal trends or trends in patient populations. Measuring daily could have you spending all of your time on data collection. There needs to be a happy medium. You also need to be able to see if an intervention is working without waiting 6 months for the evaluation. So, how frequently should you collect data? Well, this question might be answered for you. Regulatory agencies typically have a schedule that you need to adopt. That is not to say you cannot collect data more frequently, just not less. For example, the National Database of Nursing Quality Indicators (NDNQI) requires member organizations to submit data quarterly on the presence of pressure ulcers in the members' patient population. Some institutions believe this is not frequent enough to get a good picture of how well nurses are preventing these wounds from occurring, so they might collect data monthly. The greater frequency allows a better look at trends, which can enable them to more rapidly tell if an intervention is working, or whether it should be scrapped and another intervention tried. Although monthly data collection requires more resources, if it aids in bettering patient care, it is worth it. If you are strictly using run charts to control your processes, more data points are better, although the benefits need to outweigh the costs of resources, so beware of too frequent data collection. Many times when data is collected frequently, there is only a small sample. Making decisions on a very small sample is not a good practice and can lead to false evaluations and poor decisions.

Dashboards

Dashboards are a great way to present a lot of data in a little space. They are meant to cover many indicators, but are not good at supplying trending information. Dashboards are a first step to determining where there may be an opportunity for improvement. Typically, dashboards are determined by both system and departmental goals. They are somewhat comprehensive and provide a snapshot of how you are doing for the month. They usually present your data in comparison with a benchmark and, possibly, a goal. They sometimes use the red, yellow, green scheme where red is worse than goal and benchmark, yellow is worse than goal but better than benchmark, and green is better than goal and benchmark. The red, yellow, green coding is a great visual method of alerting data recipients (e.g. unit managers) to the most urgent needs. It is familiar, using the stoplight colors that everyone can relate to. Red seems to always be the color of danger, and it can be used in report cards and dashboards effectively to show dangerously poor performance on a specific indicator. Many institutions have a policy/process where if an indicator is red, the manager or leadership team for that unit must create and submit an action plan designed to better the indicators that are in the red. Some wise institutions have linked money with metrics, making managers' raises dependent on satisfactory performance on specific indicators, or giving bonuses for achieving specific quality goals determined by the performance on strategically relevant indicators.

Get IT Involved

Data collection is not a fun job. One of our colleagues did a study of the number of computer systems used in her institution. Her institution consists of a relatively small community hospital with associated outpatient services. Surprisingly, she found that the institution had over 50 distinct computer systems, but few were compatible, so data was rarely transferred from one system to another. This created breaks in the continuity of patient care as well as user frustration and frustration for those attempting to extract meaningful performance data. It seems that when institutions purchase computer systems, many do it in a piecemeal fashion, looking for something that is specialty friendly, sacrificing interdepartmental integration. So, the emergency department has a computer system that meets their needs, and surgical services has a computer system that meets their needs, both from different vendors and not compatible. A physician order from the ER does not transfer over to the OR system, so the only way to tell what was ordered is to search through a paper printout or through the caregiver report. It is easy to imagine some of the time delays and work-arounds that occur to accommodate this lack of integration, and let us not forget the threats to patient safety. So, can you fix all of your computer problems yourself? No, of course not. What you can do is first determine where your data comes from. Determine how it is collected and by whom. Then, ask the crucial question, "Is this data what I need to make decisions about PI processes and patient outcomes?" If your data is incomplete or collected manually, you will want to involve the information technology (IT) department. The questions to ask are, "Can we automate the data collection that's now occurring manually?", and "Can we get the data I need from the current computer systems?"

Many institutions have a Nursing Informatics Coordinator, typically a registered nurse that specializes in electronic nursing data input, management, and retrieval. He or she is a liaison between the IT department and the nursing department, able to determine what data can be obtained electronically and how your electronic data systems can benefit process improvement and patient outcomes. If your institution has such a person, become his or her best friend. Trust us, it will be well worth your effort. What you have done so far is retrospective, looking at how you can obtain and automate the collection of data that you already have or should have. You now want to be proactive and involve IT prospectively.

When you form a workgroup to address an opportunity for improvement, think about including an IT representative from the start, or from a strategic point where their expertise can benefit the project. This way, they may be able to design a method of data collection or a database to compliment the project and the process under scrutiny. This is precisely what we did when we tackled the CAUTIs. We realized from the data that we definitely had an opportunity for improvement. We established a CAUTI task force to design, implement, and monitor interventions to decrease the occurrence of CAUTIs. The group included an IT representative from the start, since we were certain that data retrieval and collection would be issues, as well as contemplating possible IT interventions to address the CAUTI initiative. This person proved invaluable to our efforts, designing a strategy to assist in reminding physicians and nurses to reevaluate daily each patient's need for an indwelling urinary catheter. She was also able to retrieve data that was not previously collected, but was necessary to determine a baseline for our progressing efforts. You also want to ask if you or a nursing colleague in the PI department can possibly be included in IT projects and evaluations of electronic systems for purchase.

Data Collection—Regulatory vs Improvement

When readying data for presentation and dissemination, you must consider your audience. There are typically two groups for which data is collected: regulatory agencies, for whom reporting is mandatory (external), and hospital leadership and staff (internal), for whom reporting is informational and done to improve processes and performance. Regulatory data is presented in a standard format, determined by the specific regulatory agency. For example, patient falls data are reported to the CMS as a rate (#patient falls/#patient hospital days $\times$ 1000), or in layman's terms, the number of patient falls per 1000 inpatient hospital days. This rate is meant to take patient census into account and make the data usable for comparisons among institutions. However, when reporting internally, a patient fall rate of 2.37 may be meaningless, especially to data interpretation novices. Throughout this chapter, we stress the importance of tailoring your message to your audience. It seems from our experience that this is rarely done. What we have found more frequently is that whatever is presented to the external audience is passed along to the internal audience. Sure, it is quicker just to internally send out what you are sending externally, but you might be missing an opportunity. Internal recipients may not have the maturity and depth of knowledge in data analysis and interpretation necessary to glean more than a superficial impression of the external data (is it good or bad). You, as the sender, have the opportunity to create a data message that relates much more.

Perception vs Real Data

There are truly two different types of data that, once we discuss will seem common sense, yet many a nurse leader have made the mistake of forgetting to tailor the type of intervention to the type of data. Let us explain. The two types of data are perception-based or subjective data and reality-based or real data. Patient satisfaction and nurse satisfaction data are examples of subjective data (Boxer, in press). The data you see are based on the subjective opinions of those you survey. As we know from pain assessment, another form of subjective data, perception is reality to the person, so we consider a patient's report of pain as real data and our interventions try to alleviate the pain (through medication, visualization). But what about something not as cut and dry? Let us explore your nursing staff's opinion that your benefits package is not competitive with the healthcare market. Do you run and alert Human Resources and senior leadership beseeching them to increase the benefits package for staff? No. You realize this is subjective data and before you act on it, you need to investigate whether in fact your benefits package truly is not competitive, or if it is just their perception that it is not competitive. So you do a bit of research, collecting data on competitors' benefits packages. You find out that you actually have the best benefits package of all your competitors.

Now will your intervention be the same? Will you still run and alert HR and senior management, pleading for an increase in benefits? Of course not.

What you need to do is change the perception of your staff, not increase your benefits package. What you might do is create a flyer listing your benefits package adjacent to your competitor's benefits packages and distribute this to your entire staff. This will allow them to see that they are in fact receiving the best benefits package, probably changing their perception for the better, which is a lot less costly than an upgraded benefits package. So the lesson to be learned is, when analyzing and interpreting data, first note what type of data you are dealing with, whether subjective (perception) or objective (real). If it is real data, then you can continue your evaluation and intervene if necessary. If it is perception data, you need to first find out if it is real. If it is, continue your evaluation and address the issue. If it is not, you need to work to change perceptions. That is a different goal and might require a different intervention. This exercise could save you time, money, and sanity!

Cost/Benefit Analysis

A cost/benefit analysis is usually beneficial in evaluating an intervention and achieving buy-in from others, assuming the benefits of your intervention outweigh the costs. Here is a simple algorithm for performing a cost/benefit analysis using a 2 × 3 matrix chart. The first column is titled "Cost" and the second column is titled "Benefit." The first row is titled "Tangibles," the second row is titled "Intangibles," and the third row is titled "Unknown/Conditional."

Algorithm for Cost/Benefit Analysis

- Brainstorming: List all the costs and benefits related to the topic or project. List both tangibles and intangibles.
- Placement: Place each item in the cost/benefit matrix, according to whether it is a tangible, an intangible, or an unknown/conditional.
- Determine dollars: Working with just the tangible items, determine the value of each item in dollars for the costs section and the benefits section.
- Review intangibles: Brainstorm if there are related tangibles with dollar values for these items and determine the dollars for the related costs.
- Review unknown/conditional items: Attempt to determine conditions when each would be considered a cost or a benefit, and the associated probability of that occurring. Attempt to give value to these items. These will be part of the tangible item summary.
- Report out total savings or cost in dollars.
- Report out intangible costs with associated effects and intangible benefits with associated effects.

- Report out unknown items and possible costs/benefits and possible probabilities.
- Summarize results in prose.

STATISTICS

All right, get ready for a little statistics. We just want to give you as much as we think you will need to know here. As you become more data savvy, you will need to learn a bit more, and with each new technique, you learn that you will have more resources to use and better handle on your data. We stress here that it is preferable to learn techniques as the need arises, not the other way around. If you learn a new technique and have no real use for it, 9 times out of 10, the technique will fade from memory and will need to be relearned. What is of benefit is an awareness of the techniques that are available. Many times there is no need for a formal course of study to learn what techniques are out there. These can be self-learned through reading quality related publications and practice books on quality, noting what techniques were used, why they were used, and how they were applied. It is the purpose and the application of the techniques that really count. You can relearn a technique easily or use a reference for recall if you understand what the technique is used for and how to use it. For example, we cannot, off the top of our heads create the formula for a student's t test, yet we know its basic purpose is to determine statistically if there is a difference in the mean of the scores of two groups.

To apply the t test, we would possibly need a situation where we have two like groups, one that we have done something different to. We then may want to see if what we have done has made a significant difference in what we are trying to improve. For example, what if we decided we can improve patient satisfaction by giving patients gifts when discharged. (Do not try this, your ethics committee will scream.) So you give one group of patients gifts when discharged and another group of patients receive nothing. You want to determine if giving the gift has made a difference in your patient satisfaction scores, so you compare the scores of the two groups using a t test. If you find that you are making a difference, you would most probably give gifts to every patient. If not, you can stop the gifts and save your money. So the t test can be a powerful resource.

It is time to get down to what you need to know. We are going to discuss just four things: mean, median, mode, and standard deviation. If you already have a good understanding of what they are (their differences, purpose, and application), then you can skip this section without remorse. If, like many of us, you have not used these in a while, or you only know one or two of them, it would probably do you good to read on.

Descriptive Statistics

The mean is probably the most familiar and the most used. The mean is merely the average of a bunch of values. It might be scores on a test or the number of CAUTIs for all of the units in the hospital. The mean tells you what the average is for all the scores. The mean is known as a descriptive statistic, used to describe the middle of a group of values. The mean is most frequently used for benchmarking (see next section) to compare your value or score with the middle value or score.

The median is also a measure of the middle of a group of values or scores. So we bet you are asking, "Well isn't the median the same as the mean?" Unfortunately, the answer is no, not always. Without getting into a lot of stuff about normal distributions, we will just talk about what makes them different. The mean is an average; just add all your values up and divide by the number of values. The median, however, is different. The median is the value where half the scores fall above this number and half are below it. It is the 50th percentile. So when you have some scores that are extreme, either very high or very low, you see that one might be a better, more accurate measure of the middle of the data. Let us give an example. Suppose you want to find the middle value for the salary of a staff nurse. You list all nurses' salaries, add them up, and divide by the number of nurses. If you included the CNO, VPs of nursing, and directors, you might skew the data and your middle value would be falsely high, as the senior administrators typically receive higher salaries. What might provide a better picture of the middle value for staff nurses' salaries is to look at the value at the 50th percentile: the value where half the scores are greater and half the scores are less.

You might also want to look at the most frequent value or salary. The most frequent value is also a measure of the middle and, assuming there are more bedside nurses than administrators and that most bedside nurses are similarly compensated, this value might also provide some good information on the average staff nurse's salary. This value, the most frequent, is the mode. All three of these values taken together can provide a better picture of your data than just one. It will give you a better sense of what the true salary of a typical staff nurse is.

Next we are going to show you how standard deviation (SD) can be helpful. Basically, SD shows you how much variation you have in your data. It tells you if your data is basically consistent or if there are large differences between data points. For example, patients are surveyed and asked how satisfied they are with the nursing care on your unit. Scores can range from 0 to 100. For the second quarter, the mean score was 88, up from 84 the first quarter. The median and the mode were also both 88, so you feel pretty confident that you are progressing. Delving a little deeper into that data can provide you with greater insight. The SD will tell you if all your patients basically feel the same about the nursing care, or if some are more satisfied than others. A small SD means that individual patient satisfaction scores do not vary much from the mean. This tells you that most patients feel the same about the nursing care. This is what you want. It implies that your staff is providing a consistent level of care to all (or most) patients. But what if your SD was large? Then just the opposite would be true. It would tell you that your staff might not be providing a consistent patient care experience as your patients seem to feel differently about their patient experience.

BENCHMARKING

What is Benchmarking?

You have studied two weeks straight for your advanced calculus exam. You ate, slept, and dreamt calculus. You have not left your house or answered your phone, or checked e-mail. You know it. After the test, you feel pretty good. It was challenging no doubt, but still you think you answered all of the questions correctly, some not completely though. A week goes by and grades are finally in. You hesitate to look. Your heart sinks into your stomach as you see the score: 79. You are thinking, "It can't be. I studied hard. I know this stuff." Now, why are you upset? You are probably upset because you are thinking you should have gotten a higher score. But what if I told you that the highest grade in the class was an 81? Would you feel differently? What has changed? What has changed is the benchmark. When you received your grade of 79, you were judging it against a scale of 0 to 100, where 90 to 100 is typically an A. Your benchmark was 90 to 100. With the additional knowledge that the highest grade in the class was an 81, your benchmark has changed, and with it, the evaluation of your test performance has also changed. This is the power of a benchmark. We all use benchmarks throughout our days to evaluate what we do and how well we do it. It is just not something we are conscious of. But the concept for a benchmark is the same, whether it is judging a score on a test or evaluating your unit's patient satisfaction scores or even evaluating how well you baked the cake as you use the picture in the recipe book as your benchmark.

> Benchmarking is more formally defined as the process of identifying, understanding, and adapting outstanding practices and processes from organizations anywhere in the world to help your organization improve its performance. (American Productivity & Quality Center, 2008, para. 3)

Why Do We Benchmark?

Our main reason for benchmarking is to evaluate how well we are doing. Now that does not necessarily mean that the benchmark must be our goal. They are conceptually different things, but in practice, they might be one and the same. Goals are expectations for a level of achievement. The goal also aids in evaluation, just not in the same way as benchmarks do. Goals can be based on benchmarks, or on leadership's expectation, on regulatory agencies mandates, or on your own desires. A goal is something to shoot for, something to motivate, something to strive for. A benchmark, on the other hand, is usually an average of other like data from many sources. For example, benchmarks for patient satisfaction are typically values compiled from a national database of like institutions. Many times these benchmarks are the mean or median of the scores of all the hospitals in the database. If it is a national database with many institutions, you get a better idea for how you are doing in comparison.

Just remember, on many of these databases, the benchmark is the average or the 50th percentile. If you meet the benchmark, it means you are average. That may not really be something to celebrate, unless of course, average is what you are striving for. However, being average in comparison to a database of Magnet-designated hospitals is no small feat and definitely something to celebrate. So, understanding the composition of the database is essential in evaluating your benchmark and evaluating your own performance. When you benchmark, it is best to use data from a national database of hospitals with similar demographics for comparisons with like size, area, population served, etc. A database of unlike institutions is like comparing apples and oranges.

How Do You Benchmark?

For the uninitiated, benchmarking is frequently done through companies with large national databases such as NDNQI. Participating in and using this database requires a financial outlay as well as instituting specific data collection and submission processes. Benchmarking can also be done through regulatory agencies that might establish a minimum acceptable value for specific indicators or, like the CMS, establish their own national database for specific indicators such as patient satisfaction and compliance with the core measures. How and who you benchmark against are really indicator dependent, so first determine which indicators you want to benchmark. We advise you to first find out if there are regulatory required values and start with using these as benchmarks. As you excel, you want to begin benchmarking against other similar institutions and, ultimately, you might want to use a database of Magnet-designated hospitals, to strive for true nursing excellence.

What Do You Benchmark?

Theoretically, you can benchmark anything you collect data on. Practically and typically, institutions benchmark nurse-sensitive indicators, patient satisfaction regulatory indicators, and department/specialty specific indicators like c-section rates for OB/GYN and for left-without-treatment rates for emergency departments. Nurse-sensitive indicators are indicators that demonstrate the quality of nursing care. Some are obvious, some are more subtle. When you look at the list of all the indicators you are monitoring, it is best to determine which are nurse-sensitive and which are more informational, the ones staff need to know, but really have little control over. That is basically how you determine which indicators are nurse-sensitive and which are not. The obvious nurse-sensitive indicators are nosocomial pressure ulcers and patient falls, which good nursing care can, in most cases, prevent. Nurse-sensitivity is a concept that employs a continuum from totally nurse-sensitive (totally under nursing's control) to not nurse-sensitive (not influenced by nursing). Judging which indicators are nurse-sensitive should take this continuum into consideration.

Indicators, like ventilator-associated pneumonia and CAUTIs, are less controlled by nursing care, the former needing a physician's intervention and order and a respiratory therapist's care, the latter also needing a physician's order. Then there are indicators like c-section rates and percentage of correct antibiotics ordered, of which nursing has little or no control. So again, the paradigms of a continuum are most appropriate for describing what is and is not a nurse-sensitive indicator with a graduated scale based on the amount of control nursing care has over the indicator or how much the indicator is dependent on nursing care and intervention. An indicator might be more nurse-sensitive in one institution than another. For instance, if an institution has a physician-sanctioned nursing protocol giving nurses control over removing urinary catheters when certain criteria are met, then CAUTIs shown to be related to the length of time the urinary catheter is indwelling then becomes more controlled by nursing decision and care, and thus, more of a nurse-sensitive indicator. Knowing which indicators are nurse-sensitive helps you to determine which indicators to benchmark and which indicators nursing can improve independently. It makes little sense to initiate nursing interventions to improve indicators that are not nurse-sensitive. Not that nursing cannot have an impact, it is just that they cannot greatly impact the indicator alone. It takes a multidisciplinary effort to truly achieve results.

How Often Should You Benchmark?

This is dependent on the indicator and the database that you use. Some institutions use an annual benchmark. This may be out of necessity more than anything else. It is quite time consuming and resource intensive to compile national benchmarks, and the more frequently the data is collated and benchmarks are produced, the more costly it becomes. When you look at the frequency of benchmarking, it is important to note the turnaround time from submission to the database to retrieval of a benchmark. When trying to improve an indicator, timeliness of data and comparison data is important. If it takes 3 months after data submission to retrieve a benchmark, the comparison you now have is old. If there was an opportunity for improvement, you are now 3 months late. And if you have put an intervention in place to better a specific indicator, it is not helpful to wait three months to see if you have made a difference.

What Are the Steps to Benchmarking?

1. Determine what you want to benchmark, things that will benefit most from the benchmarking process, based upon the importance, cost, and potential of change.
2. Identify the things you need to measure. What data do you need to collect?
3. Select whom you want to benchmark against: internal, external, or standard goal.
4. Obtain data from whom you want to benchmark against.
5. Measure your own performance for each variable and begin comparing the results in an apples-to-apples format to determine the gap between your firm and the best-in-class examples.
6. Look at those who are doing better than you and find out how they are doing it. Determine if these practices will work for you. If not, look at other best practices.
7. Implement these best practices by setting specific goals and deadlines, and by developing a monitoring process to review and update the program over time.
8. Monitor these best practices for improvement, and continue to benchmark.

DATA ANALYSIS

So now you have got some data and it is time to make some conclusions about what is going on. Data analysis is both a science and an art. The science of data analysis is easy: It is interpreting the data in light of the type of data and the comparisons used. The art of data analysis is a bit different: It is understanding the data well enough to know what is missing or what is superfluous. It is asking the questions about how we can get data that digs deeper, answering questions that are garnered from what you have got, but just do not go far enough. It is easier to determine how you are doing than why it is happening. To truly know what data you need, you need to know the questions to ask. The questions to ask for insight are the standard questions: who, what, where, why, when, how, and how many. You do not necessarily need to ask them all, just the ones that relate to your suppositions. Are there more patient falls around toileting issues than other issues? Are there more pressure ulcers in those with a specific diagnosis? When do most medication errors occur? These questions dig deeper than merely knowing that you have an amount of medication errors that is above the benchmark. The algorithm is for analyzing the data on the more superficial level, asking the question, "How are we doing?" This in itself is important. You need to first know if you have a problem. Then you can ask the questions and hopefully obtain the data to find out why.

Algorithm for Analyzing Data

- Look at the categories and the scale used.
- Look at the units of the numbers and how the numbers were calculated (if applicable).
- Look at the sample size.
- Look at what the sample is and how data was collected.
- Look at who you are benchmarked against.

There are two ways to interpret data. One is an absolute interpretation, where you determine how you are doing with respect to the scale used. For example, say you received a score of 93 points on your paper. Is that good? Well it is if the scale goes from 0 to 100. It is not if scores can range from 0 to 200. The second way to interpret data is to look at your data with respect to others. So, you received a score of 93 out of a possible 200 points. You are probably disappointed until you find out that the highest score received was 95. This is relative data interpretation or benchmarking as discussed previously.

DATA INTERPRETATION

- Absolute interpretation: Interpretation with respect to the scale used.
- Relative interpretation: Interpretation with respect to the benchmarking data, taking into account the sample size and method of data calculation/ collection.

CORRELATION VS CAUSATION

Causation is proving that one thing is the reason why another thing occurs. Heavy alcohol drinking causes liver damage. Shaking a baby violently causes brain damage. Talking on a cell phone while driving *causes* accidents? Working overtime *causes* medical errors? Some things can be proven beyond a shadow of a doubt; some attempts at proof leave much doubt. Austin Bradford Hill was a British medical statistician who developed nine criteria for causation. They are: temporal relationship, strength of relationship, a dose–response relationship present, consistency in the association of the two events, plausibility, consideration of alternate explanations, ability to be altered through experimentation, specificity of the relationship, and compatibility with existing theory and knowledge (Abruzzi, n.d.). For our purposes, causation can be assumed if three general criteria are met. The first is that the event causing the outcome must precede (come before) the outcome. This is straightforward enough. Talking on a cell phone after the accident cannot cause the accident. The second is that the event and the outcome must be related.

Talking on a cell phone and car accidents must be related (statistically). The third is the hard one. There must be no alternative cause for the relationship.

Wow! We have discussed a lot in this chapter. You are probably in information overload right now, so we suggest an evidence-based method of relaxing while you contemplate all of the chapter's concepts and how they apply to your quest for Magnet designation or quality improvement: Chocolate. Jennifer Copely reports in an online article that,

> [t]here are some indications that chocolate can also induce relaxation. Small amounts of the amino acid tryptophan may decrease anxiety by increasing serotonin levels. A release of endorphins in response to chocolate consumption may reduce the body's sensitivity to pain as well. (2008)

So go ahead, indulge. Then you can start on the next chapter!

CREATIVE SOLUTIONS

Creative Solution Title: *The Unit-Based Report Card*

Creative Solution Author: Bruce Alan Boxer, PhD, MBA, RN, CPHQ
Director of Quality/Magnet Program Director
South Jersey Healthcare, Vineland, NJ
Former Evidence-Based Practice Coordinator
Frankford Hospitals, Philadelphia, PA

Purpose: The goal of this project is to provide direct-care nursing staff with a focused, simplified method for obtaining timely, benchmarked data on their unit's nurse-sensitive indicators.

Legend

Overall Rating: **ADVANCED BEGINNER - COMPETENT**

Financial:

Time:

Personnel:

Other Resources:

Efficacy: **A**

Transferability: **B**

Malleability/Adaptability: **B**

Ease of Implementation: **C-D**

Synopsis: A unit-based report card was developed to address common problems in data dissemination to direct-care staff: the complexity of the data, the lack of standardization of the format for data dissemination, timeliness of the data, and the data analysis and interpretation skills of direct-care nurses. The report card standardizes the format for data dissemination to direct-care nurses throughout the institution, as well as simplifies the data, allowing for easier interpretation and analysis.

Description of Organization: Aria Health (formerly Frankford Hospitals) is the largest healthcare provider in Northeast Philadelphia and Lower Bucks County. Aria consists of three inpatient facilities and two outpatient sites. The system has 477 licensed beds and employs nearly 4000 workers with a medical staff membership of 800. They are currently not a Magnet-designated facility. They are not directly affiliated with a university, but have a diploma-granting nursing school.

The Case Study: Aria Health has a mature shared governance structure with a PI council dedicated to improving patient care and the work environment. Through council meetings and staff input, issues came to light regarding the need for unit-based, nurse-sensitive indicator data accessible to the staff on each unit, which was also easy to understand and able to be rapidly interpreted. Members of the council and the council's administrative liaison completed a literature search for best practices. The most transferrable practice was the use of a standardized data dashboard. A dashboard was currently used for hospital leadership, but was too cumbersome for staff and was missing some of the elements necessary to accurately interpret the data. The evidence-based practice coordinator worked with the PI coordinators and the nursing project manager to develop the unit-based report card. The report card format was adopted mainly because of its familiarity; nearly everyone has experience with school report cards, and their purpose is to tell you how you are doing, the same for the unit-based report card.

The report card attempts to eliminate some of the issues voiced by the staff. The first issue was the lack of standardization. Data was presented in various formats by different departments (Infection Control, Performance Improvement, Patient Satisfaction, etc.). The format of the report card is the same for each unit; only the data and indicators might be different. This format also helped to congeal the data, because staff previously stated that data was all over the place.

Many staff members were not well versed in analyzing data and wanted a tool that was easily interpretable. Through the literature review and networking with other institutions, the leaders in the development of the report card determined the data elements the report card should contain. They determined three elements essential for proper data analysis: timely data on specific indicators, benchmark/comparison/goal data, and trending data. In the report card, data is presented in two different ways. Indicator data is placed in a chart showing current data, comparison data, and whether the change (if any) was positive or negative. Accompanying this chart are 13-month trending graphs for each indicator, to show the indicator's trend over the most recent year and comparison to the same month last year. The program utilized was Excel 2002, as the report card developers were relatively well versed in this program. Macros were utilized to make data entry easier and faster.

Green, yellow, and red colors are used to convey, in a glance, how the unit is performing on each specific indicator in relation to comparison data. This helps to make the data easy to interpret for staff. The report card is limited to the four most important indicators, determined by the organization's strategic goals, staff input, applicability to the unit's specialty, and opportunities for improvement. These indicators may be changed as needs change. For example, if sustained improvement is made in a specific indicator, it would be retired from the report card while another indicator with a more pressing opportunity for improvement takes its place. The report card is also limited to one page for consistency and streamlining. That is not to say staff do not continue to receive data in various formats from various departments. This is seen as more supplementary data, accessible to all but not necessarily utilized by all. Instead of using rates in much of the trending data, staff wanted incidence data and patient days, catheter days, or whatever determined the rate overlaid as a distinct graph line. The incidence data was more meaningful and the relationship between incidence and number of days could easily be seen.

Data retrieval was coordinated among the various persons responsible for collating raw data into usable metrics. Support was obtained from those coordinating specific indicator data. A monthly timeline was established so that the persons responsible for the indicator data would send the data in a timely manner to the individual coordinating the report cards. The person coordinating the report cards was then able to produce and disseminate the report cards the same time each month. This was necessary to maintain staff and leadership buy-in, as the timeliness of data was one of the issues prior to the report card, and one that the report card sought to resolve.

The report card format was brought to leadership and staff for input and approval. The report card was rolled out with much fanfare and was distributed at shared governance council meetings. The difficulty in the unit-based report card came when the administration of the cards' contents was assigned to an administrative assistant with limited knowledge of Excel 2002, limited understanding of nurse-sensitive indicators, and limited data analysis and interpretation skills. The integrity of the report card was jeopardized as information was incorrectly placed and charts were missing data. It is crucial that one person, well versed in the report card format, in the program used to produce it, and in data analysis/

interpretation, is coordinating and reviewing the report cards before they are disseminated to assure that data is accurate and complete.

Outcome Measures:

Formative/Compliance: The report card was complete by the date projected 90% of the time in the first year. Compliance with meeting the data deadlines for those with the indicator data ranged from 70 to 100%.

Summative/Outcome: Report cards were accurate and complete 95% of the time, measured through issues with the report card reported by the unit's leadership to the report card's coordinator. Anecdotally, staff at shared governance council meetings voiced satisfaction with the report cards. Leadership also anecdotally voiced satisfaction at management meetings, stating that they are utilized extensively in quality improvement initiatives.

Evidence Supporting this Creative Solution: The use of the report card for data transmission is ubiquitous in the healthcare and business literature. There was little literature found on the efficacy of utilizing report cards. Lancaster and King (1999) discuss the use of a spider diagram to describe an innovative nurse-sensitive indicator format. Hall et al. (2003) describe the use of the balanced scorecard approach to create a nursing performance report card. Although a bit tangential, Castle (2009) found that "most consumers who used the Internet to look for a nursing home also used a report card . . . [y]et relatively few consumers primarily used report cards for the arguably more important step of comparing quality information" (p. 316).

Your collection, evaluation, and publication of report card efficacy data—how units are using the report card, which are using it as informational, and which are using it as a tool for improvement—could add to the body of literature supporting or cautioning the use of nursing report cards.

Castle, N. G. (2009). Consumers' use of Internet-based nursing home report cards. *The Joint Commission Journal of Quality and Patient Safety, 35*(6), 316–323.

Hall, L. M., Doran, D., Laschinger, H. S., Mallette, C., Pedersen, C., & O'Brien-Pallas, L. L. (2003). A balanced scorecard approach for nursing report card development. *Outcomes Management, 7*(1), 17–22.

Lancaster, D. R., & King, A. (1999). The spider diagram nursing quality report card: Bringing all the pieces together. *Journal of Nursing Administration, 29*(7/8), 43–48.

Recipe for: *The Unit-Based Report Card (Figure 5-5)*

Ingredients:

CNO/Director support

Leadership support

Figure 5-5   Unit-based report card example (colors omitted).

Unit Report Card for December 2009

Indicator	Last Month	This Month	Benchmark/Goal
# Patient Falls	3	7 [RED]	2
# Catheter Associate UTIs	2	1 [GREEN]	1
# Central Line Infections	1	0 [GREEN]	0
# Nosocomial Pressure Ulcers	4	3 [YELLOW]	2
# Patient Days	436	622	

[RED] Worse than last month
[YELLOW] Better than last month,
    Worse than benchmark/goal
[GREEN] Better than or equal to
    benchmark/goal

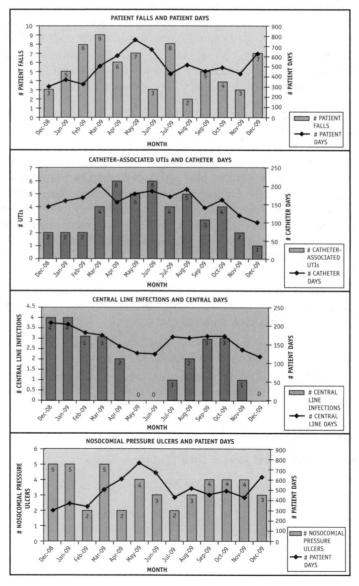

Support of stakeholders (those collecting and coordinating indicator data)

Staff buy-in

Skills to create report card, search literature, analyze, and interpret nurse-sensitive indicator data

Program to create report cards

Person to coordinate/produce report cards

Timely process to obtain data from persons collecting and collating indicator data

Timely process to disseminate report cards

Timely process to collect and disseminate formative and summative data to evaluate report card initiative

Process and people to roll out and educate staff and leadership on the report card and its use

Step-by-Step Instructions (see Figure 5-6 for Step-by-Step Instruction Timeline):

Step 1: Obtain support from CNO/Director, leadership, and staff.

Step 2: Determine needs of staff and leadership related to nurse-sensitive indicator data. Find a program to produce the report card that can incorporate the needs identified.

Step 3: Determine who will create the report card, who will coordinate it, who will disseminate it, and who will evaluate it.

Step 4: Design the following processes with stakeholder input: the process to obtain data from persons collecting and collating indicator data, the process to disseminate report cards, the process and people to roll out and educate staff and leadership on the report card and its use, and the process to collect and disseminate formative and summative data to evaluate report card initiative.

Step 5: Design the report card. Seek staff, leadership, and stakeholder input and approval.

Step 6: Establish a rollout timeline and educate prior to disseminating the first report card. Vigorously promote the report card, its benefits, and its uses. Begin producing the report cards.

Step 7: Roll out first report card and obtain feedback in various venues. Begin collecting formative and summative evaluation data. Tweak processes as necessary.

Step 8: Continue producing report cards and collecting formative and summative evaluation data.

Step 9: Collate and disseminate formative and summative evaluation data to stakeholders after 6 months of data is collected to maintain buy-in and evaluate efficacy.

Figure 5-6   Timeline for "The Unit-Based Report Card."

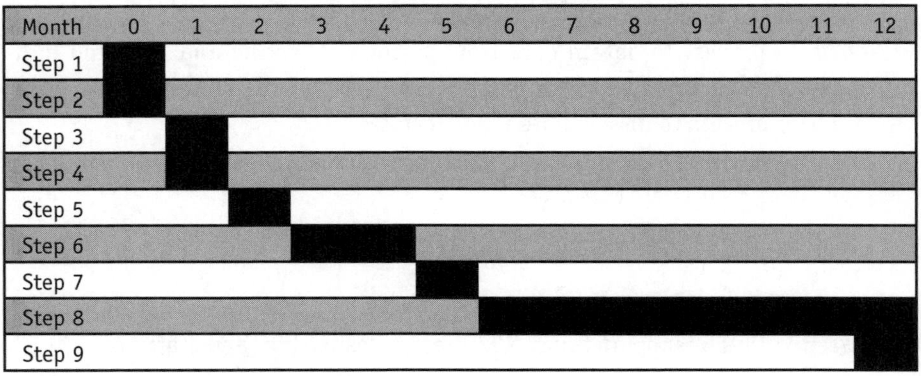

Month	0	1	2	3	4	5	6	7	8	9	10	11	12
Step 1													
Step 2													
Step 3													
Step 4													
Step 5													
Step 6													
Step 7													
Step 8													
Step 9													

Additional Outcomes to Consider Measuring:

Formative/Compliance: Consider formally evaluating the efficacy of the education provided to staff and leadership on how to read the report card.

Summative/Outcome: You might want to formally survey staff and leadership to evaluate satisfaction with and usability of the report card. Also, consider compiling how units are using the report card, which are using it as informational, and which are using it as a tool for improvement.

Insights from Original Implementation:

- You might want to search for a specific program to create the report card. It is doable in Excel, but is time consuming to create, produce, and maintain.
- Indicators need to be unit specific, yet meaningful to the institution as a whole. Focus on indicators that direct-care staff can improve, and ones that they have some control over.
- Buy-in from those who collect and collate the specific indicator data is essential.

For Further Guidance Contact:

Bruce Alan Boxer, PhD, MBA, RN, CPHQ
boxerb@sjhs.com

Creative Solution Title: *QUIFLE*

Creative Solution Author: Bruce Alan Boxer, PhD, MBA, RN, CPHQ
Director of Quality/Magnet Program Director
South Jersey Healthcare, Vineland, NJ
Idea Originated By: Interdisciplinary Patient
    Education Council
South Jersey Healthcare, Vineland, NJ

Purpose: The goal of this project is to quantify the impact of an educational poster display utilizing a nonthreatening methodology.

Legend

Overall Rating: **NOVICE**

Financial:

Time:

Personnel:

Other Resources:

Efficacy: **A**

Transferability: **A**

Malleability/Adaptability: **A**

Ease of Implementation: **A**

Synopsis: The QUIFLE is part quiz and part raffle. The idea was an attempt to measure the impact of an educational poster presentation utilizing a quiz format that, when complete, became an entry into a raffle for prizes valued in the $10 to $25 range. The QUIFLE asks questions that can only be found by viewing the educational posters. Outcomes measured are: the number of completed QUIFLEs and the number of correctly completed QUIFLEs.

Description of Organization: South Jersey Healthcare (SJH) is a Magnet-designated, multiple-hospital system. The health system encompasses two full service inpatient hospitals consisting of approximately 350 inpatient beds, comprehensive health centers, and outpatient and specialized services such as a Bariatric Center of Excellence, Wound Care Center, Sleep Center, and Balance Center. In 2008, SJH performed over 18,700 surgeries and the emergency department visits topped 97,400. The health system also serves as clinical site for nursing students from a number of local colleges and maintains a professional relationship with Cumberland County College, which is adjacent to the Regional Medical Center (RMC) campus. Also within the system is an inpatient and outpatient behavioral health facility.

The Case Study: At SJH it is common to use educational poster displays to relate information and data to staff. The poster creators typically used sign-in sheets to quantify the impact of the poster displays. However, as many of these displays went unmanned for periods of time, the validity of the sign-in sheet became questionable. It was observed that some would sign in and very quickly peruse the display whereas others would read each poster and never sign in. Contact hours are not given for these poster displays, so there was little incentive to spend time at each poster.

During Health Education Week 2009, the Interdisciplinary Patient Education Council, part of the shared governance structure at SJH, wanted to celebrate and increase awareness through a poster display focused on patient/family health education initiatives happening within SJH. A brainstorming session lead by the administrative liaison to this council, Eileen Niedzialek, RN, BSN, CDE, had the idea to create a brief quiz with questions based on each of the posters in the display. The questions were simple knowledge questions. Answers were found by reading each poster. The completed quiz was then entered into a raffle for a number of desirable gift baskets on display. Entries were picked randomly and if the answers were all correct, the person submitting won a gift basket. It was a surprising success. The announcement of the winners was eagerly awaited by staff. Not only did it help to quantify the impact of the poster display, it helped to achieve an awareness and excitement about the display and the event itself, Health Education Week. It also helped to coerce individuals to read each poster until they found the information necessary to complete the quiz.

A similar process was used during Quality Day, a celebration of the annual achievements in quality made by the dedicated SJH staff, sponsored by the Quality Council, which is part of SJH's shared governance structure. A poster display demonstrated many of the quality initiatives currently underway and the data demonstrating their effects. The administrative liaison had the idea to utilize the quiz and raffle process to entice staff to read the posters and become engaged with the celebration. He coined the term QUIFLE, and again it was a huge success. Three gift cards were raffled off amidst much excitement.

Outcome Measures:

Formative/Compliance: Nearly all submitted quizzes for the Health Education Week and Quality Day poster presentations were complete.

Summative/Outcome: Many staff submitted quizzes for Health Education Week. Because the display was open to all staff for an entire week, a percentage of staff submitting was not calculated. For quality day, there was a captive audience. Over 90% of those attending the event submitted QUIFLEs.

Evidence Supporting this Creative Solution: The QUIFLE is based on the same evaluative procedure used by many nursing organizations to provide continuing education credits used for state relicensure (where required) and recertification for national certifications. Incentives for learning and for the performance of specific behaviors (in this case, the completion of the QUIFLE), are also widely used in fields from education (e.g., classroom token systems) to health care (e.g., smoking cessation and weight loss programs).

Recipe for: *QUIFLE*

Ingredients:

Leadership support

Educational poster display

Person to create QUIFLE and answer key from posters

Person to coordinate initiative

Prizes

Box for submission of completed QUIFLEs

Computer, printer, copier, paper, pencils

Step-by-Step Instructions (see Figure 5-7 for Step-by-Step Instruction Timeline):

Step 1: Start with an educational poster display. This could be posters you create or posters others have created for a unified display.

Step 2: Create questions based on the educational posters. A rule of thumb might be to create one question for each poster. Do not make the question too obvious. Encourage participants to read through the poster to find the necessary information. Make sure you include a section for their name and possibly their unit. Make sure to also include on the form directions for completing the QUIFLE as well as information for how and when winners will be chosen, just in case some have not heard your instruction.

Step 3: Make copies of the QUIFLE and obtain the prizes.

Step 4: Vigorously promote the QUIFLE, the rules/instructions, the prizes offered, and when the winners will be announced. Make sure the prizes are tempting and desirable to most of your target population.

Step 5: Create a submission box for the completed QUIFLEs.

Step 6: Display posters with QUIFLEs and pencils for completion. Have submission box prominently displayed.

Step 7: Collect submitted QUIFLEs and randomly select one. If it is complete and correct, it is a winner. Do the same until you have exhausted your prizes. Count how many QUIFLEs were submitted, how many completed, and how many correct. If you have a defined target audience, you should calculate the percentage of the group who submitted. Of those who submitted, calculate the percent complete and the percent correct. This data could be trended to evaluate future educational poster displays. Disseminate data to all those involved in the initiative.

Figure 5-7   Timeline for "QUIFLE."

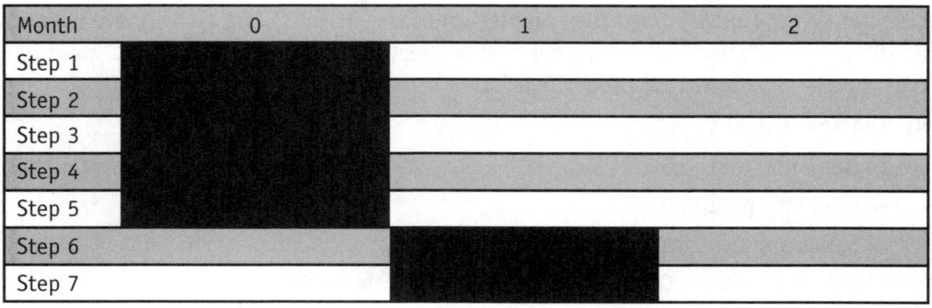

Month	0	1	2
Step 1			
Step 2			
Step 3			
Step 4			
Step 5			
Step 6			
Step 7			

Additional Outcomes to Consider Measuring:

Formative/Compliance: No additional measures.

Summative/Outcome: Formal survey of involved staff for satisfaction with the QUIFLE and the QUIFLE process.

Insights from Original Implementation:

- You could ask higher level educational questions (Bloom's taxonomy) related to material in the poster display.
- If you have a defined target audience, you may want to survey them for satisfaction with the QUIFLE and the QUIFLE process.
- Talk it up! Excite others. Make it fun.

For Further Guidance Contact:

Bruce Alan Boxer, PhD, MBA, RN, CPHQ
boxerb@sjhs.com

REFERENCES

Abruzzi, W. S. (n.d.). *Hill's criteria of causation*. Available at: http://www.drabruzzi.com/hills_criteria_of_causation.htm. Accessed December 28, 2009.

American Productivity & Quality Center (2008). *Glossary of benchmarking terms*. Available at: http://www.apqc.org/portal/apqc/ksn/Glossary%20of%20Benchmarking%20Terms.pdf?paf_gear_id=contentgearhome&paf_dm=full&pageselect=contentitem&docid=119519. Accessed December 28, 2009.

Boxer, B. A. (in press). Things are not always what they seem! A perception-based data analysis tool for nurse managers. *Nursing Management*.

Copely, J. (2008, March 5). *Health benefits of chocolate: Flavonoids help prevent heart attacks and stroke.* Available at: http://food-facts.suite101.com/article.cfm/chocolate. Accessed November 24, 2009.

George, M. L. (2003). *Lean six sigma for service.* New York: McGraw Hill.

Huff, D. (1954). *How to lie with statistics.* New York: W. W. Norton & Company.

Riding, R. J., & Rayner, S. G. (Eds). (2000). *International perspectives on individual differences.* Stamford, CT: Ablex Publishing Corporation.

Smith, J. (2008). *Parts of a chart.* Available at: http://www.jegsworks.com/Lessons/numbers/format/formatchart.htm. Accessed August 8, 2009.

Tool. (n.d.). In *Dictionary.com unabridged* (Vol, 1.1). Available at: http://dictionary.reference.com/browse/tool. Accessed August 25, 2009.

## CHAPTER 6

Implementing
Evidence-Based Practice

"One thing is sure. We have to do something.
We have to do the best we know how at the moment . . .
If it doesn't turn out right, we can modify it as we go along."
—FRANKLIN D. ROOSEVELT

"The most serious mistakes are not being made as a result of wrong answers.
The truly dangerous thing is asking the wrong questions."
—PETER DRUCKER

Okay, we are a bit biased. We admit it. One of the authors of this volume, along with a colleague, developed a program to disseminate evidence-based practice (EBP) that we think is the cat's meow. In more scientific terms, we think it is an exemplar creative solution, and not just because it is a creative solution that many can implement, but because in that specific environment with those specific supplies available, it was a truly creative use of resources to meet the institution's needs. The idea was born at a hospital located in Northeast Philadelphia, PA. The hospital was applying for Magnet designation and needed a structured way to disseminate EBP within the nursing department. At that time, the author was the Evidence-Based Practice Coordinator, a title that was newly created, with an open job description. Basically, it is one of those create-as-you go jobs, not prescriptive except for a few overall goals. After a gap analysis, the author/coordinator realized what was needed was an infrastructure to support the EBP process. There were pockets of the process happening, mostly at the clinical policy level, but the practice was sporadic and in no way systematic. There was no standard for utilizing and integrating EBP, and a definite lack of knowledge on the process components.

So with a need to be met, the author/coordinator set about using the EBP process to find ways to create a usable infrastructure for EBP use and dissemination for the institution. Nothing in the literature was directly translatable to the needs and resources of the institution, but with a bit of creativity, considering all the resource limitations both physical and cultural, he envisioned a structure to encourage, infuse, and educate on EBP. The program was called the EBP Consultant

Program (Boxer & Taylor, 2007) and successfully created an EBP infrastructure to fulfill the institution's need and help to change the culture.

The program consisted of creating in-house EBP specialists. These specialists were utilized strategically in councils, committees, and task forces to act as consultants to the groups, facilitating and teaching the EBP process as the groups tackled projects and addressed opportunities for improvement. The author/coordinator envisioned a spider web approach to disseminating the EBP process, where one is taught, he or she then teaches a group, and the group members each teach another group, resulting in widespread dissemination. Brilliant! At least we think so. You will need to judge for yourself (see the Creative Solution at the end of the chapter). The program is designed with intensive 3-day education and training on the EBP process and its use in institutional practices along with the creation of an EBP Consultants Group, which meets monthly to discuss issues relating to specific projects and for continuing education of the EBP consultants. The EBP coordinator took the roles of leader, mentor, facilitator, and educator of the EBP Consultants Group.

The first group of consultants consisted of five people: two staff RNs, two nurse managers, and one nursing performance improvement coordinator. After their graduation from the class, each was mentored on their first project by the coordinator/author, assuring proper application of the concepts and techniques learned. This also gave them the confidence to take a leadership role in their own projects and groups with whom they were working. After successful completion of the first project, they became full-fledged consultants, able to be accessed by anyone in the institution needing assistance with the EBP process. Those wanting guidance contacted the EBP coordinator, who assigned the consultants to those requesting assistance. The consultants were also required to mentor someone in the second class of consultants through their first project to reinforce their knowledge and perpetuate the dissemination of the EBP process.

The program was quite successful with two additional classes of EBP consultants prior to the author's/coordinator's leaving the institution. A culture change, although measured mostly anecdotally, was apparent through the use of the consultants, as well as the staff's verbalizations, asking more and more about the evidence behind the policy/practice changes they were exposed to. Most consultants completed their first project within four months. So, do you think you can do this in your institution? Would it help to meet your institution's goals? Are you on the journey to Magnet designation? Then this creative solution might just be what you were looking for.

WHAT IS EBP?

Evidence-based practice (EBP) seems to be the new buzzword in health care. A Google search for the phrase "evidence-based practice" conjures over three million

Internet links (as of March 12, 2006). An Entrez PubMed search of the same phrase found 1,872 citations, approximately one third of which were published within the past 2 years (as of March 12, 2006). Many definitions exist for evidence-based practice. Melnyk and Fineout-Overholt (2005) define it as,

> A problem solving approach to practice that involves the conscientious use of best evidence in making decisions about patient care; EBP incorporates a systematic search for and critical appraisal of the most relevant evidence to answer a clinical question along with one's own clinical expertise and patient values and preferences. (p. 587)

This definition illustrates the common themes found among many of the definitions of EBP. A problem solving approach relates to the nature of clinical practice, viewing the practice as a challenge to determine and use the best available procedures to achieve the best possible outcomes. "(T)he conscientious use of best evidence in making decisions about patient care" proposes the pronouncement to and responsibility for incorporating current research into one's clinical practice. The second half of the definition refers to the components of evidence-based practice: evidence from research and experts, evidence from the assessment of the patient, the clinical expertise of the clinician, and information about the individual patient's preferences and values (2005).

THE PROCESS OF EBP

1. Ask the burning clinical question.
2. Collect the most relevant and best evidence.
3. Critically appraise the evidence.
4. Integrate all evidence with one's clinical expertise, patient preferences, and values in making a practice decision or change.
5. Evaluate the practice decision or change. (Melnyk & Fineout-Overholt, 2005, p. 9)

THE VALUE OF EBP

A study by Heater, Becker, and Olsen (1988) found that patients who received care based on the best and latest research from well-designed studies experienced more favorable outcomes. Rich, Speir, Fonner, and the Virginia Cardiac Surgery Quality Initiative (2006) developed a clinical and financial database for best cardiac surgery practices resulting in best outcomes for dissemination statewide, concluding that ". . . (R)educing the incidence of complications by small fractions can yield significant savings" (p. 142). Clearly, in this litigious and economically challenged healthcare milieu, EBP is a way to satisfy both patients and providers with better, more economical care.

Pravikoff, Tanner, and Pierce (2005) found that 61% of surveyed nurses needed to seek information at least once per week, 67% of surveyed nurses frequently sought information from a colleague instead of a reference text, and 83% rarely sought a librarian's assistance in obtaining information. Studies by Shorten and Wallace (1997) and Melnyk, Fineout-Overholt, Stone, and Ackerman (2000) also found that only small percentages of healthcare providers are incorporating research findings into patient care decisions.

Basically, evidence-based practice is a process that promotes clinical decision making based on the best available evidence from research literature and clinical expertise, considering patient and family preferences and resources available. It is "(t)he conscientious, explicit, and judicious use of current best evidence in making decisions about the care of individual patients . . . [by] integrating individual clinical expertise with the best available external clinical evidence from systematic research" (Sackett, Richardson, Rosenberg, & Haynes, 1997). It encourages the clinician to problem solve in a systematic way and to seek proven methods of care in their clinical practice while concurrently individualizing care to achieve the best patient outcomes possible. Although care may be evidence-based, outcomes will vary based on patient and family values, preference, and expectations as well as the generalizability of the evidence considered.

Evidence-based practice is an overarching term that is sometimes delimited as evidence-based medicine or evidence-based nursing. However specified, the principle and process are the same. What should be stressed here is that evidence-based practice is a process, not a product. It truly cannot be a product because individual patient and family values and preferences and caregiver expertise need to be considered and integrated into the care of each individual patient. Evidence-based practice becomes something different for each patient, even though the foundation of the clinical practice might be the same literature. This distinction counters any critics who say EBP is simply cookbook medicine/nursing, or does not consider the patient or family desires. EBP is not meant to be as directive as some have believed and is more a paradigm of care than a prescription for care. Evidence-based practice does work.

- A meta-analysis by Heater et al. (1988) of 84 nursing studies determined that 72% of patients receiving evidence-based nursing care had an average of 28% better outcomes than the control patients.
- Studies by Brooten et al. (2002), Leatherman, et al. (2003), and Goode et al. (2000) show that evidence-based practice initiatives may not save money in the short term, but may result in long-term economic savings due to avoiding unnecessary procedures, better patient outcomes, and decreases in treatment complications.

THE EBP PROCESS AND THE NURSING PROCESS

The EBP process, if you look closely, is analogous to a process nurses are quite familiar with: the nursing process. In the nursing process, nurses assess, diagnose, plan, implement, and evaluate. In the EBP process, we assess the situation (assess) and formulate our problem or question (diagnose). We search and appraise the evidence to find what will solve our problem or answer our question (plan). Then we change our practice as indicated by the evidence (implement). Finally we evaluate both the implementation of the practice change and the effects, outcomes of the practice change (evaluate). When you look at the process like this, it seems much more familiar and much less threatening.

There are a few differences however within each step that we need to take note of here. In the nursing process, diagnosis consists of choosing among a list of North American Nursing Diagnosis Association (NANDA) approved nursing diagnoses. In the EBP process, our analogous task is to formulate a PICO question. PICO is an acronym for: patient, population, or problem; intervention; comparison with other interventions; and outcome. Writing a question or situation in this format probably takes as much practice as choosing a NANDA diagnosis that corresponds to your nursing assessment. The planning phase also takes on a different flavor. Searching for evidence in the EBP process requires different skills than gathering evidence from patient data for the nursing process, but analysis and critical thinking are necessary for both.

Critically appraising the evidence in the EBP process also varies from appraising evidence in the nursing process. Nurses are comfortable believing the data they see and collect, such as lab values, blood pressure readings, patient's response to treatment, etc. A different criterion is used for believing the data retrieved in the EBP process. It is not that the criteria are more difficult to understand, it is just less familiar, less intuitive, and less subjective. It takes some practice and some getting used to. Once a best practice is found, implementation typically takes more than creating an individual care plan. Instead, an implementation plan for the best practice relies on project management skills to achieve success. Stakeholder support is necessary for a successful implementation. An action plan should guide the process to meet individual objectives, thus eventually meeting the goal of full implementation. The implementation of the best practice must be evaluated along with evaluating the outcome expected. It is best to evaluate the implementation often. This is called a formative evaluation and allows you to adjust the action plan to meet the overall goals of the plan. Say, for example, you are unable to educate everyone about the new evidence-based best practice. The formative evaluation will change your timeline because you know that if not aware of the practice change, nurses cannot be compliant with the practice change. So before you evaluate the outcomes from the new best practice, you have to first make sure everyone is doing it, correctly, we might add.

OUR ALGORITHM FOR THE EVIDENCE-BASED PRACTICE PROCESS

Formulate a relevant question.
- Critically evaluate the situation.
- Use the PICO format and identify its components from the situation presented.
- Compose an appropriate practice question using the PICO format.

Systematically search for evidence.
- Identify possible sources of evidence.
- Plan and complete searches.
- Retrieve evidence from identified sources.

Critically appraise the evidence.
- Summarize each piece of evidence.
- Rate each piece of evidence as to level and quality.
- Summarize all evidence into overall findings.
- Develop recommendations specific to the situation based on the found evidence.

Change practice where indicated.
- Determine the appropriateness and the feasibility of translating recommendations into the specific situation.
- Identify all stakeholders involved and obtain their support.
- Communicate and disseminate findings and recommendations.
- Create an action plan with stakeholder input.
- Implement the changes according to the action plan.

Evaluate the implementation of the practice change.
- Evaluate the implementation process used.
- Adjust implementation process as necessary.

Evaluate the effects of the practice change made.
- Evaluate the effects of the change on stakeholders (patients, providers, the institution).
- Develop a plan to ensure integration/enculturation of change.

We were recently asked to share our expertise with the newly formed Pressure Ulcer Prevention Task Force in a 500-bed community hospital. They have had a wound care committee for some time now, but we found out through much questioning that this committee primarily deals with the care of pressure ulcers: the staging, the choice of products used in care, and determining nosocomial prevalence. However, we decided to inquire a bit further, asking what pressure ulcer outcome data they were collecting. We were told that they collect data on staging, prevalence, and whether the care guidelines are followed. What we found was that they were only collecting data to evaluate compliance measures. They were not collecting any outcome data to evaluate whether their interventions are actually making a difference in bettering patient care.

Some might argue that following guidelines implies that they are bettering patient care, assuming these are evidence-based guidelines. This is one of the fallacies of evidence-based practice, the assumption that, as long as you follow the evidence-based guidelines, you must be bettering patient care and you do not need to evaluate your efforts. Evidence-based practice is no substitute for properly evaluating the outcome of an intervention. Many factors affect patient outcomes and many are not controlled through evidence-based care. Evidence-based care is malleable. It is molded and delivered according to specific clinical and sociocultural needs, individualized for each patient, taking into account the amount and type of resources available, so it is quite likely care will vary to some extent in each individual situation.

CHOOSING AN EBP MODEL

There are many EBP models to choose from. Unlike the automobile industry where models come and go, EBP models stay around. These models are useful frameworks for standardizing the EBP process in your institution. The models basically act as algorithms for the EBP process, making it systematic and providing a common structure and process throughout the institution. We recommend that your institution adopts a single EBP model to utilize when designing policies, processes, and procedures. A single adopted institutional EBP model will also facilitate education on the EBP process and help to develop common language related to EBP.

Finding EBP models is easy. A simple Google search for EBP models will retrieve what you need. There are a few more popular models we will discuss a bit here and provide you with their Web site addresses. As with any tool or model your institutions adopts, you should get permission from its author, creator, or owner before you implement the model. This is necessary if the model is copyrighted, but a good thing to do even if it is not. The owner might have updated the model or might provide you with some insights for using the model in your specific environment.

Models vary in their complexity and their prescriptiveness. Typically and logically, the models that are less complex are less prescriptive. Which one you choose should depend on what your institution needs at its level of sophistication with EBP. To begin, you might want a more prescriptive model to guide you step by step through the EBP process. Remember that the model also needs to fit within the current structure of your institution. Establish an EBP steering committee to evaluate various models and make recommendations as to which fits best. The steering committee should consist of those that will use the model and can also evaluate its usefulness for the rest of the staff. Include staff educators, managers, staff nurses, and assure leadership support for the group. After deciding, have senior nursing leadership sign off on the choice—again make sure to contact the author/creator/owner for permission. Now you can utilize the steering committee to assist with developing a plan to roll out the model—possibly an internal PR campaign using creative solutions to promote awareness of the model and educate the staff on its purpose. This committee can also assist in deciding who will get what level of EBP education. We recommend that all nursing staff have at least an awareness of the model and what it is used for. After that, it is up to you and your committee as to how intensive the education is for those deemed appropriate.

The ACE Star Model of Knowledge Transformation

The ACE Star Model of Knowledge Transformation (Academic Center for Evidence-Based Practice, 2008) provides a simplistic visual framework to use for discovering knowledge and transforming it into practice. Its five phases are portrayed as the five points of a star, thus the title of the model. The five points are used in a continuous cycle of knowledge discovery, summary, translation, integration, evaluation, and back to discovery. This cycle guides the user in the evidence-based practice process. The model cites eight Premises of Knowledge Transformation, which provide information about the model's structure of evidence and definition of knowledge. Each phase of the model is described, albeit somewhat vaguely and briefly, requiring some foundation knowledge of the EBP process and the elements involved (Stevens, 2004).

The Web site (http://www.acestar.uthscsa.edu/Learn_model.htm) has extensive information about EBP and EBP resources, providing links to many other sites with materials to educate staff and locate evidence. This model is on the more simplistic side of the simple-to-complex continuum. Some may feel this simplicity adds to understanding, however, that understanding might be somewhat superficial, too vague to be put into practice without a thorough understanding of how to operationalize each of the model's phases.

The Johns Hopkins EBP Model

Unfortunately, when you visit the Web site that describes the Johns Hopkins EBP Model (Institute for Johns Hopkins Nursing, n.d.), you will not find a visual display of the model, but a link to purchase the book, *Johns Hopkins Nursing Evidence-Based Practice Model and Guidelines* by Newhouse, Dearholt, Poe, Pugh, and White (2007). This may be a good investment, since this model has been used, tested, and tweaked to be effective. The book also provides guidelines for using the model, which adds to its prescriptiveness, assisting the beginner in the use of the model. A perusal of the book's table of contents provides a feel for what you get. Both intriguing and impressive are the list of tools provided in the appendix. The book also provides exemplars to help guide those less sophisticated in the EBP process. The model itself can be previewed, as it was published in the *Journal of Nursing Administration* (Newhouse, Dearholt, Poe, Pugh, & White, 2005). It is definitely worth checking out.

The model is a little more toward the complex side of the continuum than the ACE Star Model, but one would certainly not call it complex. In its graphic representation, it includes factors affecting the evidence and relationships among education, research, and practice. The graphic representation elicits some understanding, but no practical prescription of the model's use. Explanation is necessary for application to real-life situations.

The Iowa Model of Evidence-Based Practice

The Iowa Model of Evidence-Based Practice (Titler et al., 2001; University of Iowa Hospitals and Clinics, 2009) is free to use, but needs to be sanctioned by the authors. You can find the form to obtain permission for the model's use here: http://www.uihealthcare.com/depts/nursing/rqom/evidencebasedpractice/iowamodel.html The Web site does not display the complete detailed model to view. Instead, it provides a graphic of the model's uses. The model is quite prescriptive, using a decision tree/process map format to guide the user through the process. So on the simplicity–complexity continuum, this is definitely the most complex of the three, but as the most prescriptive, it may be the easiest to use for the EBP beginner as a step-by-step introduction to using the EBP process. It will however probably not be as easily remembered as a simple graphic like the ACE Star Model. It is all about what works best for your institution. You can view the model and decide if it works for you at: http://www.mosescone.com/documents/public/Nursing%20Research/Iowa%20Model%201998.pdf.

NOT ALL EVIDENCE IS CREATED EQUAL

You are guilty! Yes, a preponderance of the evidence has convinced a jury of your peers that you did it, that it was you, beyond a reasonable doubt. So what does this have to do with EBP? Everything.

What EBP is looking for is a preponderance of evidence to convince you that there is an answer to your PICO question, which is certain and beyond a reasonable doubt. To do this, the evidence must be believable. "Yes members of the jury, I saw the defendant do it." How many men and women have been convicted based on these words from the anecdotal evidence of a single eyewitness? But studies have shown that eyewitness testimony can be flawed. Approximately 160 people convicted of violent crimes were misidentified by eyewitness accounts and have been exonerated by DNA evidence in the past two decades (Duke, 2006). How many juries have found eyewitness testimony believable? How did they determine that the testimony and the person testifying were believable? There has been much research in the field of criminology devoted to just that question. What is interesting is that the discipline of nursing, possibly as far removed from the discipline of criminology as one could get, is interested in much the same thing. What is it that makes evidence believable? Is it the source? Is it the content? Is it our own biases, our desire to believe it because we agree with it? Maybe it happened the same way in our practice, or maybe it agrees with what we expect. But is that good enough? No, it is not.

Eyewitness accounts are sometimes the most believable evidence without a videotape of the crime. It is the same in nursing. Anecdotal evidence, what you are seeing in your practice or someone you know telling you what works or what is the correct answer to your clinical question, is sometimes the most believable, the most trusted source. But like the eyewitness account, anecdotal evidence in practice has many flaws and ranks low on the hierarchy of evidence.

In EBP, the hierarchy of evidence relates to the believability of the evidence based on a number of criteria considered. The first of the criteria considered comes from the type of evidence we have. Research studies are always higher in the hierarchy than other forms of evidence. Conventionally, the rating given to evidence is based on principles inherent in the scientific method, a process used for example to test if one drug or procedure is better than another. Research utilizes the scientific method so its prominence in the hierarchy of evidence is truly no surprise. But the key here is believability. The whole hierarchy is in that one word. So what determines believability? Believability basically has two components, chance and bias. The key to increasing believability is to decrease chance and decrease bias. If you are a math person and wanted to describe the relationship in an equation you might write

$$\text{Believability} = -(\text{chance} + \text{bias})$$

Or you might describe the relationship: As chance and bias decrease, believability increases. Whatever way you think about it, just remember that the evaluation of any evidence in EBP is based on two questions: How much bias is there in the evidence? How much are the results of the evidence attributable to chance?

There are a number of evidence hierarchies available. Most are similar but some are more discipline specific. Hierarchies of evidence for medical decision making are a little different than hierarchies for nursing decision making, however, the difference usually lies in the complexity of the evidence under scrutiny, not the principles involved in classification. Finding an evidence hierarchy that suits your institution is important in establishing standardization and a common institutional language for discussing EBP. Some hierarchies use grading systems such as A, B, C. Some use class systems such as I, II, III. Whichever suits your institution, choosing an evidence hierarchy is necessary prior to educating the staff and establishing policies and procedures directing and establishing the institution's EBP process.

HOW TO USE THE GRADING SCALE AND QUALITY CHART PROVIDED TO EVALUATE EVIDENCE

The grading scale we have provided on the following pages is one example of the many you can find in the literature. This scale is based on the type of evidence you are evaluating. It simply asks you to identify the type of evidence, find it on the scale, and note the corresponding grade. It is based on the premise that evidence with less bias and less chance is more believable. The type of evidence and the design of a study have much to do with controlling for bias and chance. Thus, the scale will give you a relative feel for which evidence is more believable, helping you to determine the strength of the evidence's conclusions and recommendations.

So, first look at your evidence and determine what type of evidence you have. This may entail deciphering the study design of a research article. Many times a research article will explicitly state its study design. Look for this in the study. So, after you have determined the type of evidence, find it on the Evidence Grading Scale provided or another scale of your choosing. Note the grade in the Evidence-Based Practice Literature Review Summary sheet provided in Figure 6-1.

Now look at the Evidence Quality Chart provided in Table 6-1. The type of evidence tells much about the evidence's believability, but not all. There are variations in the same types of evidence dependent upon the rigor of the methodology and adherence to scientific standards. In other words, a systematic review is a high-grade piece of evidence. However, a poorly done systematic review might not be very believable, and might not be worth considering as evidence. Using the Evidence Quality Chart will require a bit of knowledge as to what constitutes a high quality study. The chart provides some guidelines, but is meant to demonstrate that believability is a continuum, and the evidence should be judged relative to the standard for excellence in the specific type of evidence and also judged relative to other pieces of evidence. The chart helps with the former; you are responsible for the latter.

Using a tool like the Evidence-Based Practice Literature Review Summary Sheet will assist you in evaluating all the evidence in total and determining which should be given more weight because it is more believable. Now that you are familiar with the evidence quality standards from the chart, rate the evidence as believable, questionable, or doubtful based on the criteria supplied, and note this rating on

Figure 6-1   Evidence-based practice literature review summary.

Author and Title	Date	Type of Study	Sample Size (if applicable)	Results and Recommendations	Limitations	Rating
						GRADE / QUALITY

Table 6-1 Evidence Quality Chart

	Multistudy Reviews	Single-Study Research	Experiential Recommendations
Believable	Search strategies are made explicit, are complete, and are reproducible. Results are consistent with sufficient numbers of appropriate studies. Methodology is consistent and appropriate for evaluating strength of studies. Review produces explicit conclusions.	Study results are consistent and have been randomized and controlled appropriately. Sample size and power are adequate. Hypothesis, interventions, and analysis made are explicit. Results are authoritative. Recommendations are consistent with and based on in-depth literature review.	Source is a recognized expert in the topic. Expertise is obvious, based on extensive knowledge of the subject matter and the evidence and/or literature written on the topic.
Questionable	Search strategies are provided but may not be complete. Results are somewhat consistent but may be lacking in the numbers of studies reviewed. Evaluation of studies is relatively consistent. Conclusions are provided by a consensus of studies.	Study results are consistent. Some controls are apparent with appropriate sample size. Hypothesis and interventions may be somewhat equivocal. Analysis is less explicit. Recommendations are not entirely consistent or are based on a somewhat superficial review of literature.	Source appears knowledgeable and credible. Expertise is believed.
Doubtful	Search strategies are not provided or are recognized as incomplete. Results are inconsistent and may be based on too few studies. Evaluation methods are not provided or are inconsistently applied. Conclusions are equivocal.	Study results are vague. Controls are not apparent. Hypothesis and interventions are unclear. Analysis is incomplete. Recommendations are not based on or consistent with literature review.	Credibility of source is questionable. Expertise is not apparent.

the summary sheet. Do the same grading and quality rating for each piece of evidence you have obtained to answer your PICO questions. Looking at all of the evidence in this framework will help you judge their relative merits and relative believability, hopefully allowing you to find a definitive answer.

Evidence Grading Scale

- **Grade A**: Evidence is from a systematic review or meta-analysis of all randomized controlled trials, or evidence is from evidence-based clinical practice guidelines that are based on systematic reviews of randomized controlled trials.
- **Grade B**: Evidence that is obtained from at least one well-designed randomized controlled trial.
- **Grade C**: Evidence that is obtained from well-designed controlled trials without randomization (quasi-experimental studies).
- **Grade D**: Evidence that is obtained from well-designed case-control and cohort studies or nonexperimental studies (no randomization and no control).
- **Grade E:** Evidence that is obtained from metasynthesis or systematic reviews of descriptive and qualitative studies.
- **Grade F**: Evidence that is obtained from a single descriptive or qualitative study.
- **Grade G**: Evidence that is obtained from the opinion of authorities and/or reports of experts.

IF IT IS EBP, DO WE STILL NEED TO TEST IT?

This question is actually moot, and we will tell you why. Many people think that all they need to do is incorporate practices that have evidence to support their efficacy. Unfortunately, this is not the case. The definition of EBP states that it takes into account "individual clinical expertise" (Sackett et al., 1997) and patients' and families' values, preferences, and expectations. So the evidence-based practice you use for a specific patient's care will vary somewhat from the evidence-based practice cited in the research. In addition, your institution, your staff, and the population of patients you serve will also vary from the institutions, staff, and patient populations in the research that shows the evidence-based practice has merit and efficacy. These are sources of variability when utilizing any evidence-based practice. What we have then are sources of variability inherent in the EBP process. Of course, the amount of this variability will differ, depending on how different your institution, staff, patient populations and the individual clinical expertise of your practitioners are from those cited in the evidence research literature. These inherent sources of variation make it necessary and obligatory to treat

EBP not as an absolute prescription, but as a recommendation, strong or weak, depending on the situational differences between the evidence research literature and your application. EBP is truly always in a state of flux with recommendations varying based on the accumulation of evidence. So, to get back to the initial question, we answer a resounding yes, you have to test it! EBP is not absolute, and just because your practice is based on evidence, it might not work with your other processes and might not have the effect you want for your specific population.

Look at Outcomes and Compliance

So, what does testing EBP mean? What do I have to do? Well, you need to have some data on the outcome you are looking to fix before you implement the evidence-based practice. This is your baseline data that told you there was a problem, and this is the data you are going to use to compare with the data you collect after you have implemented the evidence-based practice. What data will you collect after you implement evidence-based practice? You will collect the same data you collected before, the same data that told you there was a problem. For example, say your nosocomial pressure ulcer prevalence is 19%, not good no matter what database you compare with.

So, there is your problem. Now what? Well, you develop your PICO question, search the literature, find what works for your patient population and work culture, and decide to implement specific evidence-based interventions. Okay, you have implemented your interventions, and now what should you measure? Well, there are actually two things you need to measure. The first is compliance with the interventions. It does not matter how good your interventions are or how much evidence you have found to say they work. If no one is doing the interventions, your outcome will continue to be poor, and you might otherwise throw out a perfectly good, evidence-based plan to improve your nosocomial pressure ulcer prevalence. Do not do it!

First, look at your compliance with the interventions implemented. If they are good (90 to 100%), then focus on the outcome measurement you used for baseline data, the measurement that told you there was a problem (such as the nosocomial pressure ulcer prevalence). So, you are actually comparing preintervention nosocomial pressure ulcer prevalence with postintervention nosocomial pressure ulcer prevalence (apples to apples). Now you can see if your evidence-based interventions have made a difference. What happens if you look at your compliance, and you have been able to keep it at 90 to 100%, and you look at your outcome measure (nosocomial pressure ulcer prevalence) and you have not made a difference. There is virtually no change in the rate, and you have given it a chance to work. Maybe you have been monitoring it for 6 months and still no change. It is time to scrap the intervention. Yes, we said *scrap the intervention*! We know it is a radical

Table 6-2 Outcome Data vs Compliance Data

		OUTCOME DATA	
		Positive Results	Negative Results
COMPLIANCE DATA	Positive Results	You are having success. Your intervention is working! You need to sustain, enculturate, and, keep evaluating.	The intervention is not working. Stop doing it. Try a different intervention to achieve your goals.
	Negative Results	There is something else going on here. The intervention is not responsible for the outcome changes you are seeing. Investigate what could be the cause.	You need to work on achieving compliance. Until you do, you will never know if the intervention truly works.

idea, but to keep doing something that does not work is just beating the proverbial dead horse. It is time to move on, to try something new. Table 6-2 might help when looking at compliance data and outcome data in deciding what to do.

WHERE TO FIND EVIDENCE-BASED PRACTICE

When there is a need or want, someone will fill it. That is the nature of capitalism; find what people need and want and fill the void. Sam Walton did it with Wal-Mart, and Joanna Briggs did it with EBP. Joanna Briggs, as we in the EBP world know her, is the namesake of a Web site devoted to compiling and packaging evidence-based nursing. This is one of many evidence-based nursing Web sites, and it does warrant some explanation. As evidence-based practice became and becomes more widespread, there was and is the realization that ASN/BSN education really does not prepare nurses to do intensive literature reviews, integration, and analysis to find the answers to clinical questions, nor do nurses have the time to devote to this endeavor. So the need for a quick way to find the best evidence-based nursing practices was identified. To meet this need, a new service was realized. What we have is evidence-based nursing packaged, with all the quality research evaluation standards posted on the proverbial label, to answer our PICO questions quickly, possibly when we are engaged in patient care and in need of a quick evidence-based solution to our clinical problems. Joanna Briggs, like many similar Web sites, offers evidence-based nursing in the form of best practice guidelines, locating and summarizing the research literature on specific nursing questions. The hierarchy of evidence scale used to grade the evidence that helps with formulating the best practice guidelines is fully disclosed and well worth reading.

It is unfortunate that each EBP Web site uses its own literature grading scale, so to truly know how believable the recommendations are, you need to know their scale. This is definitely a drawback for the EBP novice. That is one reason why it is necessary to know research study design and the benefits and limitations for each type. It might be a bit ambitious to expect to be able to teach all nurses research study design and have them all proficient at grading and evaluating research and evidence. It is probably more realistic to teach the principles of EBP and give nurses an understanding of the criteria that evidence is graded on. This will allow them an understanding of believability irrespective of the specific grading scale used by the EBP recommendation authors. They need to understand that evidence is not dichotomous (i.e., good or bad). It is a continuum from the best to the worst. As a continuum, it must be judged against competing research on the same continuum, which demonstrates the relative nature of evidence grading.

There are many Web sites, some free, and some that require a subscription, which can be purchased by an individual or as an institution. Hospitals and healthcare organizations need to determine what is best for them. Purchasing an institutional subscription to an EBP database that no one uses or knows how to use is a waste of money. It might be more fiscally appropriate to first purchase an individual subscription for one person in the hospital who is relatively well versed in EBP and would be able to evaluate how well it meets the needs of the institution, possibly a nurse educator. After using the site and navigating through the various offerings, the nurse educator and the institution can better assess the site's responsiveness and ease of use.

There are many other venues where EBP can be found. The government also has a couple of powerful Web sites devoted to supplying EBP guidelines, recommendations, and tools for assisting with educating about EBP to enculturate EBP in your institution. We think it is definitely worthwhile to highlight one of these sites.

National Guideline Clearinghouse (www.guideline.gov) is an initiative of the Agency for Healthcare and Quality (AHRQ) and a public resource for various evidence-based guidelines. Click on the "About NGC" page and you will see the many features this site offers: PDA downloads of summaries for all guidelines, guideline comparisons, guideline syntheses, which specifically highlight areas of similarity and difference among guidelines on the same topic, as well as definitions of terms, and an explanation of the inclusion criteria for the guidelines in the database. Take some time, maybe a dateless Saturday night, and peruse the site. Look at the features and what might be most usable for your institution. We give this advice a lot. Many people think they will go to an EBP site and find what they need right away. An hour later they are frustrated. Let us set the expectation: You need to spend some time looking at individual EBP sites, getting a feel for what each one offers and how each one is laid out. The more familiar you are with the sites, the easier it will be to find what you need, when you need it.

Finding EBP through electronic databases can also take some time. You will find that different databases have different evidence-based practice guidelines. You may find an EBP guideline for wound care on National Guidelines Clearinghouse and another on Joanna Briggs. Which do you choose? Well, remember the principles of EBP. First you need to look at their literature grading scales and evaluate the number and type of studies included in their guidelines, and do not forget about age. The newer guidelines with more recently published studies will most likely be preferable to the older guideline with older studies. But you still need to look at how many studies are included in creating the guideline and the strength of the evidence on which each guideline is based.

We wish there was a foolproof algorithm or formula we could give to decide between two guidelines, but there is not. A good start is to look at the guidelines side by side and note their similarities and differences. National Guidelines Clearinghouse does this for you, but not all guidelines on all sites are included. Focus your energy on the differences, choosing the recommendations with the strongest evidence. It is fine to have a policy or procedure taken from multiple EBP guidelines. Remember, EBP is also what works best in your patient population with your institutional structure and culture. It is not right or wrong, but rather, a matter of better or worse. Think continuum, not dichotomy.

Age of the Evidence

This is probably also a good place to talk a little more about the age of evidence. How old does evidence have to be before it is too old or outdated to use? Our answer to this is a definitive "well, it depends." You have probably learned the 5-year rule in school, no research older than 5 years should be used in your references. It is a good rule to follow. But with the huge lag time between research and that research becoming clinical practice, on average, 8 to 13 years (Sackett et al., 1997), plus the time it takes to physically publish research and nursing texts, it may be wiser to reduce the 5-year rule to 3 years. This is mainly for clinical practice. For other research, like studies done on more obscure topics, there might not be any recent research.

You may have to go beyond the 3- or 5-year rules to find usable studies. That is fine. Just evaluate the study with a bit more scrutiny. Are the foundational practices the same now as when this study was done? For example, a colleague is currently undertaking a research study looking at the efficacy of a device for collection and reinfusion of autologous blood after orthopedic surgery. When the question of the efficacy of the system came up, she went to the literature to find an evidence-base supporting its use. She could find only literature older than 5 years. When she thought whether to use this research, she realized that many things have changed in orthopedic surgery in the past 10 years, such as surgical technique, guidelines for transfusion, the safety of the nation's blood supply, etc. For her purposes, she judged these changes too significant to consider this research usable. Thus, her research study was born. However, if there had been no significant changes in orthopedic surgery or the guidelines for blood transfusion, she might have decided differently. A study's age limitation is more of an evaluative process than an absolute rule. But if pressed, use the 3- or 5-year rule as a guideline.

More on EBP Web Sites

Back to the Web sites: Another government-produced EBP Web site is through AHRQ (www.AHRQ.gov). The amount of information on this site will make you feel like a kid in an EBP candy store. They publish information for clinicians as well as the general healthcare consumer. On the AHRQ Health Care Innovations Exchange page, institutions' stories of success in achieving various quality outcomes are shared. Much of this information is geared toward segments of healthcare delivery other than the hospital venue, but there is also some good information for hospitals. It is definitely worth a review.

The one page on the AHRQ Web site you should review is the AHRQ Resource Links for Nurses (www.ahrq.gov/about/nursing/nrslinks.htm). This page will show you some awesome tools to use for finding and educating others on EBP. It also demonstrates the breadth of EBP from clinical guidelines to public health preparedness. This page will also provide links to AHRQ funding opportunities, data sets, and requests for AHRQ publications.

More casual venues for EBP (and we say casual because this would probably not be a source you would go to if you had a specific PICO question that needed answered quickly) are peer-reviewed professional journal publications. A subscription to your nursing specialty journal will typically provide EBP articles along with trends in the specialty, new products, and procedures. These EBP articles, however, are usually not graded as to their strength of evidence, so that is up to you, the reader. Remember that not everything in print is true. We know this, but we tend to forget it when we read a professional publication. Remember, as we said about evidence, it is not strictly true or false but where it falls on the continuum of true and false, believable and doubtful. We need to keep a bit of cynicism in mind when we are reading and evaluating articles, constantly applying our grading and quality criteria to determine the article's believability.

Professional Conferences

Professional conferences and symposia are other great venues for learning evidence-based practices. As with publications, these are again casual sources. Here you will typically hear the latest, most up-to-date evidence on the specific topics addressed. Again you need caution in what you do with this information. You may hear about ongoing studies that have not yet shown outcomes or projects that are currently in progress. You might want to run back to your institution and try everything you hear about. Just remember that we are sometimes too quick to try things we hear about without thoroughly evaluating their merit. This can be dangerous for a number of reasons. If the practice is true research not EBP, it might possibly be outside what is considered standard of care and would need to be blessed by the IRB as a research trial. More typically, if the practice is adopted without knowing the outcomes achieved under what conditions and with which populations, it may wind up being a waste of time, money, and resources.

STRUCTURE FOR FINDING AND STRUCTURE FOR DISSEMINATING

The quality mantra "structure, process, outcomes" popularized by Donabedian (1980), a quality improvement guru, is always something to keep in mind when implementing any new initiative, especially one that you hope to enculturate. It provides a starting point for your thinking and a way to consider how the initiative will take hold. Are the things in place that need to be in place for the action (outcome) you want? First focus in on the structures necessary to support your venture. Without a solid infrastructure to support the processes of EBP, nurses will not be able to find, use, or disseminate EBP. Of course, the easiest way to support an EBP initiative is to use an existing infrastructure. Do you have access to appropriate research databases to find EBP? Where are the computers that have access located? How many do you have? Do you have a librarian, someone well versed in searching to help novices? Can you retrieve found articles either through subscriptions for full-text access or through article-retrieval services? Do you have educators and a venue to educate staff on EBP? When thinking about these questions, an internal dialogue should be taking place, questioning and answering things like, Do we need all nurses proficient at finding EBP, or can we develop specialists to utilize when needed? What do the nurses already know about EBP and what do they need to know?

There are definitely different levels of understanding the EBP process: being able to find and evaluate EBP, being able to implement EBP, and being able to utilize EBP (Hamer & Collinson, 2003). It is analogous to the research process. You can understand the research process, but that does not mean you have the skills and knowledge to perform a research study. There is a definite hierarchy in skills and knowledge associated with the EBP process, and not everyone needs to have all the skills, at least not at the beginning. It might be something you work toward, but a more realistic expectation would be to look at the institution's needs and determine the most doable, cost-effective way to meet these needs. So you are looking at your structure already in place with an eye on the outcomes you expect from your efforts to establish and enculturate EBP. Again, that internal dialogue should look at sustainability with an EBP initiative. Will the structure support a continued and continuous EBP initiative or is it inadequate for your long-term goal?

The goal of having all nurses knowledgeable about the EBP process, able to carry out the process, able to use the fruits of this process, and able to disseminate the results and outcomes of the EBP process is a worthy goal. We believe this is EBP utopia, but Wake up Dorothy! You're not in Kansas anymore! What we mean is that you need to have realistic expectations of implementing an EBP initiative. Do not set yourself up for failure by shooting for the moon. As our colleague always says when frustration sets in: baby steps . . . remember baby steps. She is right; all those steps add up. Before you know it, you are miles ahead of where you were and your eyes can be set on an even bigger goal.

So, we have discussed a bit about the importance of structure in the initiative to adopt the EBP paradigm. But what if you have no support structures or no infrastructure already in place to build upon? We think you know the answer to this. Yes, you need to build the structure. This is your first step. Much of building the infrastructure is to again look at your institution's needs and departments' strategic goals and see how an EBP initiative can help meet them. Then determine the structural components to support your endeavor and (here is the hard part), get leadership support, not just their endorsement. You need their financial support. Yes, we used the dirty word financial. Financial implications can be a death sentence for an initiative. We prefer and suggest you use the term cost-effectiveness to account for not only the financial needs of your initiative, but the financial benefit as well. This is where you need to do some homework and a little budgeting. Before you approach leadership with your plans for implementing the EBP initiative, know how much it will cost and how much you will gain. When you consider this, look both at tangible items (like computers, personnel time and salary, and other resources) and intangible items (like morale, camaraderie, professionalism, cost/benefit analysis, reputation in the healthcare community). Many times, intangible items are more persuasive than tangible items. It will help you build a stronger case for your EBP initiative if you consider both.

But do not be naïve, numbers are important. When you do your budgeting, be as realistic as possible, but only ask for what you need for the current year. You can provide further projections, but budgeting is annual in almost all institutions, so the main concern is the current fiscal year. If the budget process has already been completed, you might have to wait until the next cycle, or you might be able to use funds otherwise allocated or surplus funds.

So, now you have assessed your structure and found it to be adequate or you have created an infrastructure to support your EBP initiative. You have done your budgeting and have senior leadership's approval and financial backing. Now you will need to focus on the processes, policies, and procedures to implement the initiative. Again, familiarize yourself with the processes that already exist and use them to your advantage. For example, if you already have a process to create and approve policies and you are looking to infuse the EBP process and create evidence-based polices, modify this existing process instead of creating one anew. It seems common sense, but you would be surprised by how many institutions create duplicate processes to achieve similar outcomes. The best people to assist in creating the processes, policies, and procedures to implement the EBP initiative are those that are going to use these processes, policies, and procedures.

Also, when staff has direct input into this initiative, their buy-in will increase, and implementation might be easier than you thought. As a start to finding processes, policies, and procedures, it is wise to first search the literature. Frequently, you will find case studies on how other institutions have gone about implementing EBP. These case studies can be a valuable source of information, both for noting what worked during implementation and what did not. Remember though, this is evidence for the PICO question, "For an institution similar to mine, what are the best processes, policies, and procedures to implement an EBP initiative?" So considering this as a PICO question, you will need to consider the literature you find as evidence, rating and grading it as appropriate. Be forewarned, rarely will you find a randomized controlled trial or meta-analysis on a subject such as this. Typically what you will find are case studies, each relating one institution's journey through implementation, their successes, failures, and recommendations.

EDUCATION FOR EBP

Education for EBP is not an all-or-none choice, but a strategic planning of who needs what level of knowledge and skill. Utilizing the ubiquitous Bloom's Taxonomy (Bloom, Englehart, Furst, Hill, & Krathwohl, 1956), we recommend levels of knowledge acquisition correlated with the use of and responsibility for EBP. The more one will use and teach the EBP process, the higher the level of his or her knowledge and skill should be. The majority of the nursing staff should be at the level of application with EBP, able to apply the process and use the EBP process in new situations. If you can facilitate this, you have come pretty far. This is definitely a goal to shoot for, but in our experience, the majority of staff are at the knowledge level, able to provide a basic definition of EBP, but are unaware of the EBP process or how it relates to an individual patient. It might do you well to perform a brief assessment (a gap analysis) of your staff on their knowledge of EBP and the EBP process to see where they are and plan best how to get them to where they need to be in applying the EBP process. You should have, in your institution, one or a few recognized EBP gurus evaluate the staff's level of knowledge of EBP and the EBP process. These are the people who are the leaders in strategically planning and disseminating EBP education—the people all others use as a resource to consult if their process goes awry.

Key people, typically advance practice nurses (APN), should be at the analysis, synthesis, or evaluation stage of their knowledge and skill for EBP. Honestly, it would be EBP utopia if your entire staff were at Bloom's evaluation level. Realistically, that probably will not happen, and so, starting from scratch, we believe the strategic dissemination of EBP education is your best and most doable course of action. Begin by making a list of who, in what position, needs what type of education. Try to achieve a spider web effect for the education initiative, where someone teaches a group and those group members teach other groups and so on until everyone is exposed to the education. Look at the groups and structures already in place in your institution. The common mantra, "Don't recreate the wheel" is applicable here. If you do not have a usable venue for staff education or a structure to disseminate EBP, you might want to think about creating a structure. There are always monthly unit staff meetings, however, this is not the easiest venue to use for education since staff meetings are frequently during shift change to catch those working either of two shifts. Some are eager to go home, others eager to start the day; both groups are not ideal for teaching. Remember though, you will need to reinforce this education multiple times through multiple venues. Also consider the new hires. How will they be educated on EBP and the EBP process? Could someone present to them at new hire orientation? It is a way to indoctrinate the newbies, by enculturating EBP education into the standard new hire curriculum. Make sure preceptors also have a good knowledge of the EBP process, able to assist others in applying evidence in their practice (Hamer & Collinson, 2003).

In addition, preceptors need to be demonstrating evidence-based techniques and skills to those they are precepting, reinforcing the need to continue their education, whether it is through national certification and continuing education credits, a formal degree program, attending national conferences, or participating in local chapters of national organizations. These are all venues for acquiring evidence-based practices. And whatever one's preference, there are many ways to keep up on the newest evidence-based practices in his or her specialty. Preceptors can help set the expectation for lifelong learning and relate the relationship of continued education to evidence-based practice, keeping one's practice up-to-date and effecting patient care. It is important that this message is provided from the start of employment and enculturated as an expectation, possibly formalized as a goal on the annual performance evaluation.

We firmly believe that role modeling is one of the strongest ways to set and reinforce expectations. We could not, in good conscience, ask or tell someone to do something we could not or would not do. Why would you listen to someone voicing the need and expectation to become nationally certified, if they themselves are not certified? It is hypocritical and not very credible. This provides even more impetus to select preceptors that model the behavior and expectations for acquiring and delivering evidence-based care in an environment of learning and inquisitiveness. Asking why should be a welcome question, not a time for preceptors to become defensive about their practice.

Topics for EBP Education

We previously discussed the importance of strategically planning the education on EBP and the EBP process for those in the organization. We will not state it all again, except for noting a reminder to do it prior to starting the initiative. We will see later the importance of up-front planning in making an initiative successful. Here we would like to talk about the topics you might consider in teaching EBP and the EBP process. Topics that are intimately related to the subject are:

- The definition of evidence-based practice
- The evidence-based practice process
- PICO questions
- The hierarchy of evidence and types of evidence
- How to find and retrieve evidence
- How to evaluate evidence
- How to summarize evidence
- How to apply the EBP process in typical situations
- Where to use the EBP process

And there are some topics that are a bit tangential, but we believe necessary for successful implementation of any EBP initiative.

- Project management skills
- How to run a meeting/facilitation skills
- Cost/benefit analysis
- Data collection
- Data analysis/elementary statistics
- How and where to disseminate results of the process
- Principles of management and leadership

All of this education is not necessary for everyone and it is not necessary all at once. Some topics are essential for even a basic knowledge of EBP and the EBP process, while other topics are really only for those who are utilizing the EBP process on an almost daily basis. In every institution, there is a great deal of variability in the staff's use of and need for EBP and the EBP process. The key is to strategically match one's need with the specific education topics necessary to meet their need.

Clinical nursing staff responsible for direct patient care might only need the definition of EBP, the EBP process, and where the EBP process is used. Other needs can be handled by a sort of outsourcing, using others in the institution who are well versed in specific skills to assist with the process. The librarian can develop the PICO question and perform the search for evidence. The APN working in that clinical area can evaluate the evidence. The inquiring nurse can then be given the results to use. This limits the number of staff who need extensive education. In this model, the librarian needs to know, if he or she does not already know, how to formulate a PICO question from their conversation with inquiring staff. Their expertise enables them to search and retrieve the evidence. The APN needs to know the hierarchy of evidence, and how to grade and determine the quality of evidence. Do you see where the strategy comes into play? Developing that process and structure for finding, utilizing, and disseminating EBP is a necessary precursor to educating the staff. Once you have planned the process, determined the structure, and know who needs what education, you can develop an educational action plan to support the EBP initiative. Good planning makes good implementation!

A single individual does not need to teach all the topics. There are few individuals capable of teaching them all. Utilize your resources. Maybe the nurse researcher teaches the hierarchy of evidence and the EBP process, the finance person teaches cost/benefit analysis, the librarian teaches how to find evidence, and the director teaches how to run a meeting. You can also borrow faculty from your local college to come in and teach. There are many options. Be aware of all of them and make the most cost-effective choice. When you are planning the education timeline, some topics will need to come before others. It would not make sense to teach the EBP process prior to teaching the definition of EBP, for instance.

Another consideration when teaching is that taught individuals need to have the opportunity to practice what was taught in a real setting soon after it is taught. If you teach something, then wait 6 weeks for the opportunity when they can put the instruction into practice, they will have forgotten most of what was taught, making it a waste of time and resources. Good planning saves money. (This could be a bumper sticker!) If you remember one thing from this section, it will be the need for good planning. And the money you will save from that lesson will easily outweigh the cost of this volume and your time spent planning.

RESEARCH LITERATURE VS QUALITY LITERATURE

You should be aware that there are very real differences between research literature and quality literature. Quality literature usually contains case studies that are much less rigorous than their research literature counterparts, and more casually descriptive and experiential. Quality literature might not use statistical testing to determine success; instead, it might report a positive or negative trend or a percentage increase or decline in the outcome measures. Quality studies have a more qualitative than quantitative flavor. That does not diminish their value. You just need to think of them in a different way. As you are considering the believability of these quality case studies, also keep in mind the transferability of their strategies to your institution. This will depend upon how similar your institution is to the one in the case study. If they provide a description of their institution, patient population, staff, culture, and resources, you might get a feel for the similarities and differences. If these things are not reported, you can usually visit the institution's Web site or contact the author and inquire. It is a bit more time-consuming to contact the author, but he or she might be willing to share copies of their policies and descriptions of their processes and procedures. And, you might even make a professional contact.

WHERE TO INTEGRATE EBP TO ENCULTURATE EBP

The key to successful enculturation, in our opinion, is through massive integration. Make EBP a part of everything—and we mean everything. Let us start with the most obvious, and possibly the most difficult, patient care. We say difficult because patient care is performed by everyone. Does this mean everyone needs the same level of EBP knowledge? No. What it means is that you need to go about integrating EBP strategically. Basically, patient care starts with policy and procedures, so who creates reviews, approves, and adopts new nursing policies and procedures in your institution? It is probably not just a single individual, but probably a committee or various committees. These are the people you need to target with more intensive EBP education. Setting the expectation that all nursing policies and procedures are based on the most recent and most believable evidence available will not happen overnight, but it will happen if you are persistent and have leadership support. Remember, a culture is changed one person at a time. Education is a large part of it, but for the best effect, we believe in mentoring for those who will frequently use the EBP process. Mentoring would first consist of educating, but then actually guiding someone through the EBP process. This is probably the most effective way to operationalize the process and make it truly usable. Let us stay for a minute on the theme of setting the expectation for EBP. This could be a book in itself, but we will just provide the main principle here.

Those who champion and support the EBP initiative need to use the EBP process and expect others to do so. It means that when the CNO is in a meeting with other nursing leadership who are requesting new beds to prevent pressure ulcers, he or she should ask what evidence supports the use of these beds in preventing pressure ulcers. The first time this question is asked might send everyone scrambling for help. But he or she is setting the expectation that if you want a new product, you need to prove it works—the crux of the EBP process.

There are a number of other venues where EBP can be integrated. Many hospitals utilize guidelines or bundles. These are products of the EBP process and a way to integrate evidence-based practices into patient care. Guidelines are those step-by-step instructions we talked about previously that are based on the best available evidence. Bundles are a bit different. A bundle is not just one intervention but a bunch of interventions that, individually, has a demonstrated effect on helping to achieve a desired patient outcome (evidence), but put together, they have a synergistic effect, a total effect greater than the sum of each individual intervention. Usually, to achieve the degree of the desired outcome, all bundle elements must be implemented. These bundles are formulated using the EBP process and many of them have become a standard of care in nursing: Strive to integrate EBP in physician order sets, nurse-driven protocols using physician standing orders, performance/quality improvement initiatives, and even nursing management.

Evidence-based practice is not just confined to nursing practice. The EBP process can be used in almost all disciplines, even management. There are many management techniques and practices that have been tested under various conditions and are considered standard management practices. We suggest you read the article by Jeffrey Pfeffer and Robert I. Sutton titled *Evidence-Based Management* (2006) for more discussion on the topic. As in nursing practice, the same EBP process applies to find the most effective management processes. And as in nursing practice where the EBP process melds the proven techniques with patient preference and environmental variables, evidence-based management techniques must also consider the specific situation under which it is applied. Of course, a different set of databases will be necessary to search for evidence-based managerial practices. Keep in mind that EBP is a paradigm as well as a process, and is truly about searching for what is most effective within the specific situation under which it is applied.

CREATIVE SOLUTIONS

Creative Solution Title: *Evidence-Based Practice (EBP) Consultants*

Creative Solution Author: **Bruce Alan Boxer, PhD, MBA, RN, CPHQ**
Director of Quality/Magnet Program Director
South Jersey Healthcare, Vineland, NJ
Former Evidence-Based Practice Coordinator
Aria Health/Frankford Hospitals
Philadelphia, PA

Purpose: This program is designed to create an infrastructure to educate, utilize, and disseminate EBP and the EBP process.

Legend

Overall Rating: **Competent**

Financial: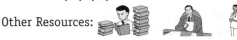

Time:

Personnel:

Other Resources:

Efficacy: **A**

Transferability: **B**

Malleability/Adaptability: **B**

Ease of Implementation: **C**

Synopsis: The Evidence-Based Practice Consultant Program is designed to use existing staff and create a group of EBP experts, able to be utilized in councils, committees, and task forces to facilitate the EBP process, and mentor and teach the process along the way. The consultants are members of the EBP Consultants Group, which meets monthly to discuss projects, progress, and problems, and addresses the continuing education needs of the group. This spider web of educating and mentoring staff on EBP and the EBP process creates an infrastructure for educating, utilizing, and disseminating EBP and the EBP process.

Description of Organization: See beginning of this chapter.

The Case Study: See beginning of this chapter.

Outcome Measures:

Formative/Compliance: Attendance in EBP classes monitored; EBP coordinator monitors attendance at monthly consultant meetings and progress in projects.

Summative/Outcome: Completion of class education; number of EBP projects completed; satisfaction of EBP Consultants and those that consult; anecdotal increase in EBP knowledge.

Evidence Supporting this Creative Solution: Arizona State University hosts a mentoring program in EBP (n.d.). Case studies of programs similar to this one utilizing a teaching/mentoring intervention to educate staff on EBP and the EBP process have shown success in the level of knowledge obtained and the successful completion of EBP projects (Cullen & Titler, 2004; Levin, 2006). The evidence for the value of teaching and mentoring to enable application of knowledge is plentiful and the credibility of these two methods for educating is well established.

Cullen, L., & Titler, M. G. (2004). Promoting evidence-based practice: An internship for staff nurses. *Worldviews on Evidence-Based Nursing, 1*(4), 215–223.

Levin, R. F. (2006). *Advancing research and clinical practice through close collaboration (ARCC): A pilot test of an intervention to improve evidence-based care and patient outcomes in a community health care setting.* Eastern Nursing Research Society Abstract. Available at: http://www.nursinglibrary.org/Portal/main.aspx?pageid=4024&pid=9083. Accessed July 30, 2009.

Recipe for: *The Evidence-Based Practice Consultants*

Ingredients:

1 EBP expert

5 to 7 BSN-prepared staff, willing to become EBP consultants

Staff buy-in

1 Program coordinator (could be the EBP Expert)

People to do education (EBP Expert may be able to do much of this)

Education plan

Classroom and supplies to teach

Secretarial support (optional, but very helpful)

Financial and time commitment from CNO, managers of staff involved and staff selected

Step-by-Step Instructions (see Figure 6-2 for Step-by-Step Instruction Timeline):

Step 1: Obtain support from CNO first, then from all nursing leadership. Work out issues of salary and time allotment for time spent in EBP Consultant role with CNO, and then get additional nursing leadership input and support.

Step 2: With EBP Expert, outline education necessary and create education plan with timeline for EBP Consultants. Identify who will teach what and obtain their commitment to teach.

Step 3: Advertise for staff RN volunteers for the program. Make the acceptance process somewhat selective based on education, skills, commitment, and availability. Emphasize the exclusivity and expertise of this group to get buy-in and set the expectation for excellence. Select 5 to 7 staff RNs for the program.

Step 4: Plan the classroom education (such as, room, supplies, people to teach, staff selected, etc.) and schedule the classes.

Step 5: Plan, in advance, what project you will assign each consultant to work on for the first exposure to an actual application of their education.

Step 6: Complete the classroom education. Award certificates for successful completion of the required education. You can present graduates with home-made business cards with title EBP Consultant. After successful completion of their first project, present new business cards with title Certified EBP Consultant. Can also make future educational/practice requirements to continue in-house certification as an EBP Consultant. All of this adds to the professionalism and expectation for excellence for the EBP consultants.

Step 7: Assign consultants to projects, committees, or task forces as appropriate. Set a schedule to meet as a group (such as monthly) to address issues. The EBP Expert will need to mentor the new consultants through their first project. These monthly meetings can be used for that purpose initially. It may help to do the mentoring in a consultant group atmosphere with individual mentoring session available as needed.

Step 8: After each consultant's first project, have them present the project and results to the group, noting what they have learned along the way. Have a small graduation ceremony: they are now in-house Certified EBP Consultants. Set up a mechanism for consultation. This can be done in many ways and according to the needs of the institution. All consults should go through the coordinator, so the program is adequately managed.

Step 9: Continue assigning projects and monitoring progress. This is the maintenance stage of the program. Can establish another class of EBP Consultants if necessary or as desired.

Figure 6-2   Timeline for "The Evidence-Based Practice Consultants."

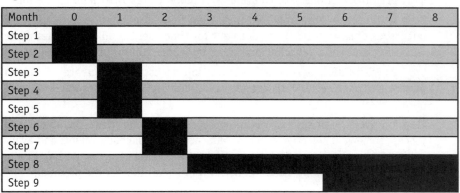

Additional Outcomes to Consider Measuring:

Formative/Compliance: No additional measures.

Summative/Outcome: No additional measures.

Insights from Original Implementation:

- CNO support is crucial to this initiative. Work out ahead of time how the consultants' salaries will be coded (i.e., nonproductive time) and how time allotment will be managed. Managers will need to know that the CNO supports this program to get their buy-in as well.
- Original hospital had two main EBP educators for this program, one a PhD, RN, knowledgeable about EBP and the EBP process, and the other was well versed in leadership education.
- Make sure that chosen staff have a firm commitment to the program, and have good availability. Staff should be aware that there are expectations of the role, and that the education is intense. Consider various methods to promote accountability, such as having consultants present interim progress reports to nursing leadership.

For Further Guidance Contact:

Bruce Alan Boxer, PhD, MBA, RN, CPHQ

bruceboxer@ymail.com

Creative Solution Title: *What Does Evidence-Based Practice Have to Do with Me?*

Creative Solution Author: **Samantha Abate, RN, BS, CCRN**
                                Assistant Nurse Manager, Cardiac ICU and
                                   Cardiac Step Down
                                South Jersey Healthcare, Vineland, NJ

Purpose: The goal is to make EBP real, valid, and tangible to staff nurses, and to increase buy-in and compliance with new EBP policies and procedures being implemented in the unit.

Legend

Overall Rating: **NOVICE**

Financial:

Time: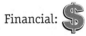

Personnel:

Other Resources: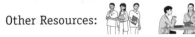

Efficacy: **A**

Transferability: **A**

Malleability/Adaptability: **A**

Ease of Implementation: **A**

Synopsis: "What Does Evidence-Based Practice Have to Do with Me?" is a binder created and utilized in Cardiac ICU to draw attention to how evidence-based practice really does impact nurses' day-to-day nursing care and activities. The binder contains each new policy and/or procedure and one short article that supports the change in practice as well as a short blurb written by a unit-based practice council (UBPC) member that ties the two together. The UBPC, with the support of the Nurse Manager, designed and implemented the binder as part of the Magnet journey.

Description of Organization: South Jersey Healthcare is a 467-bed, nonteaching, community health system consisting of three main hospital campuses and multiple outpatient satellite services. The organization received Magnet designation in February 2008 after a November 2007 survey. The creative solution was implemented in one unit, Cardiac ICU.

The Case Study: The UBPC leaders developed the idea after attending information sessions regarding EBP and meeting with the nurse manager regarding preparing for our Magnet journey. They wanted a creative way to disseminate what they had learned and the insight they had gained to their fellow staff nurses. The phrase "what does this have to do with me?" is commonly heard in response to new policies and procedures. The UBPC leaders realized the perceived disconnect between research and theory and the perception of day-to-day nursing activities and tasks, especially in an ICU setting. By titling the book after that phrase, the staff became curious about what EBP and research did actually have to do with them.

The information presented in the binder was kept short and to the point, and the evidence-based articles that were chosen were nursing and reader friendly. This project is ultimately maintained by the UBPC members, which consists of approximately six staff nurses who rotate preparing information for the binder. Basic computer skills are needed to do a literature search for an article and to prepare the summary. The nurse manager schedules time for staff to be able to work on this and other UBPC and Magnet journey projects. UBPC members, along with the Nurse Manager/Clinical Director and Clinical Nurse Specialist, identified topics for the binder. UBPC staff handled updating the binder with new topics as needed.

The binder is updated monthly or as needed. Preparing each new topic takes between 1 to 2 hours depending on how in-depth the topic is. A sign-in sheet is provided for each new topic that is added to the binder. Nurses are given in-service credit for reading the information contained in the binder, which is an incentive given that a new clinical ladder system (which requires in-service attendance) has also been implemented.

Staff nurses gained appreciation of the use of EBP in their day-to-day nursing practice. Engagement and buy-in for new projects was positively impacted. For example, compliance with pH testing of gastric tube drainage to confirm tube placement (vs confirming by air bolus auscultation) was improved and response times to rapid assessment team (RAT) calls shortened. We found that if staff understood why they were being asked to make these changes in practice, they not only got on board with the changes, they were more compliant in following the new policies and procedures.

Outcome Measures:

Formative/Compliance: Assistant manager checks book monthly to assure that updates are done.

Summative/Outcome: Sign-in sheets used to measure how many read article; better outcome of evidence-based projects; anecdotal increase in buy-in.

Evidence Supporting this Creative Solution: This creative solution has its base in Adult Learning Theory (Knowles, 1970). Learning must demonstrate real world application to be important and relevant to the adult learner. Answering the question "What does EBP have to do with me?" helps enhance this real world application.

Knowles, M. S. (1970). *The modern practice of adult education. Andragogy versus pedagogy.* Englewood Cliffs, NJ: Prentice Hall/Cambridge.

Recipe for: *What Does Evidence-Based Practice Have to Do with Me?*

Ingredients:

1 Binder

5 (approximately) BSN-prepared staff, willing to do literature searches

1 Manager/assistant manager to coordinate initiative

Time allowance for staff working on binder

Staff buy-in

Step-by-Step Instructions (see Figure 6-3 for Step-by-Step Instruction Timeline):

Step 1: Obtain support from the manager first. Work out issues of time allotment for time spent performing literature search.

Step 2: Purchase binder and gain commitment of staff members to work on the project (possibly provide some incentive or accountability). Assign coordinator (assistant manager) to monitor compliance with the initiative.

Step 3: Coordinator creates schedule for staff to update binder. Coordinator also creates process to disseminate new policies/procedures to members working on this project.

Step 4: Create binder using new policies with sign-in sheets for staff. Publicize new binder and the expectation that staff will read sheets (possibly provide incentive).

Step 5: Coordinator will monitor compliance with updating binder and number of staff reading sheets.

Figure 6-3   Timeline for "What Does Evidence-Based Practice Have to Do with Me?"

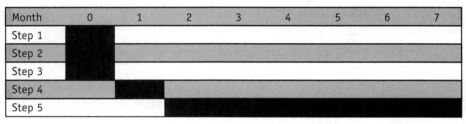

Month	0	1	2	3	4	5	6	7
Step 1								
Step 2								
Step 3								
Step 4								
Step 5								

Additional Outcomes to Consider Measuring:

Formative/Compliance: Quality of evidence placed in binder.

Summative/Outcome: Preimplementation knowledge of reason for specific policies/procedures and postimplementation knowledge to compare and determine if binder had an effect; staff satisfaction with binder.

Insights from Original Implementation:

- In the future we would like to also institute a bulletin board to make the information even more visible and accessible. A full binder can sometimes be as intimidating as the phrase evidence-based practice.
- In the future we will solicit topics from staff by asking them "Do you know why we do . . ."

For Further Guidance Contact:

Samantha Abate, RN, BS, CCRN

CCUSami@comcast.net

Creative Solution Title: *Evidence-Based Practice Process*

Creative Solution Author: Susan Langin WHNP-BC, MSN, RN
Advanced Practice Specialist
Holland Hospital, Holland, MI

Purpose: The goal of this creative solution was to develop an evidence-based process within the named organization that provides a framework for integration of evidence into all aspects of clinical practice. The vision was to assure that all patients would receive evidence-based care. The process was to be piloted in the nursing department with a long-term goal to disseminate to the entire system.

Legend

Overall Rating: **PROFICIENT**

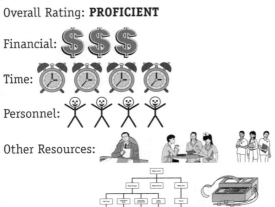

Financial:

Time:

Personnel:

Other Resources:

Efficacy: **A**

Transferability: **C**

Malleability/Adaptability: **C**

Ease of Implementation: **D**

Synopsis: Providing the highest quality of patient care is the nursing imperative and one of the strategic essentials at the named institution. Evidence-based practice (EBP) has shown substantially improved patient outcomes by providing the most appropriate intervention to the appropriate patient at the appropriate time. With a mission to promote a culture of inquiry and to create an environment for evidence-based change, the CNO commissioned a team to develop an evidence-based process within the existing organizational structure that provides a framework for integration of evidence into all aspects of clinical practice.

Description of Organization: Holland Hospital is currently a 209-bed, single, acute care hospital located in Southwestern Lower Michigan, in the city of Holland. Additional entities that constitute this system include Holland Home Health Services and the Lakeshore Medical Campus. In addition to the main campus where the majority of patient care services are provided, there are several off-campus locations where support services such as finance, information management, and marketing are housed. Other community-based services and patient service centers are in satellite locations as well. Holland Hospital consists of a broad array of inpatient and outpatient care departments along with crucial ancillary and support services. Each department provides a unique contribution to the care of patients we serve.

Holland Hospital provides services to a population of approximately 150,000 individuals from the identified primary service area. In 2008, Holland Hospital provided healthcare services for approximately 43,100 emergency department patients, over 28,600 prime care patients, and over 43,300 patient visits through Home Health Services. In addition, 18,000 babies were delivered in the Boven Birth Center and over 9200 inpatient and outpatient surgical procedures were performed. Holland Hospital was Magnet designated in 2007.

The Case Study and Evidence Supporting Creative Solution: It is well documented in the literature that the use of best evidence in clinical practice improves patient outcomes and increases patient satisfaction. Making EBP a sustained reality is, however, a difficult endeavor. This relates, among other factors, to the lack of research upon which to base implementation efforts, especially in a community hospital. The majority of research has been focused on barrier identification, implementation strategies to overcome barriers, models and frameworks. There is a lack of research designed to fully understand what it actually takes to successfully implement EBP. In an attempt to overcome this void and implement EBP, Holland Hospital developed an evidence-based practice process which included adaptation of model and framework, organizational readiness assessment, policy and procedure development, knowledge gap assessment, tool development, planned change, staged implementation, outcome measure identification, and sustainability plan development.

Essential to the development of an evidence-based process is a working definition of EBP that serves as the foundation for all educational and implementation strategies. This led to the adaption of the writing of Sackett et al. to define EBP as the conscientious, explicit, and judicious integration of best evidence with clinical expertise and patient values in making decisions about the care of patients.

There are multiple potential options and models after which to structure an EBP program. The choice is dependent on the goals and needs of the organization. Upon reviewing Holland Hospital's organizational goals, needs and values, the Rosswurm-Larabee model (Rosswurm & Larabee, 1999) was chosen. The primary components of this model are assessing the need for change, formulating a clinical question, and linking the problem with interventions and outcomes, synthesizing evidence to design a change in practice, and implementing, evaluating outcomes, and maintaining change in practice.

Organizational structure and environmental readiness are essential for the development of an EBP infrastructure. When organizations are financially stable and leaders provide the infrastructure and support, EBP will grow. Holland Hospital's assessment of their organizational structure revealed that they had the start of an infrastructure that would support EBP. The nursing department supports a shared governance model for clinical practice, which includes seven committees as well as unit-based teams. This structure embraces the councilor approach, which enhances the capability of working toward a common goal and embracing change. These committees, which are comprised of both staff nurses and nurse leaders are are the following: the Nursing Practice Executive Committee (NPEC), the Nursing Administration Committee (NAC), the Professional Advancement for Clinical Excellence (PACE) Committee, the Nursing Quality Improvement (NQI) Committee, the Clinical Education Team (CET), the Nursing Research Committee (NRC), the Evidence-Based Practice (EBP) Team, and Unit-Practice Teams (UPT). To enhance the infrastructure to support EBP, the purpose and function of the governance committees were reviewed and revised to integrate EBP. EBP was also included in the following: the definition of professional nursing practice at Holland Hospital, the nurses' job description, formal documents (e.g. policies), and strategic plans.

Leadership endorsement must be assured early in the building of an EBP program. Time and resource constraints are listed as one of the reasons for the failure to implement EBP. The nursing directors' support was critical to foster a work environment that promotes EBP, a budget and time for nurses to conduct EBP, and commitment to the strategic plan to build an EBP infrastructure. With an introduction of the initiative by the CNO, the nursing directors were provided with administrative support in their role regarding promotion of the vision, principals, and values of the project.

The literature indicates that many nurses are struggling, or lack the knowledge and skills to implement evidence-based care. As was demonstrated by our readiness assessment, many nurses lacked the knowledge or skill to assess and define a problem, formulate a question, search, critique, and synthesize the evidence. Addressing this barrier led to the development of a clinical decision tree and forms and tools to provide a guide to the steps of incorporating evidence into practice. Following a literature review, the forms and tools were developed based on the work of Newhouse, Dearholt, Poe, Pugh, and White (2007). These tools include the following: EBP Grid, Clinical Inquiry Worksheet, Clinical Inquiry Guide, Standard/Guideline Assessment Tool, Evaluation of Evidence, Evidence Evaluation Guide, Evidence-Based Practice Glossary, and Evidence Summary Worksheet. By providing a structure that guides the steps, identification of mentors, and tools and resources to assist the nurse to incorporate best evidence into practice, the growth and development of the program was fostered. A Unit-Based Practice Committee as well as the Clinical Education Team trialed the clinical decision tree and forms prior to implementation.

The EBP team and the Clinical Education Team developed multiple strategies for training and education for the directors, managers, and staff to gain a knowledge base of the EBP approach to nursing practice and to familiarize them with the structure and tools to assist them to incorporate best evidence into practice. This was implemented in fall of 2008. This was disseminated to the general nursing staff by a poster presentation at the nursing skills day, a presentation at Nursing Grand Rounds, and evaluation of evidence workshops that were conducted onsite by the EBP team and Clinical Education team. Through these workshops, the staff gained an understanding of formatting a specific clinical question, collecting the best evidence, critically appraising the evidence, integration of evidence, clinical expertise, and patient preferences to implement a decision and evaluate the outcomes. The directors, managers, and shared governance leadership were offered separate presentations that highlighted their roles. Mentors were also developed and made available on an as-needed basis for committees and unit-based practice teams.

The EBP activities that were determined to be measurable were nursing quality improvement projects, development of policies, and development of order sets. Within these activities, it was determined if the process and implementation of evidence-based practice was used, and then evidence summaries must be generated. Since the development of evidence summaries was new, the preimplementation data was zero. The expectation was that there would be four evidence summaries archived by March 31, 2009, (which was achieved) and 25 archived by March 31, 2010 (results not yet obtained). A policy audit to evaluate clinical nursing policies demonstrated that 75% of policies had references. Our goal is to increase this to 80% by January/February 2010. The audit also demonstrated that 53% of the policies with references were indicative of current evidence. The goal is to increase this to 75%.

Newhouse, R. P., Dearholt, S., Poe, S., Pugh, L. C., & White, K. M. (2007). Organizational change strategies for evidence-based practice. *Journal Of Nursing Administration, 37*(12), 552–557.

Rosswurm, M. A., & Larrabee, J. H. (1999). A model for change to evidence-based practice. *The Journal of Nursing Scholarship, 31*(4), 317–322.

Sackett, D. L., Rosenberg, W. M., Gray, J. A., Haynes, R. B., & Richardson, W. S. (1996). Evidence-based medicine: What it is and what it isn't. *BMJ, 312*(7023), 71–72.

Outcome Measures:

Formative/Compliance: Track number of nursing quality improvement projects, development of policies and development of order sets. Project/practice evidence summaries and policy reference audits.

Summative/Outcome: A survey will be conducted regarding nurses' knowledge of the use of EBP tools, location of tools, competency in appraising the literature, and mentor availability. The results of this survey will be used to continue education and integration of tool use into our process.

Evidence Supporting this Creative Solution:

See the preceding section, The Case Study and Evidence Supporting this Creative Solution.

Recipe for: *Evidence-Based Practice Process*

Ingredients:

CNO support

Advanced practice specialist team

Nursing directors/managers

Clinical education team

Computer with Web access

Step-by-Step Instructions (see Figure 6-4 for Step-by-Step Instruction Timeline):

Step 1: Adaptation of definition of EBP, EBP model, and framework.

Step 2: Assess organizational readiness assessment for development of EBP infrastructure.

Step 3: Assure leadership endorsement from CNO and nursing directors.

Step 4: Create budget allowing for nursing time to conduct EBP.

Step 5: Policy and procedure development and development of EBP tools and worksheets.

Step 6: Planned change and staged implementation including training and education of directors, managers, and staff offering information on EBP approach to nursing, EBP tools, and integration into practice.

Step 7: Outcome measurement identification.

Step 8: Sustainability plan development.

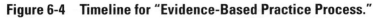

Figure 6-4   Timeline for "Evidence-Based Practice Process."

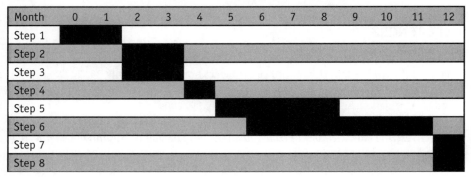

Additional Outcomes to Consider Measuring:

Formative/Compliance: No additional measures.

Summative/Outcome: No additional measures.

Insights from Original Implementation:

- Creating EBP infrastructure needs to be approached as an organizational strategy and change process.
- Implementation requires a strategic approach that includes multiple strategies.
- It is crucial to have nursing leaders buy-in and be given a role because they allocate resources that provide the necessary infrastructure to enable EBP.
- The most compelling barrier to the implementation is the need to provide the dedicated time for nurses to be away from their day-to-day clinical responsibilities to allow them to participate in this type of work.
- Initially, the support was present, but as we experienced the downward shift in the economy, we have had to reassess expectations and goals.
- Plan must be flexible to incorporate lessons learned to adapt the process to meet the needs of the nurses.
- Need to have a model and tools available.
- This is not a short-term endeavor.

For Further Guidance Contact:

Susan Langin, WHNP-BC, MSN, RN
Holland Hospital
602 Michigan Ave
Holland, MI 49423
suslan@hollandhospital.org

REFERENCES

Academic Center for Evidence-Based Practice (ACE). (2008). *ACE: Learn about EBP*. Available at: http://www.acestar.uthscsa.edu/Learn_model.htm. Accessed July 30, 2009.

Arizona State University (n.d.). *EBP mentorship tracks*. Available at: http://nursing.asu.edu/caep/mentorship/index.htm. Accessed July 30, 2009.

Bloom, B., Englehart, M. Furst, E., Hill, W., & Krathwohl, D. (1956). *Taxonomy of educational objectives: The classification of educational goals. Handbook I: Cognitive domain*. New York, Toronto: Longmans, Green.

Boxer, B. A., & Taylor, E. M. (2007). It starts at home: In-house consulting helps disseminate EBP. *Nursing Management, 38*(9), 41–45.

Brooten, D., Naylor, M. D., York, R., Brown, L. P., Munro, B. H., Hollingsworth, A. O., et al. (2002). Lessons learned from testing the quality cost model of advanced practice nursing (APN) transitional care. *Journal of Nursing Scholarship, 34*(4), 369–375.

Donabedian, A. (1980). *Explorations in Quality Assessment and Monitoring Vol. 1. The Definition of Quality and Approaches to Its Assessment.* Ann Arbor, MI: Health Administration Press.

Duke, S. B. (2006, June 12). *Eyewitness testimony doesn't make it true.* Available at: http://www.law.yale.edu/news/2727.htm. Accessed July 30, 2009.

Goode, C., Tanaka, D. J., Krugman, M., O'Connor, P. A., Bailey, C., Deutchman, M., et al. (2000). Outcomes from use of an evidence-based practice guideline, *Nursing Economics, 18*(4), 202–207.

Hamer, S., & Collinson, G. (2003). *Achieving evidence-based practice. A handbook for practitioners.* Philadelphia, PA: Elsevier Science Limited.

Heater, B., Becker, A., & Olson, R. (1988). Nursing interventions and patient outcomes: A meta-analysis of studies. *Nursing Research, 37*(5), 303–307.

Institute for Johns Hopkins Nursing. (n.d.) *Johns Hopkins Nursing and evidence-based practice.* Available at: http://www.ijhn.jhmi.edu/contEd_3rdLevel_Class.asp?id=EvidBasedHome&numContEdID=4. Accessed July 30, 2009.

Leatherman, S., Berwick, D., Iles, D., Lewin, L. S., Davidoff, F., Nolan, T., et al. (2003). The business case for quality: Case studies and an analysis. *Health Affairs, 22*(2), 17–30.

Melnyk, B. M., & Fineout-Overholt, E. (2005). *Evidence-based practice in nursing and healthcare: A guide to best practice.* Philadelphia: Lippincott Williams & Wilkins.

Melnyk, B. M., Fineout-Overholt, E., Stone, P. & Acherman, M. (2000) Evidence-based practice: the past, the present, and recommendations for the millennium. *Pediatric Nursing, 26*(1), 77–80.

Newhouse, R., Dearholt, S., Poe, S., Pugh, L. C., & White, K. M. (2005). Evidence-based practice: A practical approach to implementation. *Journal Of Nursing Administration, 35*(1), 35–40.

Newhouse, R. P., Dearholt, S. L., Poe, S. S., Pugh, L. C., & White, K. M. (2007). *Johns Hopkins nursing evidence-based practice model and guidelines.* Sigma Theta Tau International.

Pfeffer, J., & Sutton, R. I. (2006). Evidence-based management. *Harvard Business Review, 84*(1), 63–74.

Pravikoff, D. S., Tanner, A. B., & Pierce, S. T. (2005). Readiness of U.S. nurses for evidence-based practice. *American Journal of Nursing, 105*(9), 40–51.

Rich, J. B., Speir, A. M., Fonner, E., & the Virginia Cardiac Surgery Quality Initiative (2006). Making a business case for quality for regional information sharing involving cardiothoracic surgery. *American Heart Hospital Journal, 4*(2), 142–147.

Sackett, D. L., Richardson, W. S., Rosenberg, W., & Haynes, R. B. (1997). *Evidence-based medicine: How to practice and teach EBM.* New York: Churchill Livingstone.

Shorten, A., & Wallace, M. (1997). Evidence-based practice. When quality counts. *Australian Nursing Journal, 4*(11), 26–27.

Stevens, K. R. (2004). *ACE Star Model of EBP: Knowledge Transformation. Academic Center for Evidence-based Practice*. The University of Texas Health Science Center at San Antonio. Available at: www.acestar.uthscsa.edu. Accessed March 9, 2010.

Titler, M. G., Kleiber, C., Steelman, V., Rakel, B., Budreau, G., Everett, L. Q., et al. (2001). The Iowa model of evidence-based practice to promote quality care. *Critical Care Nursing Clinics of North America, 13*(4), 497–509.

University of Iowa Hospitals and Clinics (2009). *The Iowa model of evidence-based practice*. Available at: http://www.uihealthcare.com/depts/nursing/rqom/evidencebasedpractice/iowamodel.html. Accessed July 30, 2009.

## CHAPTER 7

Involving Everyone in Research

"Research is to see what everybody else has seen,
and to think what nobody else has thought."
—ALBERT SZENT-GYORGYI

"Somewhere, something incredible is waiting to be known."
—DR. CARL SAGAN

Everybody loves a party. At least that is what they thought when the Research Council at South Jersey Healthcare in Vineland, NJ, took on the task of getting more nurses aware of and involved in nursing research. Research Day was fast approaching, a day when, for the previous 2 years, the Research Council sponsored a one-day, in-house research conference. In the past, the conference mostly focused on nursing quality projects with a spattering of nursing research. But they were a bit more sophisticated now, and understood that without true nursing research, evidence-based practice would not be possible. That year would be the year that nursing research took center stage. Nursing quality would have its own day sponsored by the Nursing Quality Council later in the year.

A brainstorming session resulted in a themed Nursing Research Day with a poster contest targeted toward the development of research questions to booster awareness and knowledge of nursing research. Internal speakers discussed their nursing research and external speakers presented their nursing research, demonstrating the various types of nursing research conducted. The poster contest had entrants design a poster with the same sections as are found in a standard research proposal, facilitating the process of developing the research idea into a true research study and presenting the idea to the audience.

The theme? Let us just say that it was held the last week of October. Yes, Halloween. Their title for the conference, "Don't Let Research Scare You!" was a great way to make the topic fun and to convey that this conference was geared toward those uninitiated to nursing research. The venue was complete with Halloween décor, and of course, costumes were encouraged. Awards were presented to the best costumes as well as the best posters. The day was an overwhelming success with more attendance than in previous years, great reviews from staff, and five posters presented developed into actual nursing research projects. Now they have to top this next year!

OH NO . . . RESEARCH

The discipline of medicine, and therefore nursing, is ever changing. We can never think all we need to know we learned in nursing school. How do we acquire more knowledge as we move forward in our nursing careers? Of course, we need to read: textbooks, journals, and Internet medical sites. We can also attend continuing education courses and seminars. But how do we not only acquire new knowledge for ourselves, but also discover new information and answers to questions not addressed in current literature? In a word, research.

Most acute healthcare institutions have some form of research being conducted. Typically, it is medical research initiated by a corporation, such as a pharmaceutical vendor. The research activities are carried out by a research coordinator, usually a nurse, and overseen by a physician. Most often these activities go unnoticed by the general nursing population of the institution. Only the few involved in the care of a patient enrolled in the study are privy to the study information or even know the study is being conducted. Research lacks publicity. The queries prompting research, the process of research, and the information produced by it is not disseminated well throughout all levels of health care. Getting more people involved, such as nurses and even ancillary staff, in research will engender interest in the subject matter of individual studies as well as the process of investigating and discovering new knowledge that may enhance practice.

Nursing research is essential to the growth of the nursing profession, not to mention to the safe and effective treatment of patients. The ultimate goal of all professions is to improve the practice of its members and the effectiveness of its services. Nursing continually strives to be viewed as a respected profession. To enhance professional stature, continual development of a scientific body of knowledge is fundamental. The emergence of such a body of knowledge is instrumental in fostering commitment and accountability to the profession's clientele. Creating and extending a distinct body of knowledge will allow nursing to separate itself from other healthcare professions and better develop and define its unique role and importance in patient outcomes.

Nursing research has greatly evolved over the past century. Research in the first half of the 20th century focused on nursing education. In the 1950s, nurses researched themselves, looking to define the role and its purposes. The 1960s provided the development of nursing theories and frameworks. The 1970s introduced a change in nursing research from emphasis on education, administration, recruitment, and nurses themselves to improving patient care and the need for a scientific base from which to practice (Polit & Hungler, 1995). Today, we are still striving to improve, expand, and especially disseminate the scientific, research-based body of knowledge in nursing. All of nursing education, theory, and practice must adopt and adhere to the use of research-based information and practices (Burnes & Grove, 2001).

NURSING RESEARCH AS A PRIORITY

The need to make research and research-based care a priority in medicine and nursing has become overwhelmingly apparent in the last decade as hospitals began focusing on outcomes measurement (Harrington, 2006). Using improved patient outcomes as a motivation for nursing research necessitates a change in the paradigm of nursing research. Historically, hospital-based nursing research was pursued by nursing faculty from associated universities. The interests of academic researchers did not typically involve topics from everyday patient care. There was, and in many areas, still is, a disconnect between research studies and applicability of the information they produce in the hospital setting. Nursing researchers worked to increase the body of nursing knowledge and create, prove, or disprove abstract nursing theories. Although these are valid and important goals for research, they do not impart a great effect in the clinical setting. This is the difference between basic and applied nursing research.

BASIC AND APPLIED NURSING RESEARCH

Whereas basic nursing research is pursued to gain new knowledge without regard for the utility of the information, applied nursing research is pragmatic. It investigates questions and generates information that can be implemented into everyday patient care. Applied nursing research helps fill the gap between traditional research and practice (Harrington, 2006). Applied research does not take the place of evidence-based practice, it is a precursor to it. Applied research is the foundation upon which evidence-based practice is built. It generates practical information and strives to answer everyday clinical questions, but the actual implementation of study findings will still need to follow the evidence-based practice process (see Chapter 6).

Applied research typically is better aligned with the vision and mission of most hospitals and therefore is better accepted by administration and more easily integrated into nursing staff activities, which will be discussed further when the goals of a research program are discussed. If research topics address everyday nursing issues, research will gain the interest of the staff who endure the effects of such issues and will therefore lend to staff buy-in. It will also create the impetus for staff generated research questions and projects, the results of which can be readily integrated into practice, and the cycle continues. Research then is part of the institution's culture, the ones doing the research will also be the ones using the research (Harrington, 2006). The gap between research and practice continues to shrink as the involvement of front line practitioners grows.

As nurses, we know that every day involved in patient care or coordination of healthcare services conjures questions. A great deal of what we do as nurses is based on previous personal experience or traditions handed down from senior nurses. Although using tradition in practice offers some advantages such as efficiency, in that each individual does not have to start from scratch in their attempt to know and understand how something works or is done. Tradition allows us to not have to reinvent the wheel each time a patient care task is initiated. Tradition also provides accepted truths and may facilitate communication (Burns & Grove, 2001). However, many traditions have never been tested or validated.

In today's healthcare environment, where quality and evidence-based practice is paramount, nursing care can no longer be guided by untested stories from nursing past. Those stories, however, should not just be thought of as folklore and discarded. They can be tested to evaluate if what we think works really does work. A research project can be created and undertaken to measure outcomes when such practices are used. It can be initially a small pilot study including a small number of patients in one hospital unit and, if results are positive, the study population can be expanded. It could be the birth of a new standard of care.

Although we know that research should be the basis of all we do in health care, only a small percentage of nursing processes are research or evidence based. Nurses typically are not comfortable with the task of research. Research is often feared and thought to be a tumultuous feat. This daunting nature of research causes many important questions to go unanswered. Posing a question is the beginning. It truly is that simple. Nurses need to know that research need not be an exercise only undertaken by physicians, those with advanced degrees, or commercial institutions. Research can and should occur at every level in health care. Nursing leaders, director, managers, and educators must create a milieu in which all nursing staff feel free to question practice, voice opinions and observations, and generate researchable ideas (Ravert & Merill, 2008). A framework must then be provided to study these ideas and incorporate research into practice.

DEFINITION OF RESEARCH

What word comes to mind when you think of research? Possibly, the word experiment. You might envision a laboratory with precisely measured substances, calibrated instruments, and a scientist with a long, white lab coat. Yes, that is the picture of research, but only one type of research: basic research or bench research, as it is commonly called. In nursing, we rarely participate in bench research, but we can work to bring the information from that research to the bedside. There are several other research modalities that are used throughout the scientific community and in health care, which might be utilized to convert that basic research into applied research as we discussed a bit earlier in this chapter. Applied research is that usable research that allows us to take the newly found information and use it in the execution of patient care. So, now we need to examine all of the types of research we may use in nursing so that the type that best fits your topic of inquiry, study population, institution, and need for easy application can be chosen. Okay, so get ready to rewind back to that research class we all had to withstand in nursing school. The information might be a bit dry, but it is necessary to reach the common goal of beneficence that is central to research, as well as nursing.

Merriam-Webster defines research as a "studious inquiry or examination; investigation or experimentation aimed at the discovery and interpretation of facts, revision of accepted theories or laws in the light of new facts, or practical application of such new or revised theories or laws" ("Research," 2009). Research is an intellectual exercise undertaken to investigate a query, a problem, or a general subject matter. It is the process of collecting information about a particular subject, a method of acquiring new knowledge and correcting, refining, enhancing, validating and/or integrating prior knowledge. Research is frequently used in health care to discover, interpret, and develop methods of, and advancement in, the diagnosis, treatment, and management of patients as well as advancement in healthcare systems that support patient management. The root meaning of the word research is "search again" or "examine carefully" (Burns & Grove, 2001). In all healthcare arenas, as in nursing, it is imperative to carefully and critically examine all new practices before they are adopted and then reexamine them routinely for continued safety and effectiveness, and evaluate and reevaluate current practices to assure and enhance the quality of patient care. The most effective means of doing this is (yes, you guessed it) research. Whether it be a chart review or a series of patient interviews, in nursing, we must use a methodological system to evaluate and validate what we do, how we do it, why we do it, and if it works.

Research is a quest for answers and the journey must follow a prescribed path. Healthcare research must be scientific, but not necessarily experimental. The strict definition of scientific research is performing a methodical study in order to prove a hypothesis or to answer a specific question. It must be systematic and follow a series of steps and a standard protocol. Scientific research must be organized and undergo planning, including performing literature reviews of past research and evaluating what questions still need to be answered (Ravert & Merrill, 2008).

QUANTITATIVE RESEARCH VS QUALITATIVE RESEARCH

Scientific research is primarily either quantitative or qualitative. Both of which are frequently used in health care and can have great influence on nursing processes, but are very different in their purpose and conduct. Inherent in the name, quantitative research primarily uses numerical data and statistical analysis. This design calls for minimal researcher influence and great researcher control over the variables in the study so that extraneous factors do not influence the study outcome. This contributes to the rigor that we associate with quantitative studies and why it is known as the hard science (Polit & Hungler, 1995). A quantitative design is utilized for the purpose of comparing one thing (independent variable) to another thing (dependent variable). It simply quantifies relationships among variables with a goal of establishing associations between variables or causality. Once the relationships are understood, the goal is to be able to make generalizations about the masses regarding those relationships (Hopkins, 2000). So, if you want to evaluate the effect of nutritional education (independent variable) on blood glucose control (dependent variable) in Type II diabetics, a quantitative design would be your best modality. Or, if you want to compare the efficacy of smoking cessation counseling versus the nicotine patch, again quantitative is the way to go.

Qualitative research, on the other hand, is focused on meaning and the human experience. It is well aligned with nursing philosophy and practice, and has been used frequently by nurse researchers. Qualitative research uses observation, subject dialogue, and description. It collects subjective information with little or no investigator control. Qualitative data is in the form of words, and analysis is organization and categorization of the findings to support a meaningful theory about the phenomena being studied (Shuttleworth, 2008). It is the touchy-feely method of research, requiring the investigator to be a good, empathetic listener, which has given it the nickname the soft science (Polit & Hungler, 1995). Although quantitative research is thought to be more rigorous and robust, some research questions require a more informal method of investigation. A qualitative method is necessary to investigate issues such as how working mothers of young children cope with the demands of work and home, or how cardiac patients experience the ICU setting after cardiac surgery. Qualitative research is often a prelude to quantitative research. It helps to generate ideas that then will help create a realistic, testable hypothesis to be quantitatively evaluated.

JUDGING RESEARCH

All evidence is not created equal. Study results are only as good as the study that produced them. A good study is one that has an appropriate number of subjects, a design that minimizes the influence of the investigators, and control over environmental factors that might affect the variables. The goal of most studies is validity and believability of the results. In other words, are the results true and can they be applied to others outside of the study group? The research method used dictates these factors. Bias and chance are two concepts that define the validity and believability of a study. The study construct should allow for a little researcher opinion and emotion, which could create bias, and should work to eliminate extraneous factors from influencing the study results so that they do not occur only by chance, but are a direct product of the variables being studied.

The hierarchy of evidence rates and positions study designs based on these factors. Quantitative studies are best at minimizing bias and most feature great researcher control over variables to restrict chance from affecting the results. Qualitative studies, in their design, actually allow for researcher opinion and emotion, and therefore invite bias. As said before, there is little or no researcher control in these studies which is also purposeful, as the goal is to elicit as much subject dialogue as possible without restraint (Shuttleworth, 2008). So, qualitative design is a necessary tool in healthcare research, but it does fall short on the hierarchy of evidence. Quantitative designs are paramount in the hierarchy and qualitative typically are ranked at the bottom of the pyramid (Sutherland, 2001). However, there are many different types of quantitative and qualitative study designs all with their place in the hierarchy, again, depending upon the amount of bias and chance they allow. The magnitude of different study constructs is too great for us to review all of them in this text. We will discuss a few of the most popular or common designs, but it is advisable to have a good, easily read, nursing research text on hand to consult when a research study is being born so you can select the design that best suits your research question, study population, and resources. This will also help in becoming familiar enough with the designs to be able to accurately evaluate a completed research study, such as those published in scholarly journals, and critique them for validity and believability before you take the study's message and implement it into your practice.

RESEARCH DESIGNS

So, now let us review some types of designs and see how they rank. First, let us touch on the different quantitative designs. Quantitative studies are either experimental or descriptive. The experimental design (randomized, controlled, double-blind) is considered the gold standard in validity and believability. These studies always involve a treatment and compare the effects in different groups or the pretreatment and posttreatment effects on the same group. True experimental studies have randomization of subjects, meaning they are randomly chosen and/or randomly placed into study groups (i.e., treatment group or placebo group), which minimizes the chance that the study groups are not representative of the general population. They also provide control over extraneous influencing factors, which is usually gained by strict inclusion and exclusion criteria for study entrance as well as blinding of the subjects and possibly researchers (in a double-blind study) to who gets what treatment in the study. This study design offers the greatest amount of regulation of bias and factors that might influence the variables so that causality between the variables being studied can be accurately examined and chance eliminated (Hopkins, 2000). So, randomized, controlled, and double-blind studies are the crème de la crème on the hierarchy. These are typically medical studies; for example, drug studies in which a new medication is compared to placebo for safety and effectiveness.

Studies that lack either the randomization or the control aspect are called quasi-experimental studies. These are studies that might allow some bias or chance, as it may not be feasible or ethical to manipulate one or more of the variables in order to eliminate these factors (Burns & Grove, 2001). So, quasi-experimental design falls down to second place in the hierarchy of evidence.

Descriptive, or observational as they are also called, quantitative designs do not involve a treatment or intervention, but examine things (variables) as they are. A case study is the simplest descriptive study type. It reports data on only one subject. These are usually involving a subject with an extraordinary, rare medical condition, or a unique institutional issue. Descriptive studies of a few similar cases are called a case series. These are the weakest of the quantitative designs on the hierarchy of evidence as they do not provide any control to eliminate bias or chance, and they typically involve small numbers of subjects so that the results are not very applicable to the general public (Hopkins, 2000).

Another commonly used descriptive design is cross-sectional. In this type of study, a specific group of subjects are examined once for exposure to a causative factor or treatment and the existence of a condition and the relationships between them are determined. In healthcare research, it looks at specific factors and the health issues or medical conditions they might cause. This type of study cannot determine cause and effect. It only establishes relationships. An example would be examining a group of women who had low birth weight babies and evaluating if they drank alcohol while they were pregnant. This obviously is not as rigorous as an experimental trial and therefore falls only above a case study in the hierarchy of evidence.

Next are retrospective or case-control studies and prospective or cohort studies. Retrospective or case-control studies compare subjects with a particular characteristic, such as coronary artery disease, with control subjects without that characteristic. A comparison is made regarding possible exposure to something that may have caused the characteristic in the case/study group, for example, in this case, obesity. Case-control studies are also called retrospective as they focus on conditions in the past that might have caused subjects to become cases rather than controls (Burns & Grove, 2001). Case-control studies, just like cross-sectional, are above case studies in the hierarchy as they are only reliable in determining if a relationship between variables does not exist. They are not a strong enough construct to determine causality between variables, but might be a good place to start.

Prospective cohort studies are better at controlling extraneous factors and showing cause and effect and therefore rank higher, just under experimental design. In prospective/cohort studies some variables are evaluated at the beginning of the study, such as dietary habits and then after a period of time, the outcomes are determined such as the incidence of heart disease in the group. So, an exposure, treatment, or causative factor is known at the outset of the study and then subjects are divided in groups or cohorts based on if they have been exposed, treated, or not. The cohorts are then followed forward in time to determine if they develop a certain outcome. Although these studies rank below experimental ones, prospective cohort studies are typically less difficult, less expensive and might be more ethically acceptable than the experimental design as they do not withhold a potentially beneficial treatment from one group.

Another prospective design is that of longitudinal studies. In this type of study, one group is evaluated at several points in time over an extended period of months or years. An example is the Framingham Heart Study. This is an expensive and difficult type of study to undertake because of the time commitment required (Hopkins, 2000). There is often bias in the selection of subjects as they must be chosen on the basis of how long they will be able to be studied. Therefore, longitudinal studies rank a bit below cohort studies in the hierarchy.

Correlational studies are another means of examining relationships between variables. They look at variables that already exist to determine how they are related. They do not look at cause and effect. They are quantitative studies in that they use scoring to uncover a positive or negative relationship between the variables (Burns & Grove, 2001). For example, a comparison of income and education level could be accomplished by a correlational study. It has been shown by such studies that these two variables are positively correlated, meaning that as income increases, so does education level. Correlational studies also often explore the statistical connection between diseases in different population groups. For example, they might correlate death rates by country with estimates of exposure to certain pollutants that are common to that area. The result is typically a generalization about the variables' relationships. They employ no control or manipulation of the variables so bias and chance are not controlled, placing this type of study low in the hierarchy.

The only studies that are thought to rank above experimental, randomized, controlled studies are systematic reviews and meta-analyses. These studies combine information from all relevant trials examining the same research question. A meta-analysis is a systematic review in which the results from all of the trials included are combined statistically (Burns & Grove, 2001). Systematic reviews are actually observational, retrospective studies. So you ask how this can rank higher than an experimental trial? Well, when you combine many experimental studies looking at the same topic, you increase the sample size, which decreases the possibility of chance causing the results and increases the applicability of the results. Also, scientific methods are used in the analysis to control bias.

So, there obviously are many options when a quantitative study is your means of study. Again, the choice of which research method to use must be based on your topic of study, the variables being included, your resources available, including time available, and your hypothesis or proposed study outcome.

QUALITATIVE RESEARCH FRAMEWORKS

There are also several qualitative study frameworks. The commonly used qualitative designs are ethnographic, phenomenologic, grounded theory, historic, philosophic, and critical social theory research (Burns & Grove, 2001). We will just briefly review the goals and possible application of each design.

Ethnographic research was developed and mostly used by the discipline of anthropology. This examines and investigates cultures. Its goal is to tell the story of people's daily lives within the culture of which they are a part and develop a theory of cultural behavior so that we can understand the impact culture has on human behavior and health.

Phenomenologic research is just what it sounds like, the study of phenomena, typically phenomena regarding human behavior. It studies how each person experiences specific issues or events in their lives. The experience is recorded and then interpreted by the researcher (Burns & Grove, 2001). So, the data are the researcher's interpretation of and reflections on the participants' experiences. This is an appropriate method to study how people experience health and illness.

Grounded theory research is an inductive type of research, based on observations that are used to formulate a theory about the relationships among variables. It uses a variety of data sources, including quantitative data, review of records, interviews, observation, and surveys (Burns & Grove, 2001). It can be used to evaluate an individual patient situation, a healthcare program, or even an entire healthcare delivery system.

Historic research is an analysis of events that occurred in the recent or remote past. It is a means to evaluate past mistakes to improve and prevent them from occurring in the future (Burns & Grove, 2001). In nursing, it might be used as a means to better understand the discipline and factors that have affected nurses and nursing practice to direct improvements and enhance the future of the profession.

Philosophic research uses intellectual analyses to clarify definitions, study the nature of knowledge, identify values and ethics, or make a value judgment concerning an issue in a specific field of study. Philosophic questions guide the research. The analysis is done by literature exploration, creating questions regarding an issue, and proposing answers and then suggesting implications of those answers (Burns & Grove, 2001).

Finally, critical social theory provides an understanding of how people communicate and develop symbolic meanings in society. It investigates distortions, constraints, and imbalances in society that affect how people participate (Burns & Grove, 2001). In health care, it can uncover inequalities in care such as access to health care and might affect policy and public practices.

With the option of all of the above research modalities, it is obvious that any question or patient care issue can be molded into a research project. Once the question is composed, the means to finding the answer are defined in the research process.

THE RESEARCH PROCESS

The research process can be easily aligned with the nursing process. It incorporates similar steps and logic. Both utilize critical thinking and complex reasoning to evaluate and identify new information, discover relationships, and make predictions about what is or might occur. Both processes can be described in a sequence of five steps. First in the research process is creating a research question. In order to create a question, you must evaluate and assess a situation, process, group, or healthcare modality to uncover an issue that needs to be addressed or an unanswered question regarding the relationship of variables within the situation, process, group, or healthcare modality. That issue is what is formulated into a question that can be further analyzed. In the second step of the research process, the topic from which the question was derived must be carefully researched. This is typically by means of a literature review so that you can learn as much about the phenomena to be studied as possible and evaluate what studies have already been done and their outcomes (Zimmerman-Jones, 2009).

In nursing, we first assess a patient to gather all the necessary information about his or her current state in order to move to the second step of the nursing process, which is diagnosis of a problem (American Nurses Association, 2009). Can you see the connection? Next, in the research process, you must formulate a hypothesis, basically a guess about what the answer to your question will be. This hypothesis is based on all of the information that has been gathered thus far. It is a supposition about the cause of, effect on, or relationships between the phenomena to be studied. Your hypothesis will assist in planning your means of study and choosing your research design (Zimmerman-Jones, 2009). In nursing, once a diagnosis is found, a course of action is planned for patient care to deal with or treat that diagnosis (ANA). Then care is implemented. Likewise, in research, after the hypothesis is generated and study type planned, the hypothesis is tested. This is when the study is actually carried out (Zimmerman-Jones). Of course, any good nurse, after implementing care, then evaluates the patient again to see the outcome of the treatment and if it was successful. In research, this is done by the final step of the research process, which is analyzing the data. The analysis is done to see if the hypothesis can be supported or refuted (Zimmerman-Jones). Even if the hypothesis is not supported by the study's outcomes, the analysis can generate further research questions so the process continues and a new research project is created. This cycle should always continue as, especially in health care, information is not static. People, environments, and processes are forever changing and will always need to be analyzed for better understanding.

In a nutshell, the research process is a scientific method for formal investigation of phenomena: an issue, problem, or question. It prescribes activities to minimize the bias and prejudice of the investigator (Zimmerman-Jones, 2009). The issue, problem, or question identified in the healthcare arena, might be clinical, administrative, or ethical. It might involve one unit in a hospital or the entire nursing workforce.

Using the Research Process

So, let us focus and look carefully at how to tackle a research project using the research process. We will use an example to illustrate the process. Suppose you are an employee health nurse in a large hospital. You have worked in this position for more than 10 years. You notice that there has been what seems like an increase in the number of positive PPDs recently and you wonder why. Well, there could be several possible reasons. Is there an increase in the number of people being tested? Is there a patient in the hospital who is infected with tuberculosis, but not diagnosed or appropriately isolated? Is there a staff member who has become unknowingly infected and exposing coworkers? Have there been errors in test interpretation? Have the testing solutions changed? All of these questions are valid, but how can you go about answering them? Yes, research! But, you must first create your research question. It needs to be focused and cannot include all of the preceding questions. To narrow things down, you can first do a simple review of the employee health database to see if in fact the number of positive PPDs has increased and you can also determine in what timeframe this occurred to help focus your research even more. So, let us say the number has increased within the last year. Now you still need to find out why. It would be almost impossible to determine if there is an undiagnosed TB patient in the hospital or staff member and you would know if any of those with a positive PPD had active disease as they would have had further testing. So, what else could be the cause? How about the testing solutions? Does the solution used have any impact on the test results? This can be your research question. Because there are two different solutions used for PPDs, and in your preliminary research and literature review you found that one (solution X) has a higher false positive rate than the other. So, your hypothesis is, the number of positive PPDs has increased secondary to the use of solution X.

The first three steps of the research process are already completed. A research question was created after the topic of interest was narrowed by doing some preliminary investigation and eliminating some questions that would be difficult or impossible to answer. With the introductory, small-scale research project that you will be pursuing, a literature review was done to gather more information about the topic, and from that information a hypothesis was created.

Now it is time to plan the study. You need to choose a study design. All of that not so exciting information about quantitative and qualitative studies that was reviewed now becomes important. You need to think about how you can best answer your initial question. You must consider your budget, timeframe, personnel resources, and from where you will be gathering your data. Because the topic of interest involves a specific product and the results (positive or negative) that occur after the product is used, a quantitative study would fit best. Although it is possible to utilize an experimental design for this study, randomization, and blinding of the participants and/or researcher would be difficult, time intensive and an expensive endeavor for a solo researcher with a full-time job that does not include research in the job description. Also, PPDs are not routinely offered to the general population. It is a screening method for those at high risk for TB such as the immunocompromised, residents of areas where TB is endemic, and public service workers, which of course includes healthcare workers. So, you would not be able to gather subjects from the general population and you have an appropriate population at your fingertips, the employees at your hospital.

Healthcare workers from a specific hospital who have had PPD screening is a cross-section of the population, so a cross-sectional design could work, but because you have existing records of the screening and results of these healthcare workers, some with a positive (case) result and some negative (control), a retrospective, case-control design would be appropriate and not terribly difficult or costly. So, you can review all of the employee health screening records from the past 12 months. Those with a positive PPD will be your cases and those with negative PPDs will be the controls and you will then extract from the records which solution was used to perform the test. Of course, before accessing those records you will need to write a study proposal and submit it in a prescribed form to the Internal Review Board (IRB), which is described in detail later. After the study proposal is reviewed (and hopefully accepted) you can get started. You will not need much in the way of financial support as chart reviews will not incur much cost, but you might want to recruit a few people from your department to help with the chart reviews and data collection.

So, if they do not volunteer, you might need to offer a little incentive. You can petition your department for financial support, showing the positive effect of knowing if solution X is causing an increase in positive and possibly false positive PPDs in hospital employees, which will incur more cost for the institution, not to mention stress and possibly health effects if prophylactic medication is taken by these employees. You will have to name the people working on the study with you before submitting to the IRB, so that all those that will have access to the private, protected information of the subjects will be identified and approved. You will not need to consent each individual subject with this type of study design, hopefully the IRB will agree, as you are not implementing any treatment or altering care, but simply reviewing records. You must be sure to not identify the subjects when collecting or reporting the data. Now the data will be collected and your hypothesis tested.

Next, you will need to analyze the data with (yes, you knew it was coming) statistics. As it is way beyond this text, we will not review statistical analysis, but again a good research text can be of great help. You can do the analysis yourself with the assistance of a statistics computer program such as Excel, or you can recruit the assistance of a statistician, which might incur more costs. Once the results are uncovered, if supported, this can be used to petition a change in practice and have solution X no longer used for PPD screening at your institution and then you might bring this to a higher level, such as to the attention of the CDC. If your hypothesis is not supported, do not fret, you can evaluate your data and study design, and possibly continue with another study expanding on the possibilities that might be causing your initial observation.

NURSING RESEARCH PROGRAM DESIGN

As Magnet designation is being sought by many hospitals to prove the superior status of their nursing staff, it is becoming evident that in a large number of those hospitals nursing research is lacking. Nursing research is a requirement for achieving Magnet designation and therefore nursing research programs are now frequently being implemented (Turkel, Ferket, Reidinger, & Beatty, 2008). Aside from the Magnet journey, the drive for quality, evidence-based nursing is paramount in today's healthcare environment especially with scrutiny of the Centers for Medicare and Medicaid Services (CMS). Nursing research evaluates direct patient care measures and works to improve them by implementing research findings as appropriate to improve quality of nursing care and patient outcomes. Nursing research occurs infrequently if there is not a formal nursing research initiative within the hospital, hence, the birth of nursing research programs. A hospital-based nursing research program typically begins with and is driven by a nursing research council (NRC).

The council should include a leader or director, who might be an advanced practice nurse or ideally a doctorally prepared nurse with experience and interest in clinical nursing research. The research director might be active in an adjoining university and dedicate part-time hours to the research program or, as the program progresses, this may become a full-time position within the hospital. If a doctorally prepared nurse is not available on a full-time basis to chair the council, the institution might contract one as a consultant (Ravert & Merrill, 2008). Other members of the council are clinical nurse managers, nurse educators, or staff nurses representing each clinical area in the hospital, and possibly a librarian and ideally an instructor or representative from a partnering college or university (UNC Healthcare, 2009).

In many institutions, the nursing research program is created under the direction of the chief nursing officer/executive (CNO/CNE). The NRC should either include the CNO/CNE as a member on the council, or at least must maintain a good working relationship with the CNO/CNE as this is the person who will have most success lobbying hospital administration for staff and financial support (Turkel et al., 2008). Ad hoc members should also be invited. They could include other healthcare professionals that are involved with clinical research projects and staff from a clinical setting in which a project is being conducted or implemented (UNC Healthcare, 2009). They may offer insight when a project is being reviewed for approval. It is also helpful to open the council to interdisciplinary personnel as they could be a resource for project creation, conduct, and implementation. This also allows nursing to build a strong relationship with all disciplines, which is necessary to positively affect overall patient outcomes.

Although nursing research programs typically do not have any physician involvement, it might behoove the council to have a physician who is involved in and an advocate of research to serve as a resource for clinical information that could impact a nursing research protocol and also for additional lobbying support for funding. Once well established, the research program might want to integrate commercial research projects and possibly partner with medicine on some projects to maintain staff interest and financial viability. Nursing involvement in commercially funded research will provide experience with the research process and might translate into the initiation of independent nursing research.

As nursing research expands, the council might develop into a Center for Nursing Research (CNR) that will be a stand-alone department that will direct, track, educate, and provide resources for all nursing research in the institution. The CNR will include the research council and staff, or might collaborate with a statistician who will serve as a resource for data analysis, and an evidence-based practice coordinator who will educate and assist nurse researchers in implementing their study findings into patient care in accordance with evidence-based practice guidelines. As funding allows, it would be advantageous to have a financial manager to assist in securing funding from the hospital or associated college or university for research projects and to chair and assist in the grant writing process to attempt to gain external financial support. This person would also assist in delineating the financial resources needed for each research project. Another possible position in the CNR would be that of an IRB administrator. This person would be a liaison between nurse researchers and the IRB, and would assist with IRB submissions, track the progress of submissions and the need for updates and annual reviews. This will be a great resource and will allow the nurse researcher more time to focus on the study protocol and data collection. The CNR will be the central source for the provision of nursing research education for clinical staff.

If partnering with a college or university, education might be offered through them via classroom instruction or, if a professor is on the research council, he or she could act as an educator to the staff. In order to accommodate all interested clinical staff in the research program, and to properly educate them, a more formal means of education might be needed. This could be in the form of a nursing research fellowship, which will be described in the next section of this chapter. The fellowship would be housed in the CNR and directed by members of the NRC (Turkel et al., 2008).

The CNR and NRC should develop bylaws to define their purpose, membership and member responsibilities, meeting schedule, and decision-making processes regarding the implementation and maintenance of the research program and individual research projects (UNC Healthcare, 2009). A nursing research program that is to be implemented into a hospital or healthcare system must be well aligned with the mission and vision of the institution. The research program needs to be tailored to fit the institution, not vice versa. Careful evaluation of the priorities of hospital administration and staff is necessary to shape the program for acceptance by the masses. Again, as part of the Magnet journey, a research program will not only be welcomed, but will be necessary to achieve and maintain Magnet designation. Buy-in from administration is needed to allow for funding and access to needed facilities and personnel to create the program, and ultimately, buy-in is needed from practitioners who will be creating, executing, interpreting, and utilizing the research projects and findings.

A RESEARCH MISSION AND VISION

To this end, a mission and vision should be created for the research program that exhibits the values of the institution as well as nursing. In an article by Harrington in which the development and implementation of a nursing research program is described, the mission and vision of the program was created using the concept of applied research and the hospital's mission in which the program was to be implemented (2006). In concordance with this view, the mission and vision may include statements such as "Our mission is to utilize research to address and answer staff generated ideas and questions from the bedside and support evidence-based practice to improve patient care and advance nursing practice in accordance with the mission of the hospital," or "Our vision is to be a program that brings bedside clinicians to research and research to the bedside."

Harrington also talks of creating a philosophy of the nursing research program. The philosophy should talk of embracing staff ideas and inquiries regarding clinical practice, promoting the enterprise of applied research, and supporting the integration of such research with evidence-based practice to ensure the best possible patient care (2006). The creation and use of a mission, vision, and philosophy might seem unnecessary and frivolous, but it will institute a standard and a focus for the program and remind everyone of the values on which the program is based. It will allow for consistency in the program despite any possible turnover of its administrators. It will ensure that the efforts put into the program will not be in vain and the fruits of the program will persist.

RESEARCH PROGRAM GOALS AND ACTION PLAN

The overall goals of a hospital or healthcare institution–based nursing research program are to generate new knowledge, advance the practice of nursing, and to improve the quality of patient care (Harrington, 2006). To accomplish this, the program needs to ensure the continued support and interest of the nurses as well as hospital administration. The program must be designed to get nurses to do research, read research, practice using principles from research, and to overall love research. Well, maybe that is going a bit far, but truly, a research program needs to get people excited about research. This is the initial battle in developing a research program as research is typically seen as extracurricular, time consuming, and difficult to perform. Turkel et al. (2008), in describing the creation of a nursing research fellowship program, note the top five barriers to nurses performing and utilizing research:

- the nurse does not have time to read research,
- the nurse does not feel she/he has enough authority to change patient care procedures,
- there is insufficient time on the job to implement new ideas,
- the nurse is unaware of the research,
- physicians were not cooperative with implementation.

The greatest of those barriers was insufficient time. So, a nursing research program must serve to introduce, educate, and facilitate the process of nursing research while allowing protected work time for research activities.

It is also important to define the types of research to be undertaken, and focus on nursing research that is synergistic with nursing practice. If it is a teaching hospital or academic institution, a program that includes both basic and applied research might be welcomed. In a community hospital setting, applied research is usually a better fit. In any institution, applied research will most likely garner the most interest from nurses, as it will allow current and practical issues to be studied. Also, applied research typically works to improve patient care by collecting and analyzing clinical as well as administrative data that will impact decisions made by all levels of personnel in the hospital (Harrington, 2006).

From the mission, vision, and philosophy, specific goals for the program need to be delineated and molded into an action plan. The goals and action plan should include: methods of conveying information about the research program to all staff; providing initial and ongoing research education for those who will coordinate the program and for all clinical staff; creating policies, procedures and guidelines for research activities; providing information on and assistance with implementation of research findings using the evidence-based practice process; and encouraging and assisting with preparing publications and presentations from research study results (Harrington, 2006).

Communication and Dissemination of Research Program Activities

To communicate and disseminate research information, an Internet or intranet site can be composed for the research program that displays current nursing research activities and research projects that are ongoing and might need references for patient enrollment. It should have links to resource sites and could include research tips (similar to clinical pearls) each week. It should also provide information and a link for evidence-based practice sites. The Web site might also feature published research projects from within the institution. Updated information on upcoming research events within and outside of the institution should also be featured on the site. Another means of communication might be a monthly newsletter featuring current research activities, ongoing projects, educational events, publications, and presentations. The newsletter could also include fun but educational activities, such as crossword puzzles, to entice readers and possibly increase interest in research. Flyers, posters, and mass e-mails listing ongoing studies might also be used to inform all clinicians in the institution of research projects. To advertise current projects, you can create laminated pocket cards introducing and detailing each study and attach them on a ring for easy portability and reference. This process is detailed in one of the creative solutions at the end of this chapter. Again, make it fun. Use vibrant colors, catchy slogans, and encourage interaction. On all media regarding the research program, attach phone numbers and e-mail addresses where more information can be accessed.

Research Day is another activity that can surely spread the word about research. It is essentially a party celebrating research in general and focusing on what research is currently being done and has been done in the institution. It can be as elaborate as the coordinators would like, but the main goal is to gain the attention of the masses. Its purpose is to show that research can be fun and fulfilling while improving how we do what we do. It is also a venue for showcasing the research work that has been done and any acknowledgments received by the individual researchers and the hospital. This is further detailed in the introduction to this chapter and in a creative solution at the end of the chapter.

EDUCATION FOR RESEARCH

As stated previously, to educate nurses about research, readable information can be made available on a Web site or newsletter, but more formal methods of education should be offered as well. A curriculum should be established covering basic research information and instruction on the research process, as well as evidence-based practice processes. A conference can be organized during which advanced practice nurses who are well versed in research can present on varied topics in clinical research. Continuing education credits can be offered if the conference is approved by the American Nurses Association. Novice and expert nurse researchers can present current projects that are active or can share results of their studies in breakout sessions. Referrals to texts and external conferences or classes can be offered. You might even consider partnering with a college or university and arrange for all first-time researchers to attend a research class. Another offering might be periodic small sessions with a doctorally prepared nurse or other APNs from within the institution, or consultants lecturing on a specific research topic or clinical issue that needs or is currently under further research (McNett, Fusilero, & Mion, 2009). This might help those who are assisting in study coordination and those coordinating commercial studies that might have more complicated clinical backgrounds.

The IRB also typically offers some education sessions that usually focus on issues specific to IRB structure, function, and study reviews, and this can be invaluable as all human subject studies need to be submitted to the IRB for review and submission. This can be a tedious process. Monthly research workshops can be implemented where achievements in nursing research, publications, and presentations are showcased, and issues regarding ongoing projects are reviewed and discussed. Ultimately, a research internship to a fellowship program can be created and implemented which will work to produce clinical nurse researchers (Turkel et al., 2008). From this, a teach-the-teacher approach can be taken for continued research education and mentoring. A great example of this is the nursing research fellowship program described by Turkel et al. (2008). They illustrate a fellowship program created in a community hospital in which there was a nursing research council (NRC) that studied barriers to direct-care nurses participating in research. Those barriers were "lack of professional writing experience, knowledge deficit related to conducting a review of the literature, inadequate awareness of research methods, lack of statistical support, and no available mentor" (Turkel et al., 2008, p. 27).

They, with the approval and support, both procedural and financial, of the CNE, developed a program to eliminate those barriers. This nursing fellowship program allowed for protected time away from the bedside for staff nurses to conduct research studies of clinical relevance from observations they made while caring for patients. The fellowship required an application to enter, and would be available to only six to eight nurses. The year-long program allotted a specific amount of time each month for the nurses to dedicate to their research studies. Educational symposia, a PhD consultant, and a statistician were made available to the fellows. This was an exemplar program and was recognized as such by the American Nurses Credentialing Center (ANCC) (Turkel et al., 2008).

In addition to education regarding the research process, there should also be attention paid to reading and evaluating current healthcare literature. A journal club can be organized in which research from peer-reviewed journals are studied, dissected, and discussed. Not only will this educate participants on how to evaluate a research study for validity and reliability, and how to interpret the findings, but it will also engender knowledge of current clinical and social healthcare information and issues. It is so important to be well versed in current literature as it helps to improve patient care, but it might also prompt better relations with physicians, as it enables nurses to talk the medical talk and helps to advance the nursing profession as a whole.

RESEARCH PROGRAM POLICIES AND PROCEDURES

Policies and procedures for the program and research activities need to be created and placed on the Web site as well as on hard copy and placed in a manual that will always be located and accessible in the research office. The policies and procedures need to address the hierarchy of staff in the research program and each position's role and responsibilities; the process for submitting research ideas; the process for evaluating if the idea is suitable for the institution, department and/ or patient population; the process of IRB initial submission and annual renewal; HIPPA policies that must be followed during research on human subjects; the process for study implementation; the process for data review and analysis; evidence-based practice processes that will allow for implementation of study results within the institution; and the process for writing up study results for publication and or presentation.

There are inevitably many forms that are necessary to complete during the research process, some enforced by the IRB, and some only specific to your program. It makes it much easier for the researchers, especially the novice and occasional researchers, to have readily available templates of all the required forms. The IRB forms are typically on the institution's or external IRB's Web site, but a link to them can be placed on the research program Web site for easy access.

Additional forms that might be needed are those to streamline submissions of research protocols, data collection tools, statistical analysis tools (either a link for such tools or possibly a statistical computer program that could be lent out or used in the research office as requested), and budgetary/financial planning forms such as Excel spreadsheets to track study personnel and equipment costs and possibly generated revenue if participating in commercial studies. Also, resources for possible funding opportunities for noncommercial studies should be made available.

A checklist should also be provided that is comprehensive and includes all possible tasks that need to be completed from initiation to completion and publication of a research project. Ethics and ethical treatment of research subjects, although typically included on most IRB Web sites or in IRB manuals, should also be included in the policy and procedure manual for each individual research program. This will hopefully demonstrate to all involved in research that the ethical treatment of research subjects is of utmost importance and if the rights of subjects are not able to be protected or are compromised in any way in a research study, then that study must be aborted.

IMPLEMENTING A RESEARCH PROJECT

Once the research project is reviewed by the NRC and the IRB and approved, the study protocol is then implemented. This is easier said than done. The research council should provide assistance with accessing the needed patient population and/or records as well as the personnel needed to complete the data collection and analysis. The NRC chairs as well as the doctorally prepared nurse consultant should be available for mentoring and assistance through regularly scheduled meetings, as well as by e-mail and phone (McNett et al., 2009). Research liaisons may also be secured by the research council and assigned to projects in specific areas. The liaisons would be those ad hoc members of the research council. They might be staff nurses that have experience in research and who will assist with studies being done in their clinical area. They could be advanced practice nurses, such as clinical specialists or educators in specific clinical areas that dedicate time to help with research activities. Implementation might also occur as part of a fellowship program as described previously, in which staff nurses are given protected working hours to carry out their study protocol. Another method that can be initiated by the NRC as part of the plan for project implementation might be debriefing sessions during which the nurse researchers can openly discuss any issues they have encountered during study implementation and possibly help each other with creative ways to overcome these obstacles.

The time for implementation of nurse driven clinical studies really depends upon what type of research is being performed, on what population, and in what venue. A timeframe should be decided upon for all studies at the outset.

Turkel et al., (2008) states that a 12-month period was given to fellows in the research fellowship program to develop, implement, and disseminate findings from their studies. However, they also note that several obstacles were encountered by some of the fellows that lengthened the time to complete a study. For example, in two of the studies mentioned in the article, it was difficult to reach the number of needed subjects for the study. One study took 2 months longer than anticipated, and in the other study, enrollment time exceeded the time allowed in the research fellowship (2008). The NRC needs to have a plan in place for instances such as these. They might have backup nurse researchers who will be able to take over a study if the primary researcher is not able to complete it, so that the work put into the study and the information the study would produce is not lost. Another possibility is to have research partnerships. In the fellowship program, more nurses wanted to participate that the program could handle, so they created four fellow positions and four partner positions. In that case, the fellows were completing, from design to dissemination of findings, a nursing research study, and the partners were responsible for completing a literature review, evidence-based practice project, and dissemination of findings. This partnership structure could work in many ways. Different parts of one study could be tackled by each nurse or one nurse could complete the actual study protocol, while the partner could work to implement the findings via the evidence-based practice process. There are endless possibilities. You have to use what fits your institution and research program, and always be open to needed change. The research process, although prescriptive, is subject to variation, especially during the implementation phase and in clinical research when human subjects are being studied.

PUBLICATIONS AND PRESENTATIONS

All of the efforts placed into a research project will be in vain if the findings are not disseminated so that they can be utilized appropriately to improve practice. We must never let research findings sit in a dusty binder on a shelf in some hospital administrative office. We must publish, publish, publish, and present, present, present. Writing up the findings of a study is not usually very difficult, but writing the results so that they will be published in a peer reviewed journal or presented at a clinical seminar of healthcare professionals is very different. However, it is important for a nursing research program to include protocols in their action plan to provide for assistance with writing for publication and to find venues for dissemination for the newly discovered information. Writing workshops can be included in the research education workshops. The college or university with which the research program associates may offer classes on professional writing. Also, the council should have several resources for writing, such as the doctorally prepared nurses and other APNs who should have great experience in this area and can mentor the nurse researchers in the hospital (Ravert & Merrill, 2008). Presentations can be planned for Research Day and possibly during nursing ground rounds. The NRC should create lists of contacts for popular nursing publications and seminars, and should provide information on how to submit for publication and offer assistance to the researchers when doing so.

HOW TO FIND A RESEARCH PROJECT

How do you find a research project? Look around you. Observe the unit in which you work. Observe your patients and their family members. Monitor their responses to your care or to the environment or treatments they are receiving. Do you find practices that just do not seem to work or that seem to possibly cause harm? Are there recurrent patient issues such as falls or skin ulcers? If you can say yes to any of these questions, you can establish a research project. You might wonder if a specific testing modality is reliable, such as the PPD solutions in the example study presented in this chapter. You can do a chart review to evaluate the results of each person who has had the test and how well it accurately predicted an outcome. You may think of an intervention that might increase patient comfort, such as music in the preoperative area, which has currently received a lot of attention, or by extending family visiting hours. Alternatively, you might have an ingenious, innovative idea on how to prevent falls or skin breakdown. Do a literature review and determine if your idea is truly new or adequately studied. From there you can create your own research proposal (Beyea, 2000).

Regardless of the problem you have identified or the idea you have thought of as a potential research project, never embark on the project until you do a thorough literature review on the topic. Use the library or online searches, and discuss your idea with department chairs or experts in the field. If you find the topic has been researched before, determine if there is enough data and if that data is reliable and valid. If you feel the topic is adequately covered, you might move on to a new topic or use the findings from the research you read to create an evidence-based practice project to see if the findings can be implemented in your work area.

Most importantly, read nursing journals. You might come across an interesting nursing research study that might not present definitive results. Most research articles have a section on the need for further research. Reviewing that section can offer several ideas for research projects. Remember research is a cycle. No one study is definitive. You can expand on that study or maybe test the intervention in a different population. Studies often need to be replicated to assure validity and reliability of the results. You might study the same topic as another researcher, but use a different study design to improve the outcome (Beyea, 2000). In addition, any one of those supposedly tried and true nursing interventions that have been passed down from senior nurses for many years but never formally studied for effectiveness, can be the subject of your research project.

Regardless of where you find your impetus to do a research project or what topic you choose to research, you must find interest in the topic. If it is a topic that is forced upon you or one that you simply settle for, you will most likely not have the continued motivation to see the project through to completion. Research, although necessary and rewarding, takes a lot of time and effort. As you have found in this chapter, it requires a lot of reading, planning, and writing. So a strong interest must be present to successfully complete the project.

THE INSTITUTIONAL REVIEW BOARD

The National Research Act of 1974 was created by the National Commission for the Protection of Human Subjects of Biomedical and Behavioral Research (NCPHS) to oversee and regulate the use of human experimentation in medicine (National Institutes of Health, 1979). The act defines institutional review boards (IRBs) and requires them for all research conducted or supported by any federal department or agency. IRBs are themselves regulated by the Office for Human Research Protections (OHRP) within the US Department of Health and Human Services (HHS). IRBs were developed in direct response to research abuses that occurred in the 20th century. In the United States, IRBs are governed by Title 45 Code of Federal Regulations (CFR) Part 46 (National Institutes of Health, n.d.).

For those of you unfamiliar, the IRB is the body that oversees research in an institution. Research studies are required to be approved by an IRB to ensure the safety of study subjects. The IRB typically meets monthly and its members are required to be a diverse group to ensure that people from different points of view are utilized.

The purpose of the IRB is twofold: primarily, to ensure that subjects are put in as minimal a risk for bad outcomes as possible, and secondarily, to validate that the study design and methodology will answer the research question. If the study design and methodology is not sufficient to answer the research question, there is little reason to do the study and to expose subjects to even minimal risk. The IRB will look at consent forms and study protocols to determine if the study merits their blessing.

It is essential to develop a good rapport with the IRB administrator. He or she will most likely be your point person for readying nursing proposals and completing IRB paperwork. They might also be willing to help educate the nursing staff on what the IRB does, and the procedures it follows. All investigators are also required to have education in human subjects protection. Some institutions offer their own course, and others use an online course such as from the NIH Office of Extramural Research, available at http://phrp.nihtraining.com/users/login.php (Accessed August 1, 2009).

We suggest familiarizing those contemplating a research study with the necessary IRB forms and requirements. Although there is one governing agency, each IRB is a bit different in its policies and procedures. If you do not have an IRB in your institution, you can utilize a local IRB to review your study. There will most likely be a charge for this, but it is truly necessary, especially if you plan on publishing your study. Most publishers want to ensure the highest ethical standards of the research they publish. IRB approval helps to validate that ethical research standards were met.

CREATIVE SOLUTIONS

Creative Solution Title: *Don't Let Research Scare You!*

Creative Solution Author: Roseanne M. DeFrancisco, MSN, RN
Clinical Outcomes Manager
South Jersey Healthcare Elmer Hospital, Elmer, NJ

Purpose: The goal of this project is to introduce research to South Jersey Healthcare (SJH) nursing staff and to highlight nursing research.

Legend

Overall Rating: **COMPETENT**

Financial:

Time:

Personnel:

Other Resources: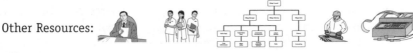

Efficacy: **B**

Transferability: **B**

Malleability/Adaptability: **B**

Ease of Implementation: **C**

Synopsis: See beginning of this chapter.

Description of Organization: South Jersey Healthcare (SJH) is a Magnet-designated, multiple-hospital system. The health system encompasses two full service inpatient hospitals consisting of approximately 350 inpatient beds, comprehensive health centers, and outpatient and specialized services such as a Bariatric

Center of Excellence, Wound Care Center, Sleep Center, and Balance Center. In 2008, SJH performed over 18,700 surgeries and the emergency department visits topped 97,400. The health system also serves as a clinical site for nursing students from a number of local colleges and maintains a professional relationship with Cumberland County College, which is adjacent to the RMC campus.

The Case Study: South Jersey Healthcare's Research Council is an integral component of Shared Governance in the hospital system. One of the goals of our Research Council is to educate our staff on the research process and also expose our bedside nurses to the wonderful world of research. Our creative solution was to organize and present a day filled with research: a day to teach, to learn, and to spotlight nursing research. The council envisioned the Research Day to be both educational and entertaining. The third annual Research Day was entitled "Don't Let Research Scare You!" and was held the week of Halloween.

The Research Day was opened by SJH's president and CEO, and chief nursing executive. Nursing staff were encouraged to attend in costume and prizes were offered for the best futuristic nurse, nurse of the past, scariest nurse, funniest nurse, and cultural nurse. Each unit throughout the system was encouraged to develop a research question, and the Research Council announced a call for posters relating to the research question. Prizes for the most creative and informative poster were awarded. Poster criteria was established and specified by the Research Council. Criteria included size of poster, the creator's responsibility for presenting to colleagues, as well as a sample poster layout. The sample poster layout mimicked those sections commonly found in a research proposal. The presenters were asked to include and state the research question, what the literature revealed on their topic, what methods would be used to implement it on the unit, and what benefits and outcomes would possibly be derived from the research project. The posters were judged by SJH's chief nurse executive and the VPs of Patient Care Services. The response was overwhelming and great ideas were generated from this exercise.

The conference also featured two keynote speakers who are experts in the field of research, one from Columbia University and another from Wilmington University. Topics included "Nursing and Clinical Research" and the "Role of the Nurse in Clinical Research." Sessions were also offered on library resources and review of literature, a hands-on research activity involving literature searches, the Institutional Review Board, SJH's Magnet Journey, and current research studies at SJH. Contact hours were awarded for this conference.

The project was lead by a subcommittee of the Research Council, which included SJH's Director of Quality and Magnet, the chair of the Research Council, and members of the council including our administrative assistant. Members of the subcommittee met frequently as we prepared for Research Day. These planning meetings consisted of brainstorming sessions, decorating sessions, and weekly updates on the planning.

SJH leadership provided support and actively participated in the event. The Research Council members and our administrative assistant were the founders of the event, but our staff was the most important participants of this great day. The Research Council has sponsored this research conference for the past 3 years, typically scheduled in the fall. The Research Council considered a Halloween themed research day and the council ran with this idea.

The Research Day was offered to SJH staff throughout the hospital system. Participation for this event was outstanding. Specialties throughout the system participated in the conference.

The conference was held on hospital grounds. Catering and decorations were incurred expenses. The keynote speakers were provided with an honorarium. Expenses were also incurred for the prizes for best poster and best costume. The hospital's own computer and projector equipment were used, so no additional costs were incurred.

Approximately 75 staff members attended the conference. Research council attendance has increased since the Research Day. Twelve research questions/posters were presented. Five have been developed into full-fledged research studies, four with IRB approval, and one scheduled to present to the IRB. There was no baseline data for comparison other than staff participation in the conference, which has increased over the past two years.

Outcome Measures:

Formative/Compliance: Attendance at planning meetings; progress toward goal according to pre-established timeline.

Summative/Outcome: Number of Research Day attendees; number of posters submitted; number of posters developed into research projects; attendee satisfaction; subsequent number of Research Council members.

Evidence Supporting this Creative Solution: Research and specialty conferences are a standard venue in the nursing profession to share information and raise awareness of specific and pertinent issues. Encouraging research questions that are rooted in clinical practice makes it pertinent to clinicians, utilizing principles of Adult Learning Theory (Knowles, 1970).

Knowles, M. S. (1970). *The modern practice of adult education. Andragogy versus pedagogy.* Englewood Cliffs, NJ: Prentice Hall/Cambridge.

Recipe for: *Don't Let Research Scare You!*

Ingredients:

CNO support and budget

Staff buy-in

Established Nursing Research Council/Planning Committee

1 administrator and council chair to coordinate initiative with skills in project management/event planning

Time allowance for staff working on conference

Venue to hold conference/catering

Supplies for flyers, advertisements, and programs

Ability to provide continuing education hours (optional, but important)

Speakers for conference (internal and external)

Audio/visual equipment

Step-by-Step Instructions (see Figure 7-1 for Step-by-Step Instruction Timeline):

Step 1: Obtain support from CNO first. Work out issues of time allotment for staff time spent working on conference. Estimate costs and agree on budget.

Step 2: Administrator and council chair obtain commitment from Nursing Research Council/Planning Committee and brainstorm for theme, contests, program, speakers, and posters.

Step 3: Administrator, council chair, and council members create timeline and action plan specifying who is responsible for what and by when. Meet every 2 weeks.

Step 4: Book venue, estimating number of participants. Book caterer. Reserve audio/visual equipment. Find out what is necessary for continuing education credits (optional). Plan where posters will be displayed and who will judge and criteria.

Step 5: Invite and obtain commitment from internal and external speakers. Ask speakers for objectives, CV, and all necessary items for continuing education credits (if applicable) and apply. Create evaluation form for attendants to complete.

Step 6: Develop a mechanism to accept registration for the conference. This will allow better prediction of attendance. Ask unit managers and directors to encourage attendance.

Step 7: Publicize! Advertise the conference featuring the speakers and continuing education credits (if applicable). Call for posters and publicize the contest (Figure 7-2).

Step 8: Plan logistics, assigning duties to council members/planning committee members, such as set-up, coordination of day (registration, speaker assistance and introductions, evaluation, and clean-up). Make sure to have someone acting as photographer to document the event.

Step 9: Have the event! Possibly present an honorarium to speakers. Distribute continuing education credits to attendees (if applicable).

Step 10: Share evaluations and other outcome measures with council members/planning committee. Congratulate all who contributed. Disseminate results of the event throughout the institution.

Figure 7-1   Timeline for "Don't Let Research Scare You!"

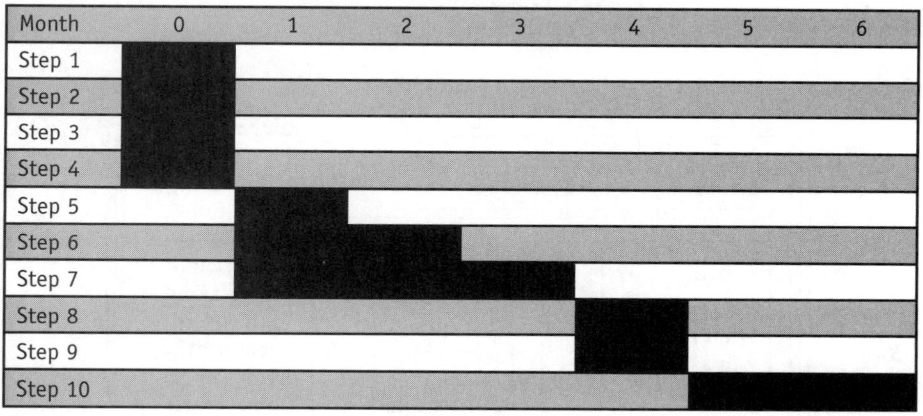

Month	0	1	2	3	4	5	6
Step 1	█						
Step 2	█						
Step 3	█						
Step 4	█						
Step 5		█					
Step 6		█					
Step 7		█	█				
Step 8				█			
Step 9				█			
Step 10					█		

Additional Outcomes to Consider Measuring:

Formative/Compliance: No additional measures.

Summative/Outcome: No additional measures.

Insights from Original Implementation:

- Commitment of the research council members was an integral part of the success of the research conference.
- Encourage members to be creative and innovative, and make it fun!
- Enlist the support of leadership and watch the staff's love of research bloom.

For Further Guidance Contact:

Roseanne M. DeFrancisco, MSN, RN
defranciscor@sjhs.com

Figure 7-2   Sample flyer for nursing research conference poster criteria.

Nursing Research Conference Poster Criteria

1. Poster should be 1 standard size poster board.
2. You should be able to speak about the poster and present it (briefly).
3. Notify administrative assistant if you will be preparing a poster.
4. Posters should be submitted to the administrative assistant by Friday, October 24.
5. Make sure the names, credentials, and units are on the poster.

Sample Poster Layout
(Yours can be different. Just include all components.)

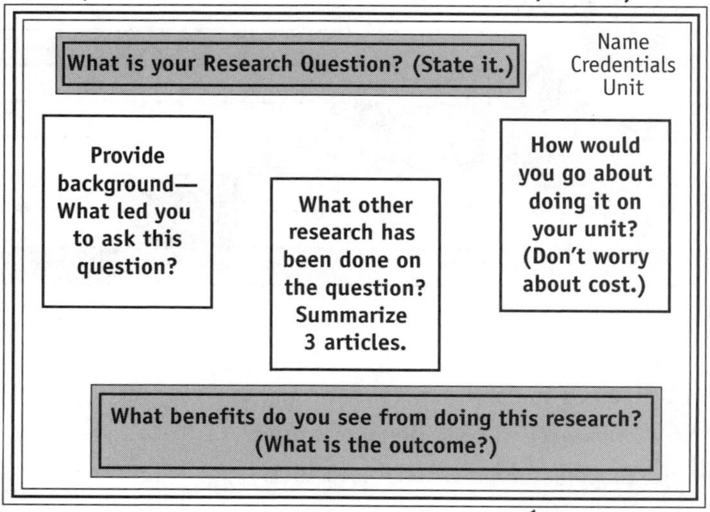

	Name
What is your Research Question? (State it.)	Credentials
	Unit

Provide background—What led you to ask this question?	**What other research has been done on the question? Summarize 3 articles.**	**How would you go about doing it on your unit? (Don't worry about cost.)**

What benefits do you see from doing this research? (What is the outcome?)

Prize for Best Poster
Choice of -
~$100 Restaurant Gift Certificate~
~Pizza Party for Your Unit~
~$100 Spa Gift Certificate~

Creative Solution Title: *Research Reference Pocket Cards*

Creative Solution Author: **Ellen Boxer Goldfarb, MSN, CRNP**
Cardiology Nurse Practitioner
Penn Presbyterian Medical Center

Purpose: The research pocket cards were created to allow easy access to and portability of current research information and facts about research projects being conducted in the hospital to increase staff awareness of and encourage staff involvement in research.

Legend

Overall Rating: **ADVANCED BEGINNER**

Financial:

Time:

Personnel:

Other Resources: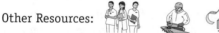

Efficacy: **A**

Transferability: **A**

Malleability/Adaptability: **A**

Ease of Implementation: **A**

Synopsis: The laminated research reference cards are simply a pocket guide to research activities occurring within the hospital setting. As many nurses love to stock their many pockets with reference material to assist with patient care, this was seen as an easy, acceptable addition to their pocket guide collections that would assist in disseminating research information. Each card represents a current research project or study being conducted in the hospital. It provides the title, purpose, and a brief background of the study. It lists inclusion/exclusion criteria for subject entry (if applicable) and any information that might assist staff in collecting needed data. It also provides contact information for the study investigator so that further information can be sought or assistance with the project can be offered.

Description of Organization: This creative solution was implemented in Thomas Jefferson University Hospital (TJUH), which is a large 957-bed, multidisciplinary, tertiary care hospital. It is part of a multihospital system, offering both inpatient and outpatient care at four different locations. TJUH is a university, teaching hospital. At the time this creative solution was implemented, the hospital did not have

Magnet designation, but it currently does. TJUH operates several major programs in a wide range of clinical specialties such as the HeartCARE center, Jefferson Hospital for Neuroscience, the Rothman Institute for Orthopedics, Kimmel Cancer Center, and Transplantation Services which offers liver, kidney, pancreas, and heart transplantation. In the past year, TJUH has had over 47,000 admissions and over 106,000 emergency room visits. TJUH employs over 5000 full-time staff, with almost 2500 of them being registered nurses. TJUH is associated with Thomas Jefferson University (TJU) and serves as a clinical site for nursing students and medical students from TJU as well as many surrounding colleges and universities.

The Case Study: Research reference pocket cards were originated and utilized by a nurse coordinated research program at a TJUH. The idea was born primarily out of the need to increase awareness of the research studies that were currently enrolling patients so that referrals for possible study subjects could be made to the research team. The cards were also a means to entice hospital staff to participate in research. The cards were originated by the research director and initially created by the director and individual research coordinators with assistance from the research center's administrative assistant. Each researcher made new cards as necessary to update existing study information or when a new study began.

The cards were well received as they conveniently fit into nursing uniform or lab coat pockets, were color coded, and easy to read. Staff also appreciated being involved in the research process. The cards created a buzz about research around the hospital. The cards were also helpful to the primary researchers as quick reference guides for their own studies, as well as to their colleagues, which enabled the researchers to help each other in gathering data. The cards were fairly simple to produce with little cost involved, and they yielded a great return. Several contacts were made with staff suggesting patients for enrollment or inquiring about the research that was being conducted and how to get involved. Subject enrollment increased in existing studies and new researchable ideas were suggested, which yielded new studies. The pocket cards proved to be both cost and time effective as a continually reproducible intervention that fashioned positive outcomes for the entire research program.

Outcome Measures:

Formative/Compliance: Periodic assessment of percentage of staff members carrying the cards with them during working hours; survey staff to evaluate utility of cards.

Summative/Outcome: Comparison of the number of staff participating in research before and after distribution of the cards; increase in number of study subjects enrolled.

Evidence Supporting this Creative Solution: Everything from critically important nursing and medical information such as CPR instruction to wildfire information for firefighter safety are available in pocket card format. Pocket cards provide concise, usable information and can always be readily available for quick reference. The use of pocket cards as part of an educational intervention for fourth year medical students was studied to evaluate if they had an impact on knowledge, attitudes, and self-efficacy of the students and the relationship of these attributes to patient care practices. There were significant improvements in all three areas after the implementation of the module, which included pocket cards (Carson, Gillham, Kirk, Reddy, & Battles, 2002).

Carson, J. S., Gillham, M. B., Kirk, L. M., Reddy, S. T., & Battles, J. B. (2002). Enhancing self-efficacy and patient care with cardiovascular nutrition education. *American Journal of Preventive Medicine, 23*(4), 296–302.

Recipe for: *Research Reference Pocket Cards*

Ingredients:

> 8.5″ × 11″ hard-stock, multicolored paper
>
> 1 Computer with a word processing application
>
> 1 Printer
>
> 1 Laminator
>
> 1 Hole puncher
>
> 1 Pair of scissors or a paper cutter
>
> 1 Metal ring for each group of cards
>
> 1 Research coordinator/assistant

Step-by-Step Instructions (see Figure 7-3 for Step-by-Step Instruction Timeline):

Step 1: Obtain synopses of all nursing research projects being conducted, including purpose, enrollment criteria or data to be collected, timeframe for the study, and personnel conducting the study and their contact information.

Step 2: Organize the preceding information in easily readable bullet format in a word processing document on the computer. Format and size the information so that four duplicates can fit on one piece of 8.5″ × 11″ paper. Each card should be approximately 3.5″ × 5″.

Step 3: Print each study synopsis with investigator contact information on hard-stock paper. Make it double sided if necessary to fit all of the study information. Use a different color paper for each study or all studies of a certain type so that their cards are easily identified in the pack.

Step 4: Cut out the four cards from each piece of paper.

Step 5: Laminate the cards.

Step 6: Punch a hole in the left upper corner of each card; place the hole in the same area on each card.

Step 7: Organize the cards by study type, chronologically, or alphabetically, whatever works for your study collection.

Step 8: Place all cards on the metal ring and secure it in the closed position.

Step 9: Distribute the cards to all nursing units and all hospital departments.

Step 10: Update card packs periodically by adding or removing cards from each card pack. This can be done by having drop off and pick up boxes placed on each unit for staff to trade in cards as necessary.

Figure 7-3   Timeline for "Research Reference Pocket Cards."

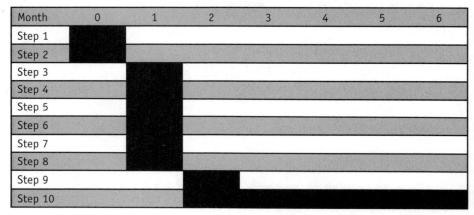

Month	0	1	2	3	4	5	6
Step 1							
Step 2							
Step 3							
Step 4							
Step 5							
Step 6							
Step 7							
Step 8							
Step 9							
Step 10							

Additional Outcomes to Consider Measuring:

Formative/Compliance: No additional measures.

Summative/Outcome: No additional measures.

Insights from Original Implementation:

- If you have a shared governance council structure, you may use this structure to help disseminate the cards.
- Need to obtain buy-in from all research investigators.
- Might want to integrate the process of producing these cards into the approval process for beginning a nursing research study. This will help enculturate the practice.

For Further Guidance Contact:

Ellen Boxer Goldfarb, MSN, CRNP
Ellen.Goldfarb@uphs.upenn.edu

REFERENCES

American Nurses Association (ANA). (2009). *The nursing process: A common thread amongst all nurses.* Available at: http://www.nursingworld.org/EspeciallyForYou/StudentNurses/Thenursingprocess.aspx. Accessed June 28, 2009.

Beyea, S. (2000). Getting started in nursing research and tips for success. *AORN Journal, 72*(6), 1061–1062.

Burns, N., & Grove, S. K. (2001). *The practice of nursing research conduct, critique, and utilization.* Philadelphia: W.B. Saunders Company

Harrington, L. (2006). Implementing a hospital based nursing research program in 30 days. *Nurse Leader, 4*(1), 37–55.

Hopkins (2000) Quantitative Research Design. Sportscience 4(1), sportsci.org/jour/0001/wghdesign.html. Accessed July 10, 2009.

McNett, M., Fusilero, J., & Mion, L. (2009). Implementing programs of nursing research and selecting doctoral nurse leaders. *Nurse Leader, 7*(1), 42–46.

National Institutes of Health (NIH) (n.d.). *Office of Human Subjects Research.* Available at: http://ohsr.od.nih.gov/. Accessed August 1, 2009.

National Institutes of Health (NIH) (1979, April 18). *Regulations and ethical guidelines.* Available at: http://ohsr.od.nih.gov/guidelines/belmont.html. Accessed August 1, 2009.

Polit, D. F., & Hungler, B. P. (1995). *Nursing research principles and methods.* Philadelphia: J.B. Lippincott Company.

Ravert, P., & Merrill, K. (2008). Hospital nursing research program: Partnership of service and academia. *Journal of Professional Nursing, 24*(1), 54–58.

Research. (2009). In *Merriam-Webster Online Dictionary.* Available at: http://www.merriam-webster.com/dictionary/research. Accessed August 2, 2009.

Shuttleworth, M. (2008). *Qualitative research design.* Available at: www.experiment-resources.com. Accessed June 16, 2009.

Sutherland, S. E. (2001). Evidence-based dentistry: Part IV. Research design and levels of evidence. *Journal of the Canadian Dental Association, 67*(7), 375–378.

Turkel, M. C., Ferket, K., Reidinger, G., & Beatty, D. E. (2008). Building a nursing research fellowship in a community hospital: Original program construction: Nursing research fellowship program. *Nursing Economics, 26*(1), 26–34.

UNC Healthcare. (2009). *Nursing research council bylaws UNC.* Available at: www.unchealthcare.org/site/Nursing/sharedgov/researchcouncil/index_html. Accessed July 22, 2009.

Zimmerman-Jones, A. (2009). *Introduction to the scientific method. Overview of the scientific method.* Available at: http://physics.about.com/od/toolsofthetrade/a/scimethod.htm. Accessed June 30, 2009.

## CHAPTER 8

Turning Nurses into Writers

"The pen is the tongue of the mind."
—MIGUEL DE CERVANTES

"The skill of writing is to create a context in which other people can think."
—EDWIN SCHLOSSBERG

The ability to write well is one of the characteristics of a well-rounded nurse, since skill in writing demonstrates both intelligence and the ability to think critically. As professionals, nurses need to be able to write well, since being a professional requires effective communication. Nurses communicate with other healthcare team members through progress notes and other clinical records, and important information regarding patient care is passed on through such records. For the best care of our patients, this information must be clear and concise, yet thorough and accurate, since these records may also serve as legal documents. Nurses also communicate with our own professional audience, as well as other disciplines and the public, by writing in various publications. As nurses, we possess unique knowledge and skill, and we should share these with others. Since the role of nurses is ever changing and expanding, we need to let the public and the entire medical community understand exactly what nurses do. Through our writing we can make others aware of "what we know to be true" and provide "evidence for what we do" (George Mason University, 2010, para. 1–3).

This poignant quote from the George Mason University's Web site sums up why it is imperative for nurses to write. It speaks of the many important reasons why nurses should write: to communicate what you know and learn to others with the general goal of enhancing the pool of nursing knowledge, to enhance the professionalism of nursing and the public's view of the nursing profession, and, of course, to ultimately improve patient care.

Communication of information is key to the viability of any profession. In nursing, communication is often the whisper down the lane type. This is evident in the method of educating nurses. Nursing is somewhat unique in its method of rearing its young. Practice principals are introduced in the classroom, reinforced by a nursing text, but ultimately relayed and adopted in the clinical setting, from one nurse to another during preceptorship. The novice nurse takes what the senior nurse tells him or her as scripture, but often is not obligated to reference the scripture, that is, nursing literature. Medical education also utilizes relayed information from one physician to another, but medical text and current literature are core to the profession. Medical students, interns, and residents are expected to not only reference and memorize the principles of medical literature, but to also contribute to the body of medical knowledge by publishing. With the advent of evidence-based practice and Magnet designation, the nursing profession is heading in that direction.

How should nurses learn the essential information required to take care of patients? We must read and study what nurses before us have written. The foundation of what we know in nursing should come from published writings by nurses that are based on research and proven methods of practice. So, you say that writing is only for nursing scholars, those who work in academia and participate in research, and therefore you do not need to be skilled in writing as a bedside nurse. Well, much of what will make a difference in bedside care is information communicated by those who provide bedside care. Nursing knowledge should be continually enhanced by contributions to nursing literature from all levels of nursing. The best way to communicate and disseminate information that might bring about necessary change in patient care is by writing and publishing. Nurses can write anything from articles for peer-reviewed journals, chapters for healthcare texts and editorials, to abstracts for evidence-based practice projects, or simply a letter to your local politician or hospital administrator. Regardless of what you write, it must be professionally written to be read and acknowledged. There is technique, skill, and art in writing and it must be learned and practiced in order to be perfected (Price, 1988).

A nursing school principle that we will never forget is, "if it wasn't written, it wasn't done." This was preached in school so that we would learn to always document what was observed about a patient and what was done while caring for a patient. Despite these preachings, writing skills are not formally taught in nursing school. Even nursing documentation, although not publishable material, should be in professional language and well organized for the rest of the patient care team to easily understand. Therefore, it is important for nurses to develop good writing skills to be used in everyday practice. These skills, if developed during the basic education of nurses, can translate into professional writings that are routinely produced by nurses. Until writing becomes a standard part of nursing education, we must educate nurses on the job and assist them in sharing their everyday experiences to improve the experiences of their successors (Price, 1988).

That same principle, "if it wasn't written, it wasn't done," is true not just for documenting daily patient care, but also for documenting principles of patient care that are learned or discovered in practice and should be communicated so that all nurses and patients might benefit. So, if you participated in an evidence-based project to decrease patient falls on your unit, write about it. Share the insights you have gained from the project and allow others to benefit from this important work. Write a description of your work and the research behind it. You can collaborate with colleagues on your unit and jointly write an abstract or an article for your hospital newsletter or Web site. Start small to become comfortable with the task of writing. Then the goal of writing for publication will not seem so daunting. You might expand on a hospital-based manuscript and eventually submit it for publication in a nursing journal. We know most nurses feel that writing and publishing are unreachable goals. This was true for us at one time. We never imagined when beginning our careers in nursing that we would some day be publishing the book that you are reading. We each separately began by writing a short article for a nursing journal on a topic with which we were familiar from our daily work. One of us was then invited to write a chapter in a healthcare book. The other tapped into school writings that were well received and found them to be publishable material. We then realized that we could do more. With some research into the process of book proposal writing, we collaborated on an idea and here we are. If we can do it, so can you.

Barbara Hafer, former Pennsylvania treasurer, states, "While writing is as indispensable a tool to the professional nurse as the stethoscope, thermometer, or BP cuff, it is more powerful because of its ability to bring about change—its ability to remedy" ("Dear Abby," n.d.).

You may feel that you entered into the nursing profession only to care for people and writing is not the act of caring. You may believe, as many others do, that professional writing is not within the scope of nursing practice. However, as in all professions and in the profession of nursing, there is a great responsibility to the people for which you care as well as the community of nurses with which you work. That responsibility is to do no harm and to work toward the greatest good for the greatest number. If we do not lend to others the lessons we learn in practice then we will not be honoring either of these responsibilities. Suppose a medical researcher discovered the cure for the common cold, but did not share the findings with the rest of the medical community. Maybe that person verbally told a few of his or her colleagues, who might tell a few others. This verbal, "whisper down the lane" communication would not only take an inappropriate amount of time for the information to reach the community, but it might not be seen as legitimate as the process and specifics of the discovery were not documented. So, we must remember, sharing is caring. Disseminating important information that can improve the health and well-being of the community is caring for the community. As a nurse, your patient population does not just include the patients assigned to you on a typical work day, it includes all of your fellow citizens. When you write about healthcare policy in a journal article or to a local, state, or national politician, you are caring for those affected by the decisions made according to that policy. When you write a hospital policy prescribing fall prevention procedures or visiting guidelines, you are caring for all of those who will be affected by the policies—patients as well as their families. Writing patient education materials provides care for all those affected by the disease, process, or health concern you are addressing (Saver, 2006). Even when you write an editorial about a previously written piece on nursing practice, you are caring for other nurses as well as the profession of nursing. Caring, the overarching duty of the nurse, can be accomplished in many ways. Kathleen Heinrich, PhD, RN, in an article for American Nurse Today, writes a true and poignant statement, ". . . by writing a single article, you can reach more people than you could over a lifetime of nursing practice" (2009). So, keep doing what you do best in practice, but do not keep it to yourself. Share your pearls of wisdom as previous nurse writers have shared them with you.

WHY DON'T THEY WRITE?

Shifts that last for 12 hours, during which a bathroom visit is not always feasible and only a few morsels of food are inhaled while documenting in a patient's chart, is a typical work day in the life of a nurse. When not fulfilling their full-time work duties, home and family responsibilities, continuing education seminars for mandatory credits, and overtime shifts occupy a nurse's days. So, it is obvious that time, or lack thereof, is the most common reason that nurses do not write professionally. Work schedules typically do not allow for dedicated time to write for dissemination and publication. Writing must be fit into that busy schedule. As expected, writing, if not required for work or school, usually is what is eliminated from the to-do list, or at least put on the very bottom and rarely checked off. In addition to lack of time, lack of skill and knowledge about the process, and intimidation by the thought of writing for publication are the typical barriers preventing nurses from writing. Spear (2006) describes "the fear factor" that prevents many graduate nurses as well as nurse colleagues from writing for publication. Many are fearful of having others read their work, as they believe it will not be not good enough. Also, the fear of rejection once a writing endeavor is pursued holds some nurses back. Nurses might also think of scholarly papers they were required to write for school and are reminded of the distress they caused. Because of the prescribed detail required in academic writing, many view writing as a chore. Professional writing does not have to be like writing that research paper for which the professor picked the topic and gave you ten pages of requirements you must meet in order to get a passing grade. In practice, there are so many different types of writings and venues for your writings that are possible, that you can actually write about what you want and how you want to write it, as long as you adhere to some standard guidelines. Lack of knowledge of all the possible writing opportunities available might also add to intimidation as it is often thought that only primary research can be published in nursing journals and the like (Spear, 2006). Although research is very important to the nursing discipline, there are many other types of writing that are informative and of value, such as description of an evidence-based practice protocol used on your unit. Professional writing is a skill that is typically not well developed in undergraduate, nursing education programs. Yes, we all are required to have completed English classes, but neither the goal of, nor the outcome of those classes is the development of a professional writer. Even in graduate programs, with the exception of those with a literary focus, writing is not formally taught. The lack of formal training in professional writing is a one of the several reasons why the majority of nurses do not write. Writing well is a skill that must be learned, and it takes time, effort, and lots of practice to develop. Most science-based programs, like nursing, do not require any writing classes. Most nurses have not been exposed to any literary direction since freshman English class, which typically reviews the classics and maybe introduces personal journal writing, but it does not prepare future nurses for writing for publication in a medical journal. So how then are we supposed to know how to compose a letter, proposal, abstract, or article to relay information in our professional community?

Also, while those in many other professions regard publishing articles that offer important information for the profession an act of generosity as well as a shared responsibility, nurses give mixed messages to their publishing colleagues. Some believe that writing for publication is in a sense bragging, calling attention to yourself (Heinrich, 2009). Possibly they are comparing telling others the good things you do as a nurse to telling people when you help an elderly, vision-impaired person across the street. Perhaps it seems to take the altruism out of nursing. Some might feel that those who are publishing are reaping a secondary benefit. These nurses probably are benefiting, not necessarily financially, but it does feel good to see your name in print and have your work accepted and printed in a respected publication. So what? Just because the publishing nurse benefits, that does not remove the benefit that might be given to others from the information shared (Saver, 2006).

Ultimately, the biggest problem and global barrier to nurses writing is the lack of encouragement and mentoring. There is no general expectation for nurses to write and therefore, it is not a developed or encouraged activity for most nurses. Hospital educators typically do not enforce the need for nursing written contributions and do not offer guidance in this endeavor. So, even if a nurse came upon a writing opportunity, she most likely would not have the necessary support to pursue it. Mentoring nurses and beginning writers is so useful and needs to be incorporated into the agenda of nurse educators in all hospitals. It gives direction, encouragement, and support that helps allay the typical fears and breaks down the barriers to writing (Spear, 2006).

TYPES OF WRITING

Writing is literally defined as the representation of language in a textual medium with the use of signs, and symbols or words. Practically, it refers to the creation of meaning and the information generated by written words. Writing is a vehicle for expression of factual information, personal thoughts, and beliefs as well as lessons learned from personal and professional experience. There are several types of writing. The type chosen by an author is dependent upon the overall message to be conveyed and the avenue by which the message is to be delivered. In other words, your writing type will be based primarily on your topic of interest as well as the venue for which you are writing.

All writing is primarily categorized as fact or fiction, but there may be some overlap. Healthcare writings are all mostly factual and categorized as nonfiction. Healthcare pieces also may have some elements of persuasion to encourage the reader to adopt a practice, use a product, or better understand a process or theory that is being represented.

It is important when producing nonfiction, and more specifically, pieces on healthcare topics, to employ simplicity, clarity, and directness. The information that a nonfiction work provides should not need interpretation. Nonfiction works are typically sources of reference for accurate information. The facts need to be plainly stated.

Your audience is also very important to consider in any literary endeavor, but it is probably most important in nonfiction. Understanding potential readers' use for the work and their existing knowledge of a subject are both fundamental when writing nonfiction healthcare pieces. For example, when writing an article for a general nursing journal such as the *American Journal of Nursing* (AJN), you must remember that nurses from all levels of experience and from many different specialties could be reading your work. Therefore, you should write a general account of your topic. Including too many specific details might lose the reader's attention and/or be over the heads of readers not currently practicing in the area about which the article is written. So, for example, when writing about prevention and treatment of deep vein thrombosis (DVT) in a general nursing publication, you should describe the general pathophysiology and risk factors for DVT and modalities of prevention and treatment, but you would not want to present the specifics of the intrinsic and extrinsic clotting cascade and the chemical properties of the medications used to target areas of the cascade to prevent and treat DVT. That type of information would be better suited for a more specific journal or text about hematology or vascular medicine. The reader can be directed to a textbook or pharmacology text if further information is needed.

After determining your topic and the audience you will be targeting, you need to decide the message that you want your writing to convey. If you are describing a person, place, or thing, you will write a descriptive paper that creates an impression, image, feeling, and overall effect about the topic. It essentially paints a picture with words. This might be appropriate when writing about a new healthcare product, such as a dressing that promotes hemostasis at puncture sites. You might choose to recount an event in your practice which would call for a narration piece in which you would re-create the incident, including specific details, the mood of the event, and the overall effect and emotional experience of the event. Description of an educational experience, such as a conference or a patient experience such as an end-of-life event would fall into this category. Your topic may be strictly informational, providing a definition and explanation of a disease state or instructions and explanation of a process. An example of this would be an article on the pathophysiology and presentation of ventilator associated pneumonia (VAP) or an article providing instruction for patient positioning to prevent VAP. You might also define a nonclinical process, such as how to arrange and lead unit council meetings as part of quality improvement measures and the Magnet journey. You might want to analyze and compare and contrast something in your writing such as nursing theories or processes, for example, the use of observation versus physical or chemical restraints to prevent patient falls. Finally, you may feel strongly about a policy or procedure and want to write an argument paper in which you explain your position on a topic to prove your point. Your topic and your intended message should come together to form your thesis statement, which will focus your paper and tell your audience what to expect from your work. Once you have determined these pieces: your topic, audience, purpose for writing, and message to be conveyed, you will need to decide how and where (in what type of venue) to present it (Zilm, 2008).

VENUES FOR DISSEMINATION

Do not be fooled into thinking that the only publishable nursing information is that from large clinical trials and the only place to publish is a peer-reviewed nursing journal. You may conduct a small pilot study or evidence-based practice initiative on your unit and whether the results were positive or not, you can write a piece describing why you felt the study or initiative was needed, how you designed and implemented it, the results, and why you believe it was or was not successful. This can be submitted to a local, in-hospital newsletter, a general nursing journal or EBP journal, or you could create a poster and submit it for presentation at a nursing conference. There are multiple venues in which nurses can present and to which they can submit their work (Nettina, 2006).

So, what are the types of writing venues that nurses most commonly pursue? A fairly comprehensive list would include newsletters, posters, PowerPoint presentations, abstracts, articles including informative/educational articles, quality improvement articles and research articles, research proposals and grant proposals, editorial letters, nominations for nursing awards, and, probably less often, textbook chapters and entire books. This list progresses from least to most difficult and most to least likely writing endeavor to be pursued by nurses. We should now categorize these venues as internal and external.

Internal Publications

The best place for a novice nurse writer to start is internal publications. They are typically less formal and have fewer restrictions. There are flexible criteria for submissions to internal publications, which is more inviting to the novice writer. Publishing internally also allows for direct access to feedback from readers (good or bad, but hopefully constructive), which will help the new writer improve the skill in preparation for external, scholarly publications.

Internal publications include institutional, departmental, or maybe even unit-based or council-based newsletters, policies and procedures, PowerPoint presentations, and posters. A hospital Web site might also be a venue for submitting a writing project. The pieces in internal newsletters are usually editorial or short articles describing a hospital or unit-specific event, project, or initiative. You might even describe a specific patient encounter that offered a learning experience for the staff, such as a novel illness or extraordinary outcome of treatment. An important and mandatory consideration when writing pieces such as this, or any publishable material, is to be sure not to include any patient names or identifiers in your writing (Trotter & Rasmussen, 2006).

Newsletters

You can have some fun with internal publications, which can help to get nurses involved and excited about writing. You can create a newsletter for any organized group or initiative, such as the research newsletter talked of in Chapter 7. In a newsletter, you can include, in addition to an educational and informative article, a gossip column that discusses current happenings involving hospital or unit staff. You can have a kudos section, in which you highlight staff with accomplishments such as awards, graduations, and publications. You can get all staff involved, including ancillary staff such as nursing assistants and unit clerks. This may help to unify the staff and offer more credence to the ancillary positions. Give the newsletter a catchy, maybe comical name and disseminate it in meetings, mailboxes, online, and of course in the infamous staff bathroom where you know everyone will at least get a glimpse of it.

PowerPoint Presentations

PowerPoint presentations can be utilized to teach unit, department, and hospital staff about new initiatives, evidence-based practice protocols, and disease processes. You usually see clinical nurse specialists or nursing educators doing this type of activity, but getting general nursing staff to participate will offer experience with creating the PowerPoint project, which is an invaluable skill, as well as experience with public speaking, which we all can use. Doing small, unit-based presentations can inspire nurses to take presentations on the road to nursing and healthcare conferences. You can create a PowerPoint club, similar to a journal club, in which you meet periodically to share knowledge through presentations. These presentations can be for nurses, by nurses or even by nurses to physicians such as interns and residents. Do not let this replace journal club as that is also another means of not only sharing information, but also introducing and enticing staff to read, write, and disseminate.

It is important to note here that there is a difference between presenting and teaching. We all have sat through presentations, those with and without PowerPoint or visual aids, and have come out knowing very little more than we did before the presentation began. Presenting is simply that, presentation of information. It does not imply that the information is learned by the recipients. Teaching involves methods that work toward understanding and learning of information and concepts (Samuelowicz & Bain, 1992). So, a novice nurse writer or presenter might need the assistance of a nurse educator to teach as opposed to just present to the audience. This is when clinical nurse specialists (CNS) can team up with nurses to create and disseminate. Rather than having one CNS present to and teach all of the nurses on a unit or in a department, it can be more efficient and better accepted if the CNS worked with staff nurses to research, organize, present, and teach to their fellow nurses and peers. A teach-the-teacher model can work well here.

Policies and Procedures

Policies and procedure writing, although not as exciting as newsletter contributions or PowerPoint presentations, is a great way to get nurses more comfortable with the writing process. It can be made a bit more inviting if it is incentivized. Policy and procedure teams can be created, and scheduled. Paid time should be offered to create the policies and procedures. Acknowledgment of individual nurses for their work on the policies and procedures and publishing the documents with the names of those who created them might be enough incentive to get nurses involved in the process.

External Publications

Posters

Posters and poster presentations can actually be internal or external. A poster is a pictorial or graphic depiction of a project such as a quality improvement project, a clinical study, or a principle supporting or originating from such a project. In health care, posters typically portray hospital and nursing initiatives and are usually, if internal, displayed in the hospital or submitted for display externally at a healthcare or nursing conference. A poster is sometimes accompanied by a verbal presentation, but usually the poster does most of the work. Posters are a communication tool that should be able to stand with or without the creator to send a message to viewers. It must be clear and concise in its message, and viewer friendly. In other words, it must be organized well with an easy to follow sequence, contain minimal text so that it is not cumbersome to read, display understandable graphs, and, if possible, should avoid mathematical equations that can complicate the poster. Posters should follow specific guidelines similar to those used in writing a scholarly article. The poster should have a succinct title, a review of literature proving the need for the project being described, a purpose, the project description and methodology, outcomes, implications for nursing, and recommendations (Ulrich, 2007).

What makes a poster a good starting place for the novice nurse writer is that it has little need for eloquent prose, which is typically the intimidating feature of writing and publishing. A good understanding of the subject and some creativity are the needed ingredients for a good poster. Also, posters are amenable to group projects. So, the members of a unit-based council could all work together to create a poster describing an evidence-based practice project done on their unit or the force of Magnetism that their unit represents. It is for the most part easier to begin an endeavor such as writing and publishing with a partner or group, again making posters a good place to start. Posters are frequently utilized and needed for display to support a hospital mission such as infection control and decreased falls. The Magnet journey and its forces are also frequently depicted on poster presentations, which helps spread the word, offer information, and rally support. A poster that is created for a specific hospital or even a school project may later be submitted for acceptance to a widely recognized conference such as the ANCC National Magnet Conference. Although you might believe a poster is simply an arts and crafts project, once you do it, you realize that it entails a good deal of effort, and a poster that is accepted for display in any arena is something to be proud of. So, take credit for your work. A poster presentation, whether displayed internally or externally, should be added to your resumé or curriculum vitae (CV). Poster templates can be found on the Web at http://evidencebasednursing.blogspot.com (Bogert et al., 1992).

Abstracts

Abstracts are another writing endeavor to be approached by the nurse writer, both novice and experienced. An abstract is a short, concise, self-contained piece that describes a project, experiment, or topic that is detailed in a larger work, most often a journal article. Abstracts are written when submitting articles to journals, submitting poster presentations, applying for research grants, completing a master's thesis or PhD dissertation, writing a proposal for a conference paper or presentation, and writing book chapters or whole book proposals. There are three types of abstracts: descriptive, informative, and critical, but for scientific works such as those in health care, an informative abstract will most often be needed. An informative abstract does not critique a work; it simply presents all of the main arguments and results. It is important that an abstract contain the topic of the research or project, the main objective or purpose, methodology, main findings or conclusions, and recommendations. Essentially, it includes all of the components of the complete work, but in a greatly condensed form. This is the challenge of an abstract. You must fit all of your information in a specified amount of words, typically 100 to 200 words, or no more than 10% of the complete work. It is very important to be close to the number of words prescribed by the publisher to whom you are submitting. You should never go over the limit, nor should it be severely short on words. An improper length may actually cause an abstract to be rejected despite content ("Language Center," n.d.; "The Writing Center," n.d.). Although counterintuitive, the abstract, as you will see in the next section describing the writing process, is usually written last, after your complete work is finished.

Journal Articles

The production of journal articles is a common goal in writing and publishing for many nurse writers. Journal articles are seen as the pinnacle by many. Writing a journal article can be daunting, though. You can start with an informative or educational article describing a disease process, nursing procedure, or a nursing principle. This type of article is less formal than a research or experimental article and more easily approached. It requires some clinical experience in the area being reviewed as well as some library or Internet research to learn the background and current facts about the topic. Next, you might attempt a quality improvement or EBP article. Inevitably, if your hospital is seeking Magnet status or is already designated, there should be several active nursing quality improvement projects. You can write an article describing a project, the background, and why the project is needed, detailing the initiatives and procedures involved, delineating the results or outcomes, and finally, relating any recommendations for the readers. The next and perhaps more difficult endeavor is a research article. This will include an introduction to the research topic, review of literature proving the need for the research, a description of the research protocol, the methodology, and results, which usually entails some description of statistics used and the final outcome and recommendations. It might sound cumbersome, but if the individual steps of the project have been recorded as the project proceeded, formulating it into a journal article takes only some organization and the addition of some prose. Before writing any article or paper for publishing, though, it is helpful to choose a journal to which you will submit. Each journal will have author guidelines that are necessary to follow for your article to be considered for publication. These guidelines can also assist you in writing as they typically prescribe the amount of words allowed, the organization of the piece, and the formatting required (Jenkins, 1995). You can write a query letter first, if you have not yet written the article, to determine if a piece about your topic is desired by the journal. If your article is already written, you might submit the abstract as previously discussed. If your article is not accepted by the first journal to which you submit, do not fret. There are several others that might accept your work. Learn from any feedback that is obtained from the first journal to revise your work for future submissions. Again, do not forget to make appropriate changes to the text and to formatting as prescribed by each journal's submission guidelines. Some professional scientific writers, editors, and publishers would tell you to always choose your journal for submission before you begin any writing. Although it is best to know where you are going to submit and their requirements, you can write a piece and later decide it is worthy of submission and simply reorganize it as needed for a specific journal. You might also take a piece that you wrote for school or work and later submit it by making some minor changes.

As said, changes may need to be done several times before your article is accepted, but do not let a rejection or two stop you. Keep trying and resubmitting, there surely is a journal out there for your work. It can help to have a colleague review the piece, especially someone who has published before. He or she might offer suggestions for changes that can help you conquer the rejections and become a published author.

Abstracts and articles can be submitted to a general nursing journal such as *The American Journal of Nursing* (AJN), as well as other medical and healthcare journals that have a specific interest in your topic, such as *The Journal of Public Health Management and Practice*. There are also several online or electronic publications to which you might submit. For a fairly extensive list of healthcare publications, journals, and newsletters or papers, you can reference Pam Pohly's Net Guide (http://www.pohly.com/admin2.html).

Research Proposals

A research proposal is obviously needed before the research is initiated and therefore would be written before the research article previously described. The proposal and article are similar in content, but the proposal is the plan of action for the research project, whereas the article tells the readers what occurred during the research project, the outcomes, and results. The research proposal presents the research problem and its significance, states the research question and hypothesis, and delineates the methods that will be used to answer the research question and/or test the hypothesis, which is the research design. This will include the population to be involved in the study, inclusion and exclusion criteria, the sample size, the variables to be evaluated, and the methods of data collection and analysis. In addition, the proposal provides a timetable and outline for conducting the study, and estimates the financial and personnel costs of the protocol. The research proposal must also include an ethical review of the study if it is including human subjects, and a consent form that is used to inform potential subjects about the study and allow them to make an informed decision whether or not to participate (Carlson, Masters, & Pfadt, 2008). This is necessary for approval from the Institutional Review Board (IRB), otherwise known as the ethics committee, for the venue in which the study will take place. (You can learn more about the IRB and its functions in Chapter 7.) So, the proposal is the preliminary step in your research. It is essentially a road map of your study. The proposal is needed to delineate your research intentions to the powers that be that will allow you to pursue the inquiry. These powers are the IRB, hospital and/or university administrators, and medical and/or nursing staff of the venue at which the research will be performed. There is also a research council or evidence-based practice council in most teaching and in many community hospitals. Such councils have become more prevalent with the advent of Magnet status, which appropriately charges nursing with the responsibility to propose, initiate, and complete research activities.

Grant Proposals

If the proposed research will require funding over and above what is available from your institution, you might need to apply for a research grant. Writing a grant proposal is similar to the research proposal, but must be edited to the specifications of the granting body. Several and varied agencies offer financial support for nursing research. Some examples are the federal government, National Institutes of Health (NIH), national and local foundations, industries such as pharmaceutical and medical equipment companies, and nursing organizations such as AACN and ANCC. Each entity that offers funds for healthcare research has specific criteria that must be met by the study, along with a specific application form and process. You want to choose an agency that will have interest in your topic of study. So, for an ICU nursing protocol, AACN would be an appropriate sponsor to target. In general, you can access the Web site of the funding agency and follow the guidelines for grant application. The typical components of a grant application are a cover letter, application form, abstract, the body of the research proposal as previously described, an ethical review, budget, biographic sketches of the personnel involved in the protocol, any appendices that support the research, such as graphs, and references. As it is not within the scope of this book, detailed information on what to include in each of these sections can be obtained from the specific organization. It is important in the grant application process to pay close attention to the application instructions and guidelines as you can be denied a grant due to any deviation. To be successful in obtaining a grant you must have a good and interesting research idea, so review yours with other more experienced researchers and those with expertise in the area of your proposed research before you pursue the grant research proposal process. You must be able to prove, when writing your proposal, that there is a gap in nursing knowledge that will be filled by the answers to your research question and how the results will impact nursing practice. Grant and research proposal writing skills are not innate. They must be developed with practice and active participation in research.

You also must set aside enough time for writing a research proposal and/or grant application. At least 6 months is needed to prepare an application, although this needs to be individualized to the writer's ability, comfort level, and other professional and personal commitments (American Association of Critical Care Nurses, 2003). So, determine your topic of interest, do the background research and literature review, determine to whom you need to submit your proposal, and determine to whom you will apply for financial support. Seek out someone, preferably in your institution or at least local who has experience writing proposals and work with that person throughout your proposal writing process. Determine the deadlines for proposal and grant application submission, and create a doable timetable. Be sure to include time to review, revise, and have colleagues review your work.

Letters to the Editor

A work that is much less formal and strict in criteria than a journal article or research paper, but is publishable in most nursing journals, is a letter to the editor. This can be a short piece that requires minimal or no research. It is usually fun to write as it is in response to an article or column about which you have a passionate view. You can approach this in two ways: decide on a topic that interests you and find a journal with a piece on that topic and write a letter in response to it, or you can choose a piece that you already read and found to be interesting and write your opinions in the letter. Although there are not many rules in writing a letter to the editor, you will need to follow some instructions that are typically delineated on the editorial page of the journal. Your letter might be one of hundreds sent to the editor, especially if you are submitting to a popular, well-read publication. To ensure your letter will be read and published, you should keep the letter short, clear, and focused. Include your major points in the first few paragraphs. Use concise, poignant phrases and sentences, and refrain from using clichés. You want your letter to stand out from the crowd, so think of novel ways to approach the subject of interest. You might be controversial or you might disagree with the author's views, but do not personally attack the author. Keep your letter in good taste. Be sure to include your name and contact information as most publications verify, by phone or mail, the authenticity of the author. As with any piece you submit, make sure it is typed, double-spaced, spell checked, and proofread. Send your letter only to the publication in which you really want it to appear, but if you do not get a conformation call in 7 to 10 days, then you can try submitting it elsewhere (eHow, n.d.; PageWise, Inc., 2002).

Nominations

A novel writing endeavor for nurses is nominations for nursing awards. Although these are not publishable works, they do attract positive attention to not only the nominee, but to the writer as well, if the nominee wins the award. Nominations also help to get the hospital or entity at which the nominee works known in the professional nursing community. They can be used as PR for the hospital. Writing nominations is more creative than scientific writing and of course, no scientific research is needed. You need to interview the nominee to understand what makes him or her eligible for the award in question. You also have to follow the requirements for the nomination set forth by the awarding committee. You must include in your description of the nominee the characteristics that the award exemplifies, such as caring, compassion, commitment to teaching, education, and excellence in nursing. It is in how you present these criteria that your creativity prevails. The use of eloquent, possibly poetic prose will elicit the attention of the awarding committee and will win the award. Although the nominee should be (and hopefully is) truly worthy of the award, it is the worthiness of the nomination that is most important in the application process, as it is all the reviewing committee has to evaluate the candidate. Again, although writing nominations will not get you published, they will get you more comfortable with writing, and will get you recognition at least within your institution and possibly within the nursing community in which the award is being presented.

Books

Although it may seem like an unobtainable goal, writing book chapters or a complete book is possible for the nurse writer. The opportunity for contribution of a book chapter might present itself while working with a senior nurse, nursing educator, or administrator as it is often necessary to have many contributors to nonfiction, healthcare texts. If you have an original idea for a complete book that you think will be marketable and desirable, you can write a query letter to a publisher to see if there is interest. If the feedback is positive, you will need to detail your idea in a book proposal. A typical nonfiction book proposal consists of the proposed title of your book and how it is unique, an overview of the book idea with a synopsis of the book content, the author's background (which is essentially biographic information and qualifications that enable the author to produce the proposed book), reviews of competitive works, discussion of market potential of the book, a marketing plan, an annotated table of contents, chapter outline, and possibly a sample chapter.

Each publisher may want slightly different components for the book proposal, so be sure to request their required format before submitting your proposal. Further detailing the components of a book proposal is beyond the context of this book, but there are several online and print resources to reference when you are ready for this undertaking.

THE WRITING PROCESS

As we discussed previously, writing is met with trepidation by many people. Many nurses believe writing to be a chore, but if it is viewed as an opportunity to learn and expand your profession and career, it will be more palatable. Just like any new task, writing can be daunting, but if you have an idea that you are interested in and passionate about and you follow a systematic approach, writing will produce much less anxiety. Also, the more you do it, the better you will get and the more confidence you will have in your writing ability, which will lend to a comfortable relationship with writing. Think of it in comparison to learning to how to place an IV. The first few times, it was probably very intimidating. After many attempts, following a step-by-step protocol, and achieving successful placements, you became a pro and now it is a routine procedure for you. This can be the same for writing. You need to adopt a protocol for writing, implement it, repeat it several times, and then it will become routine.

The writing process actually begins before you put a pen to paper. First, you need an idea, a topic, or an inspiration. The development of an idea for a written work is prewriting, the first step in the writing process. In this step, you will organize your thoughts and brainstorm. Think about the message you want to convey in your writing. Decide in what format you want to present it, such as a hospital newsletter article or a peer-reviewed journal article. If you choose to write something for an outside publication, choose two potential publications to which you will submit before you start writing. Read and evaluate the author guidelines for those publications so that you can create your work within those parameters. With that in mind, commit to an approximate length that your work should be and the tone in which it should be written (formal, instructional, editorial). Also, remember to identify and think about the audience for which you are writing so that you can tailor your writing to fit their knowledge and understanding of or familiarity with the topic (The Writing Process, n.d.).

Once you have decided what you want to write and know the guidelines within which you must present your writing, you must schedule the time to write. Remember this is the biggest barrier to writing: lack of time. If you evaluate your work and home schedule and carve out times within that schedule during which you will write, even if it is 30 minutes a day, you will be successful.

Now you can begin working on the meat of the piece you are going to write. You might first want to document all of the main topics that you will want to cover in your work. To do this, it might be helpful to draw a picture or diagram, make a collage from newspaper clippings on your topic, verbally brainstorm with a colleague (just make sure to write down what comes out of your brainstorming so that you do not forget any points), make a bulleted list of all of your major points that you want to include, or create an outline with headings and subheadings. The latter is typically a good exercise even if you choose other methods to initially sort out your thoughts. An outline will really bring organization to your writing and might also allow you to better schedule your writing as you can choose a time frame for each section of your outline (The Writing Process, n.d.). When you create an outline and break down the writing task into pieces, it will not seem as cumbersome. You can then tackle one piece at a time.

Once you have categorized and arranged your thoughts into some semblance of order, you can begin to gather facts to support your thoughts. Do a literature search. Take each topic, heading, or subheading, and research it individually. Assess what you already know about the topic and look for resources to support and further your knowledge. You can do an online search and obtain some full text articles for free, others you may be requested to buy. (But before you get out the credit card, contact your hospital's library or a local college or university library. They typically can pull most articles and/or books for you or at least help you to locate them.) Then collate the information into batches corresponding to the heading or subheading to which the information pertains. After gathering the information, read through it all and extract the key points and facts that you will want to include in your article. Writing the article is then simply wrapping prose around the information, facts, and statistics you have gathered. This is the next step in the writing process: creating your rough draft.

In the rough draft, you will put all of the thoughts or facts you have collected into sentences. You will organize your paper into paragraphs. First should of course be the introduction, which should give the reader a glimpse of what the piece is to be about and should include some type of thesis statement (i.e., the purpose of the piece). Then you would include possibly several paragraphs describing the review of literature and facts about the topic. If it is a research article, you will include a methods section, and you will then have several paragraphs describing your thoughts, opinions or results. You might need to complete additional literature reviews to gather facts and statistics to support your assertions in the paper. Finally, you will write your conclusion in which you basically sum up what you have said in the paper and answer the thesis question that you presented (The Writing Process, n.d.).

Once your rough draft is complete, you can begin to revise and edit. You may want to restructure some sentences, check that you have not been repetitive, correct or add information, reorganize sections, and refine your language to improve your paper. You might also need to update some facts if new findings have occurred since you first began your work. At this time, you should have a peer read your paper and share feedback or advice. You might also want someone from the general audience for which your paper is written to read it and assure that it is understandable and enlightening. You should then revise again as necessary and reread. Finally, do not forget to check spelling and grammar. Throughout the writing process, if you have a thought about your topic or an epiphany about how to convey an idea, write it down. Even if you are not in front of your computer, are in the bathroom, or awaken from sleep at 3 a.m. with a catchy phrase in mind, write it down. Sometimes your best ideas come at the oddest times.

The following is a quick, reference list for the essential steps to completing and submitting a journal article. You can use this as a checklist as you proceed through the process so that you are sure not to miss any steps. Following the list is a basic outline of a research article with brief synopses reiterating what is needed in each section.

Steps to Completing an Article

1. Settle on the idea, and choose two possible publications.
2. Look at author guidelines for publications.
3. Schedule the time to write.
4. Literature search: What has been done? Successes?
5. Start writing.
6. Literature search: Statistics and facts to back up what you are positing.
7. Keep writing.
8. Edit . . . revise . . . edit . . . revise . . .
9. Have a colleague read it. **Always!**
10. Edit . . . revise . . . edit . . . revise . . .
11. Get all the extraneous paperwork completed: CV, copyright form, contract, etc.
12. Pray and **submit!**

Basic Research Article Outline

I. Introduction:

The introduction should resemble a 'V', where you start with a broad problem facing a large population and narrow it down to the specifics of what you are going to tackle in your paper. This will ultimately conclude with your thesis statement (Figure 8-1).

Figure 8-1   The introduction funnel.

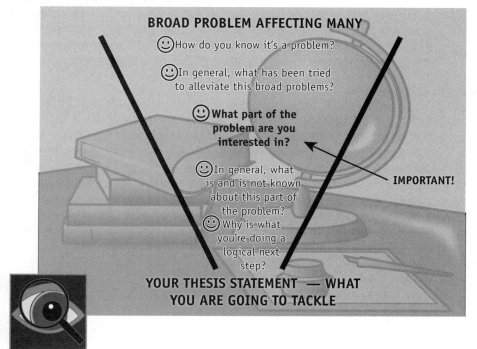

II. Literature Review

This is where you talk about what others have found concerning your topic and things related to your topic. A good literature review tells the reader what is and what is not known about the topic, and what should be the next logical step in tackling the problem.

III. Methodology

In this section, discuss how you designed your intervention, the sample you used, how you collected the data and what measures were used to determine if your methodology worked, and the detailed description of what you did and how you did it.

IV. Results

In this section you will describe the outcomes of your intervention in terms of findings per number of subjects, the statistical evaluation of the study findings, and what the statistics mean.

V. Discussion

In this section you will review the limitations of the study that might have affected the results, the overall finding of the study (the answer to your research question), the implications that the findings have for the general population and healthcare practices, and future research that is needed to expand on your work (Carlson, Masters, & Pfadt, 2008).

VI. Abstract

The abstract comes first in your submission, yet it is written last. As noted earlier, abstracts contain a very brief summary of the background, methods, results, and conclusions of your project. It is usually limited to 100 to 200 words. This is the hardest part: getting all of the needed information in without writing too much. It may help to go back to the outline you created before writing the article and write a sentence about each category or heading in the article. The abstract is very important to your publication as it is often how the article is categorized as a reference and how it will be accessed online. Keywords from the abstract are typically what is used to find an article when searching online. Also, if the reader does not like the abstract, he or she will usually not even attempt to read the article. Sometimes there is only access to the abstract when an online search is done and many times, the researcher will use only the information from the abstract rather than accessing the whole article. So, the abstract must be comprehensive, but concise and well written to attract readers.

HOW TO HELP NURSES WRITE

As with any skill, writing is learned and continually improved with practice. Most nurses, especially those in traditional bedside care positions, do not routinely write anything other than nursing notes (George, 2005). Even writing nursing notes has declined with charting by exception and computer charting programs requiring check marks rather than narrative. Scholarly writing is not included in undergraduate nursing curricula, nor is it an expectation of student nurses. However, in many graduate programs, there is a requirement to produce a publishable written work and writing for publication is an expectation of master's and doctorally prepared nurses working in any area of the profession. So, there we find a gap in preparation and expectations in the nursing profession. Nurses are not routinely educated on how to write professionally and submit for publication, but are increasingly expected to do so. How can we fix this? How can we fill in this gap?

Ideally, we need to start in school. Nurses need to be reared with writing instruction and repetitive practice in producing written works as well as reading, scrutinizing, and evaluating published, professional works such as peer-reviewed journal articles. Reading and writing professional, published, or publishable papers needs to become part of the culture of the nursing profession. Many graduate nursing programs do incorporate a research class that typically spans two semesters and requires production of a research manuscript. A class such as this focuses on the research process and does give some instruction on how to organize a manuscript and perform a literature review, but it typically does not provide intense instruction on and guidance with the actual writing process, which is truly needed by the novice writer. A course dedicated to the process of professional writing, encompassing all of the types of writing discussed previously needs to be incorporated not only into graduate nursing programs, but should be included in the undergraduate nursing curriculum. Introducing writing and publishing early on as part of the expectations of the profession is the only way it will be enculturated into the profession. It is up to professors of nursing and those on each state's Board of Nursing, who creates and prescribes nursing school curriculum, to adopt a mandate and process for the introduction to and instruction for writing. Do not fret; the revamping of the nursing curriculum does not have to be done immediately. We can start small and work our way up. For instance, writing workshops can be incorporated into most school programs, as well as in hospital education programs. Heinrich, Neese, Rogers, and Facente (2004) describe a writing-for-publication workshop that was developed for graduate students in nursing and introduces them to writing for publication, including sequential steps in the publishing process and peer editing. The article describing this workshop outlines the systematic process for introducing writing for publication. This can be a good resource for nurse educators and nursing administrators, especially those involved in the Magnet journey, as having nursing staff involved in research, information sharing, and publication is important for Magnet designation.

Most of us, from novice to seasoned nurses, have some written work that we completed for a prior school assignment that can be publishable. It may need a little reworking or embellishment, but it might be a good start to the publication process. Established nurses might tap into their portfolio of papers previously done for college assignments or work projects and reconfigure it to fit the prescribed guidelines of the venue in which they want to publish. Reversely, current students can write papers that can not only satisfy a class assignment, but also be presented for submission, possibly to a hospital newsletter for a clinical site at which the student is practicing. It might surprise you what you can uncover in things you have already written that can be publishable material. Nurse educators, professors, and clinical educators need to relay this to their students, so that all they write or have written can be evaluated and shared with the nursing and healthcare community.

In addition to having formal writing education incorporated into the nursing curriculum, mentoring should be instituted in schools and healthcare work places because writing skills should be developed over time. As discussed previously in this chapter, many nurses have fears or reservations about writing professionally and sharing their writing with others. Again, nurses currently have little formal instruction in writing for publication and would not even think they are capable of such a thing (Nettina, 2006). So, as it is tradition in nursing for senior nurses to precept the novices when they are coming into clinical practice, it should be tradition for nurse writers to mentor novice nurse writers so that the goal of publication and information dissemination can be met by the majority rather than a few.

Mentoring is extremely important to inspire others to write and create a new generation of nurse authors. Mentoring not only teaches the skills and process of writing, but it helps to build confidence in writing ability and familiarity with the process. Mentors first need to address the barriers to writing that nurses encounter: fear, intimidation, and lack of time. To do this, a mentor needs to break down the process of writing (specifically, writing for publication) into steps or attainable goals. This will demystify the process and make it less cumbersome to the nurse writer. The mentor needs to guide the author-to-be through each step of the writing and publication process, giving clear direction, support, and encouragement. The novice writer needs to know that each writing endeavor is a work in progress, that it will need to be revised and rewritten, and that is okay. It does not have to be perfect after the first attempt. Several drafts may be needed until the final product is ready for publication. Ultimately, the mentor needs to sit down with nurses and write. Immediate feedback about their writing, tips for improvement, and developing thoughts into words on paper together with novice writers will eventually enable them to do it themselves. Once a nurse achieves his or her first publication, confidence will be boosted and for many it will entice a passion for publishing and lead to repeated efforts and future publications. Help to get nurses to that first successful publication, and it will be a powerful motivator for future writing (Spear, 2006).

The mentor needs to be someone who has written and published before and feels comfortable with the process. In the hospital setting, unit educators, who are typically clinical nurse specialists and those in the education department, and Magnet directors, who are typically masters or doctorally prepared nurses, are typically well suited to be writing mentors as they most likely have had exposure to and experience with scientific writing for their master's thesis or doctoral dissertation. Even a staff nurse who has previously published can serve as a mentor to a peer. You must ensure though that the person who will be mentoring is skilled specifically in professional, nonfiction writing. There may be nurses who are excellent creative writers, but they might not have any idea how to write an abstract in which you must get a large amount of factual information in a very concise and structured format. Mentors, therefore, need to be carefully selected.

To promote writing and publishing in your institution, you might establish a writing group, for which time is secured to discuss the writing and publishing process, to write, get feedback, and submit for publication. This group can institute the teach-the-teacher method; each nurse who successfully publishes can then mentor other novice nurse writers. Participation is typically voluntary and time spent with the group might or might not be paid time for staff nurses. Meetings might be habitual, every month or quarter, or as needed when a nurse has a project to be developed. Criteria should be developed for entry as a mentor for two reasons: to ensure that the mentors are sufficiently experienced, and to have staff view entry into the group as a privilege or an honor.

So, how do you ensure continued involvement in the group by staff nurses? You need to publicize the group and let everyone know that writing can be fun and exciting. Exemplify the nurses who have published and publically acknowledge those who mentor. Relay how good it feels to see your name in print. You might also seek out staff nurses with ideas for evidence-based projects or those who want to share clinical experience stories or exemplars related to clinical practice or professional issues and develop them within the group.

An example of a writing group is one that was constructed by a few staff nurses, spearheaded by the Magnet director of a local hospital and was called GAS (Group for Abstract Submissions). The members of this group were those who had experience publishing. They would identify nurses in the hospital who had completed evidence-based practice projects or who had an idea for a project and developed it with them and guided the nurse through the writing and publishing process until he or she had a finished, submitted product. Once the abstract was submitted, that nurse was essentially set free and the next nurse with aspirations for publication was embraced by the group. For a more detailed description of the group and its construct, see the creative solution at the end of this chapter.

Another means of getting staff involved in the writing process is the organization of intensive writing retreats. Such retreats allow for isolated, focused time during which experienced and novice writers can work together to develop writing skills and produce written pieces for publication. One such retreat employed principles of servant leadership and incorporated mentoring and peer learning. Many benefits were realized, such as increased participation of staff in publication activities, positive effects on collegial relationships and team building, and the production of publications submitted to peer-reviewed journals (Jackson, 2009). Retreats like this can be as formal or informal as your institution would like. It can take place at a participant's house or in a comfortable place in the hospital that is conducive to this type of interaction. If finances allow, an outside facility could also be used such as a hotel conference room. The retreat can last a day or possibly even a weekend. Evaluate what the participants favor and try to construct the retreat with those factors in mind. This can be a fun excursion from the daily routine of healthcare work with a positive and long-lasting outcome.

As there is an increased expectation that academic as well as clinical nurses will contribute to the profession through scholarly writing, there must be multiple efforts within the hospital setting to promote and develop an interest and skill in writing. In addition to the smaller scale efforts described previously that are typically initiated by individuals in education and staff development positions, the hospital as a whole needs to show support of writing and publishing initiatives. As nurse leaders and administrators, you can develop institution goals for writing and publishing, and create incentives for writing and publishing. Of course, financial incentives are always welcome and usually effective in motivating staff to participate in activities, and this could be used to motivate nurses to write by attaching a dollar amount to a completed publication. Since financial incentives are not always feasible and might be viewed negatively by some, there are several other means to incentivize writing. An annual contest for poster presentations, written works, and publications can be developed in the hospital. Movement up the clinical ladder can be enhanced by writing initiatives and successful publications. You might work with the continuing medical education (CME) department to accredit approved, completed written works as continuing education exercises that will grant Continuing Education (CE) credits to those who produce them. Mandatory, annual education might include information about the writing and publishing process, as well as evidence-based practice exercises and how to disseminate their results. There are a multitude of ways to get nurses involved in and excited about writing; however, they need the commitment and support of the institutions, nurse leaders, and administrators to be successful.

Historically, professional writing and publication has not been a routine or expected endeavor by nurses other than those in academia. Today, the drive for the enhancement of nursing as a profession, the pressure for accountability of nurses for excellence in practice, the requirements for the implementation of evidence-based practices, and the goal of Magnet designation for hospitals has begun to create expectations for all nurses to be involved in knowledge acquisition and information dissemination. This means that nurses at all levels will be expected to participate in evidence-based practice activities, original research, and dissemination of the results. The problem that arises is that there are many barriers for nurses that prevent them from participating in these activities. As nursing leaders, we need to provide services that help to eliminate the barriers to writing and publishing. First, we need to provide instruction to develop writing skills, and guidance and coaching through the publication process to alleviate the fears of first time writers. Then we need to allow for the time required to learn, as well as produce, publishable works. Finally, we need to ensure continued interest in and commitment to writing, publishing, and information dissemination so that it is seen not as an extracurricular activity, but rather, as a core objective of the nursing profession.

CREATIVE SOLUTIONS

Creative Solution Title: *A Care Center Newsletter*

Creative Solution Authors: Terri Spoltore, RN, MSN, CCRN
Director, Medical Care Center and Transitional Care Unit
South Jersey Healthcare, Vineland, NJ

Bruce Alan Boxer, PhD, MBA, RN, CPHQ
Director of Quality/Magnet Program Director
South Jersey Healthcare, Vineland, NJ

Purpose: The goals of this project are to encourage and provide a venue for staff nurses to write in a professional capacity, to improve communication through enhancing interpersonal relationships with interdisciplinary team and care center specific staff, and to improve staff engagement and ownership of the five standards that align with the organization's strategic plan/goals: quality, patient/family satisfaction, fiscal responsibility, employee satisfaction, and patient length of stay.

Legend

Overall Rating: **NOVICE–ADVANCED BEGINNER**

Financial:

Time:

Personnel:

Other Resources: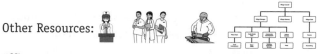

Efficacy: **A**

Transferability: **A**

Malleability/Adaptability: **A**

Ease of Implementation: **A**

Synopsis: Each care center at South Jersey Healthcare–Regional Medical Center is specialty specific and composed of multiple units. The Medical Care Center consists of the Medical Intensive Care Unit, the Medical Stepdown Unit, and the Medical Acute Unit. Encouraging the professional development of staff can be difficult. The Medical Care Center newsletter was developed to provide encouragement and a venue for nurses to write in a minimally critical environment. Nurses who wrote for the monthly newsletter were assured that the text would be edited to correct grammar, and the nurses were mentored through the writing, if necessary, by more experienced staff. Writing was mainly factual, conveying information that was otherwise just known to individual units. This internal writing was seen as a stepping stone to writing for external nursing publications such as nursing magazines and journals, as well as abstracts for poster presentations at professional conferences. In addition, it was hoped that by sharing and publishing the information, there would be better communication and engagement throughout the care center.

Description of Organization: South Jersey Healthcare (SJH) is a Magnet-designated, multiple-hospital system. The health system encompasses two full service inpatient hospitals consisting of approximately 350 inpatient beds, comprehensive health centers and outpatient, and specialized services such as a Bariatric Center of Excellence, Wound Care Center, Sleep Center, and Balance Center. In 2008, SJH performed over 18,700 surgeries and the Emergency department visits topped 97,400. The system contains an inpatient behavioral health facility, Bridgeton Health Center. The health system also serves as a clinical site for nursing students from a number of local colleges, and maintains a professional relationship with Cumberland County College, which is adjacent to the Regional Medical Center (RMC) campus.

The Case Study: As a Magnet-designated organization with a commitment to the professional development of nurses, SJH recognizes the need to contribute to the collective knowledge of the nursing profession. Professional writing seems to be difficult for nurses, yet is the main venue for disseminating practices, information, and research to others in the profession. To develop the professional writing ability and confidence of direct-care nurses on the Medical Care Center, the director had the idea for a care center newsletter and brought the idea to the care center leadership and the unit-based practice councils. The newsletter also seemed a good intervention to engage staff and to disseminate the enormous amount of information that needed to be shared. The participants in this initiative were: the clinical director, nurse manager, assistant nurse managers, clinical outcomes manager, performance improvement manager, patient relations representative, unit-based practice councils, and direct-care staff.

With limited resources, the Medical Care Center newsletter seemed a cost-effective method to address all of the issues previously noted. The template design was borrowed from internal newsletters already circulating. One staff member volunteered to assemble and format the newsletter. Writing was done by the care center staff, encouraged by the unit-based practice council members. Editing was done by the care center leadership. Copying and distribution were completed by unit-based practice council members. The monthly process, including deadlines, was established for writing, editing, compiling/formatting, copying, and distribution.

From the first edition, the newsletter was and continues to be a great success. Direct-care staff are more likely to read the newsletter than multiple posted notices with the same information. Staff look forward to new newsletter issues, and more staff have volunteered to write. The next step is transitioning these writers to submit for external nursing publications and presentations. We also plan to incorporate contests to increase readership and engagement, and listings of internal and external educational offerings so staff will be aware of the many internal and external professional development opportunities. Additionally, the newsletter communicates the positive accomplishments of staff; having their name and accomplishment in print to share with peers, supports ongoing positive professional growth and employee satisfaction, which we believe will ultimately benefit our patients' care.

Outcome Measures:

Formative/Compliance: The number of writers for the newsletter and the newsletter's readership is steadily increasing.

Summative/Outcome: The communication areas of the annual Employee Opinion Survey have increased. Anecdotal staff satisfaction and opinions of better communication is expressed frequently, and staff awareness of newsletter content through casual conversations is apparent.

Evidence Supporting this Creative Solution: Nursing newsletters are used frequently by various nursing organizations to relay information to their constituents. For example, *MedSurg Matters!* is the official newsletter of the Academy of Medical-Surgical Nurses (AMSN), and contains clinical information and news relevant to the membership of AMSN (n.d.). Although it is designed as a venue for communication, the AMSN encourages members' written contributions. Arizona State University College of Nursing and Health Innovation also publishes a newsletter for communicating news and events (http://nursingandhealth.asu.edu/files/n2n/newsletters/summer2009.pdf retrieved December 24, 2009). Adopting a similar format internally is an innovative way to bring a similar professional atmosphere to the care center milieu. Transitioning to external writing is the next logical progression for care center newsletter writers.

Academy of Medical-Surgical Nurses (AMSN). (n.d.). *MedSurg Matters!* Available at: http://www.amsn.org/cgi-bin/WebObjects/AMSNMain.woa/1/wa/viewSection?s_id=1073744080&ss_id=536873298. Accessed December 24, 2009.

Recipe for: *A Care Center Newsletter*

Ingredients:

Director/Manager support

Staff buy-in

Writing skills

Staff member accountable to compile and produce newsletter

Time allowance for staff with salary

Computer/word processing/printer/paper/template

Shared-governance structure to implement initiative (optional)

Step-by-Step Instructions (see Figure 8-2 for Step-by-Step Instruction Timeline):

Step 1: Obtain buy-in from staff and leadership, identify one staff member accountable for compiling and formatting newsletter, establish writing, production and distribution process, and timeline. Assign a unit/care center leader to be the primary editor, ensuring appropriate and accurate content.

Step 2: Establish format and content of newsletter with both leadership and staff input.

Step 3: Get all resources necessary: newsletter template, computer, paper, and copier. Recruit writers through the unit-based practice council or staff meetings.

Step 4: Set deadline for first issue and begin the writing, production, and editing process. Keep to the established timeline. Tweak the process if necessary to fit within the specific schedule/culture of the unit or care center.

Step 5: Produce the first issue. Zealously promote it. Make it ubiquitous. E-mail an electronic copy to all staff, if able. Have hard copies available in multiple locations throughout the unit/care center. Talk it up; make it fun!

Step 6: Continue production, continue recruiting writers, and tailor the newsletter's content to meet the needs and interests of staff.

Step 7: Mentor writers to write for external nursing venues.

Step 8: Measure staff satisfaction with the newsletter, number of writers monthly, and number of writers who subsequently write for external nursing publications. Share success with other units/care centers.

Figure 8-2   Timeline for "A Care Center Newsletter."

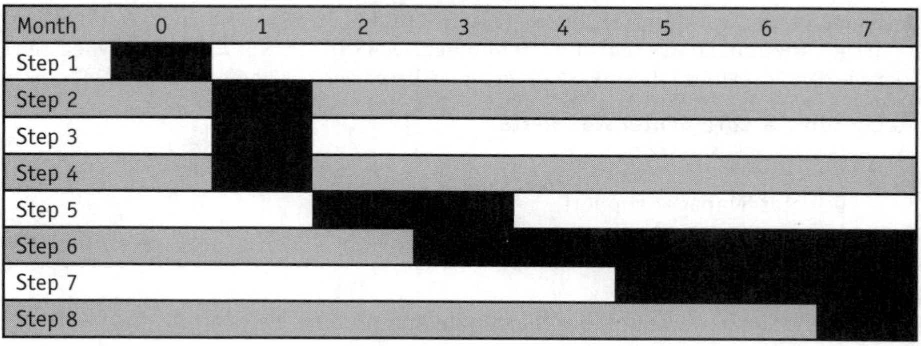

Month	0	1	2	3	4	5	6	7
Step 1								
Step 2								
Step 3								
Step 4								
Step 5								
Step 6								
Step 7								
Step 8								

Additional Outcomes to Consider Measuring:

Formative/Compliance: No additional measures.

Summative/Outcome: Measure the number of contributing writers that publish in external nursing venues; formally survey the staff for their satisfaction with the newsletter as a communication device.

Insights from Original Implementation:

- Organizing information is critical, and having a template designed into which information could be inserted would make it easier to assemble; select key contributors to seek out information; keep to timeline.
- Commitment of the staff is essential.
- Choosing the right person to compile and format the newsletter is crucial to keeping to the timeline and continuing the initiative. Choose someone who is detail-oriented, a stickler for deadlines, assertive, and respected by staff.
- Give writers credit for their writing; always have their name and credentials as the byline to an article or informational column. Also give credit in print to the person formatting the newsletter. This provides both incentive and recognition.
- Placement of the newsletter is important. The employee restroom and break room are terrific places to put a supply of newsletters.

For Further Guidance Contact:

Terri Spoltore, RN, MSN, CCRN
spoltoret@sjhs.com

Bruce Alan Boxer, PhD, MBA, RN, CPHQ
boxerb@sjhs.com

Creative Solution Title: *GAS*

Creative Solution Author: **Bruce Alan Boxer, PhD, MBA, RN, CPHQ**
Director of Quality/Magnet Program Director
South Jersey Healthcare, Vineland, NJ

Purpose: The goal of this project is to mentor nurses to write research and quality improvement project abstracts for submission to professional conferences to promote and disseminate the patient care improvement projects undertaken at South Jersey Healthcare (SJH), and to create the expectation for professional dissemination when any nursing research or quality project is undertaken.

Legend

Overall Rating: **NOVICE–ADVANCED BEGINNER**

Financial: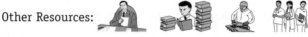

Time:

Personnel:

Other Resources:

Efficacy: **A**

Transferability: **A**

Malleability/Adaptability: **A**

Ease of Implementation: **A**

Synopsis: A group of leaders committed to nursing professional development formed a group within the shared-governance structure to mentor and facilitate nurses writing research and quality project abstracts for submission to professional nursing conferences. The group is known as GAS, Group for Abstract Submission, and strategically targets the coordinators of nursing research and quality projects to submit abstracts based on received calls for abstracts from professional nursing conferences. The group has been quite successful in mentoring nurses in writing and submitting abstracts and has raised the bar, creating the expectation to professionally disseminate the results of every research or quality project undertaken. Anecdotally, this has also raised both the internal and external perception of professional excellence of SJH nursing.

Description of Organization: South Jersey Healthcare (SJH) is a Magnet-designated, multiple-hospital system. The health system encompasses two full service inpatient hospitals consisting of approximately 350 inpatient beds, comprehensive health centers and outpatient and specialized services such as a Bariatric Center of Excellence, Wound Care Center, Sleep Center and Balance Center. In 2008, SJH performed over 18,700 surgeries and the emergency department visits topped 97,400. The health system also serves as clinical site for nursing students from a number of local colleges and maintains a professional relationship with Cumberland County College, which is adjacent to the RMC campus.

The Case Study: As a new employee of SJH, the Director of Quality/Magnet Program Director saw some amazing nursing practices occurring at SJH, yet the nurses at SJH thought this was just business as usual. They did not believe they were setting new standards or creating new ways of delivering high quality patient care. As a personal goal, the director was determined to get these nurses to realize the contribution they were making to patient care and to share this contribution with others in the nursing profession. The first call for abstracts received, provided a venue to demonstrate the value of SJH nurses' innovative practices. The director saw a nursing practice at SJH that met the requirements for the abstract submission, and with the collaboration of those that initiated the project, wrote an abstract to submit. The acceptance of this abstract brought an amazing change in the self-perception of SJH nursing.

At his former institution, the director developed a group to mentor nurses in professional writing. The initiative described here is a bit more proactive and strategic, utilizing professional conferences' calls for abstracts as impetuses for forming a group to strategically brainstorm which projects would fit abstract requirements. The group formed at SJH used the acronym GAS, the Group for Abstract Submissions. This group not only strategically picks projects for submission, but mentors the projects' coordinators to write the abstracts, and facilitates the submission process. The group is formed from members of the Nursing Research Council, part of the shared-governance structure at SJH. As such, the group is promoted at all research council meetings and within the shared-governance structure. As part of the shared-governance structure and because of the positions of the group's members, they are privy to many of the quality initiatives and research projects ongoing at SJH. The membership of GAS includes: the Director of Quality/Magnet Program Director, the Director of Behavioral Health, the Outcomes Manager/Chair of the Nursing Research Council, the Administrative Assistant to the Director of Quality/Magnet Program Director, and the cochair of the Nursing Research Council. Ad hoc members are also recruited when necessary.

The process is as follows. When a member of GAS receives a call for abstracts from a local, national, or international professional nursing conference, he or she calls the group together to brainstorm which projects meet the criteria for submission. The coordinators of these projects are contacted and invited to participate in the writing and submission process. If agreeable, the project coordinator and GAS members meet and write an abstract according to the call for abstracts criteria and submit. If successful, GAS members assist the project coordinator in developing the poster or presentation. GAS has been quite successful. In 1 year, more than 15 abstracts have been accepted at various local, national, and international professional nursing conferences. Anecdotally, this initiative has instilled an air of professionalism and has elevated the self-perception of SJH nurses. It has also instilled a bit of competition, and has raised the bar in expectations to be innovative in patient care initiatives.

Outcome Measures:

Formative/Compliance: On average, 75% of members are available and willing to meet when calls for abstracts are received. Project coordinators were all 100% amenable to writing and submitting abstracts when contacted.

Summative/Outcome: Approximately 80% of submitted abstracts were accepted for presentation. Anecdotally, when a quality or research project is undertaken at SJH, professional dissemination of results has become an expectation of project coordinators.

Evidence Supporting this Creative Solution: The author based this creative solution on a variation of the project in the article *Filling in the Gaps* (Boxer, in press). Here, the group assembles only when a call for abstracts is received and strategically brainstorms for internal projects to fit the notice's requirements. Mentoring in itself has an abundance of supporting literature. In nursing, mentoring is seen in many aspects of professional development. Professional writing is merely an extension of this concept.

Boxer, B. A. (in press). Filling in the gaps. *Nursing Management.*

Recipe for: *GAS*

Ingredients:

CNO and leadership support

Staff buy-in

Willing group members with mentoring and professional writing skills

Time allowance for project coordinators and mentors with salary

Shared-governance structure

Call for abstracts

Step-by-Step Instruction (see Figure 8-3 for Step-by-Step Instruction Timeline):

Step 1: Obtain support from CNO, leadership, and staff. Make nursing professional development a strategic initiative.

Step 2: Utilize shared-governance structure to recruit those with experience in professional writing and mentoring. Also recruit those who are privy to the research and quality improvement projects ongoing at your institution.

Step 3: Form the GAS and set the process for meeting, brainstorming, contacting project coordinators, mentoring, and abstract submission. Establish a timeline for the submission process from receiving the call for abstracts to submission. You can use a different name for your group. Just make the acronym catchy and memorable. Have fun with it.

Step 4: Promote the GAS vigorously. Establish, distribute, and promote the group's contact information for those receiving a call for abstracts unknown to the group's members.

Step 5: Have members search for or join organizations that disseminate calls for abstracts for professional nursing conferences.

Step 6: Assemble as needed, meeting call for abstract deadlines for submission.

Step 7: Follow up with project coordinator, meeting and mentoring for conference poster/presentation if submission is accepted.

Step 8: Disseminate the notice of acceptance of the submission throughout the nursing department, creating an expectation for the professional dissemination of research/quality initiatives. This also incentivizes the professional dissemination of projects and rewards those who have done so successfully. Keep track of the number of submissions and the number of submissions accepted.

Figure 8-3   Timeline for "GAS."

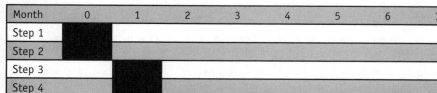

Additional Outcomes to Consider Measuring:

Formative/Compliance: Survey staff to determine awareness of the GAS.

Summative/Outcome: No additional measures.

Insights from Original Implementation:

- Make sure there is a member of the group who either regularly searches for, or is connected enough to receive as many calls for abstracts as possible. This might consist of an awareness campaign to inform staff to send any calls for abstracts that they receive to a member of GAS.

- Select group members who are committed and ready to mentor.
- Commitment of the CNO, leadership/management, and staff is essential. Professional development of staff should be a strategic initiative.

For Further Guidance Contact:

Bruce Alan Boxer, PhD, MBA, RN, CPHQ
boxerb@sjhs.com

REFERENCES

American Association of Critical Care Nurses (AACN). (2003). Writing a successful AACN grant proposal. Retrieved from http://www.aacn.org/AACN/research.nsf/Files/GP/$file/Writing%20a%20successful%20grant.pdf. Accessed March 10, 2010.

Bogert, S., Rutledge, D., Morrison, V., Smith, J., Dureault, K., Norman, V., & Ulrich, T. (2010, April 14). *Nursing Research: Show me the evidence!* Available at: http://evidencebasednursing.blogspot.com. Accessed March 10, 2010.

Burnard, P. (1992). Why nurses do not write. *British Journal of Nursing, 1*(5), 221.

Carlson, D. S., Masters, C., & Pfadt, E. (2008). Guiding the clinical nurse through research publication development. *Journal of Nurses Staff Development, 24*(5). 222–225.

Dear Abby (n.d.). *Some good advice.* Available at : www.word-crafter.net/CompIpn/DearAbbyPN.doc. Accessed April 11, 2010.

eHow. (n.d.). *How to write a letter to the editor.* Available at : www.ehow.com/how_8921_write-letter-editor.html. Accessed November 7, 2009.

George, A. K. (2005). Review of the book *Writing in the health professions*, by B. A. Heifferon. *American Journal of Pharmaceutical Education, 69*(5), 2.

George Mason University (2010). *Introduction.* Available at: http://chhs.gmu.edu/writing/introduction. Accessed April 11, 2010.

Heinrich, K. T. (2009). Why nurses should write for publication (but don't). *American Nurse Today, 4*(8).

Heinrich, K. T., Neese, R., Rogers, D., & Facente, A. C. (2004). Turn accusations into AFFIRMATIONS: transform nurses into published authors. *Nursing Education Perspectives, 25*(3), 139–145.

Jackson, D. (2009). Mentored residential writing retreats: A leadership strategy to develop skills and generate outcomes in writing for publication. *Nurse Education Today, 29*(1), 9–15.

Jenkins, S. (1995). How to write a paper for a scientific journal. *Australian Journal of Physiotherapy, 41*(4), 285–289.

Language Center. (n.d.). *Writing up research: The abstract.* Available at: http://www.ait.ac.th/education/LanguageCenter/ait-writing-services/guide-book/the-abstract.html. Accessed October 23, 2009.

Nettina, S. M. (2006). Nursing publication: Get involved. *Topics in advanced nursing eJournal, 5*(4).

PageWise, Inc. (2002). *Writing a letter to the editor.* Available at: http://www.essortment .com/all/lettertothe_rvet.htm. Accessed November 11, 2009.

Price, P. J. (1988). Nurses need to be taught to write. *AORN, 47*(2), 457.

Samuelowicz, K., & Bain, J. D. (1992). Concepts of teaching held by academic teachers. *Higher Education, 24*(1), 93–111.

Saver, C. (2006). Reap the benefits of writing for publication. *AORN Journal, 83*(3), 603–606.

Spear, H. J. (2006). Nurses and publication success: the value and importance of mentoring. *Nurse Author & Editor, 16*(3).

The Writing Center. (n.d.). *Abstracts.* Available at: http://www.unc.edu/depts/wcweb/ handouts/abstracts.html. Accessed October 23, 2009.

The Writing Process. (n.d.) *The writing process* (graphic). Available at: http://www.franklin .ma.us/auto/upload/schools/fhs/285-writing-process.gif. Accessed October 23, 2009.

Trotter, C., & Rasmussen, N. N. (2006). Writing for publication: Supporting the neonatal nurse practitioner student. *Neonatal Network, 25*(2), 75–76.

Ulrich, T. (2007, April 10). *Making a poster presentation* (blog entry). Available at: http:// evidencebasednursing.blogspot.com/2007/04/making-poster-presentation.html. Accessed March 10, 2010.

Zilm, G. (2008). *The SMART way: An introduction to writing for nurses.* Philadelphia: Mosby, Inc.

## CHAPTER 9

Institutionalizing Nursing Autonomy and Professional Development

"Professionalism: It's not the job you do, it's how you do the job."
—ANONYMOUS

"Unless we are making progress in our nursing every year, every month, every week, take my word for it we are going back."
—FLORENCE NIGHTINGALE

Autonomy is essential to professionalism. Nursing has continually strived to achieve professional status and with that, gain autonomy in practice. But what do we mean when we say we want to be autonomous as nurses? Wade (1999) refers to a general dictionary definition of autonomy as "the right of self-government; personal freedom; freedom of will; and a self governing community." In nursing, the desire for self-government and freedom of will does not refer to the individual nurse, but to the profession as a whole. This is the difference between personal autonomy, which is independence of the individual, and professional autonomy, which is independence of those within a profession to practice without the control of a governing body external to that profession. Numerous definitions and descriptions of the concept of professional nursing autonomy have been created, but it is difficult to find an all-inclusive definition, so we will evaluate several sources to develop a comprehensive description and understanding of what makes nursing an autonomous profession.

Most definitions speak of independence in decision making within the nurses' scope of practice and responsibility for one's actions. Some, more recent definitions, appropriately address the role of education of the professional nurse, the responsibility of the nurse to the patient as an advocate and in decision making regarding their care, and the inevitable need for interdependence with other members of the healthcare team to assure the best care of the patient. The following is the definition used by Wade (1999) to describe the concept: "professional nurse autonomy is . . . belief in the centrality of the client when making responsible discretionary decisions, both independently and interdependently, that reflect advocacy for the client." This definition is fairly comprehensive, but it does neglect to address two aspects that are very important to the development and maintenance of professional nursing autonomy: education and scope of practice. Education of the nurse is highly important as it is what enables the nurse to make appropriate, independent, and interdependent decisions in patient care. Nurses' knowledge of areas such as human anatomy and physiology, pharmacology, etc., their confidence in that knowledge, and their awareness of the abilities and limitations of their licensure allows nurses to choose necessary nursing interventions as well as evaluate the advanced practitioner prescribed interventions and decide if they are appropriate and in the best interest of the patient. Nurses can and must challenge advanced practitioners to ensure only safe and necessary interventions are prescribed and never unquestioningly enact practitioners' orders. Nursing knowledge must be combined with their values, and their decisions should be based on reason and deliberation to exhibit true autonomy in practice.

A complementary definition to Wade's is one by Schutzenhofer (1987), stating that professional nurse autonomy is " the practice of one's occupation in accordance with one's education, with members of that occupation governing, defining and controlling their own activities in the absence of external controls." Directors of nursing have defined autonomy as "freedom to practice," "independence in nursing and decision making," and the "ability to self-govern." (Kramer & Schmalenberg, 2003). Various other, more recent definitions recognize autonomy as simply "control over work," "freedom to act on what you know," and "freedom from bureaucratic restraints" (Kramer & Schmalenberg, 2003). Obviously, it is difficult to find one definition that speaks to all of the essential components of professional nursing autonomy. This is because professional nursing autonomy is a dynamic process in a complex healthcare system that is ever changing. Despite these inevitable changes in health care, we must have some constants that make evident autonomy in our profession as nursing autonomy is essential to the forces of magnetism and strongly relates to nurse job satisfaction (Kramer & Schmalenberg, 2003).

Essentially, to be autonomous, the nursing profession must be able to provide care for patients within their scope of practice and in accordance with their education without the rule of physicians/advanced practitioners or hospital bureaucracy. The historic view of the nurse as the physician's helper has caused much difficulty for the nursing profession to be viewed as an autonomous profession. There is no doubt that we as nurses need to work with physicians and advance practitioners as well as the plethora of other healthcare team members to provide for the best and highest quality patient care. However, although there is clearly overlap with medicine, nursing has its own body of knowledge and a unique scope of practice. This is evidenced by the American Nurses Association Standards of Nursing Practice and the Professional Practice Model, both of which will be described later in this chapter. In addition, nurses are taught by nurses and use texts written by nurses. Nurses are also governed by nurses. State boards of nursing, not boards of medicine, delineate licensure requirements and grant nursing licensure. In most healthcare facilities, nurses are directly managed by nurses. So, to recap, as nurses, we have our own body of knowledge, a defined scope of practice, and nurses call the shots for nursing practice. These are the components of the equation that equal professional autonomy (MacDonald, 2002).

Nursing autonomy and independence as a profession is increasingly being acknowledged by those outside of the profession. It is gaining recognition from some government institutions. Many state nursing practice acts define nursing in broad terms that do not include dependence on physicians or other practitioners. A great example of a nursing practice act that represents nursing as an autonomous profession and incorporates many of the essential components of this distinction is that of Massachusetts. The act defines nursing as

> assist[ing] individuals or groups to maintain or attain optimal health, [including] administration of procedures "prescribed" by advanced practitioners, clinical decision making based on nursing theory to develop and implement care strategies, evaluating responses to care and treatment, coordinating care delivery, collaborating with other members of the healthcare team and management, direction and supervision of the practice of nursing. (The Center for Nursing Advocacy, 2006)

It also states that "each individual licensed to practice nursing in the commonwealth shall be directly accountable for the safety of nursing care he delivers" (The Center for Nursing Advocacy, 2006).

Accountability and Autonomy

Accountability is also key to autonomy. We must know that the outcome of every action we take in patient care, whether prescribed by a physician or other advanced practitioner, is our responsibility. With that, we must be sure that we know why we are doing what we are doing. We must have some base knowledge that enables us to know and be sure that our actions are appropriate and in the best interest of the patient. Finally, we must take ownership of our actions and accept the consequences of those actions. This, ultimately, is accountability (Maas, Specht, & Jacox, 1975). In other words, we cannot blame the physician in defense of an action that might have caused harm to a patient. If we carried out a prescribed treatment, we are as responsible for the result as the ordering party. Before carrying out any order, we need to have a rationale for why we are doing it and how it will help the patient, and know the possible risks. From that, we must decide, independently, to either proceed with the prescribed treatment or not. Nurses must be able to say, "I did that and this is why," and the explanation should be evidence-based. Nurses need to be legally and morally responsible for their practice to be autonomous in their profession.

State laws clearly define nursing's responsibility for managing itself. They define nursing practice including a wide range of critical prevention and care functions that do not require or depend on physicians or other advanced practitioners (The Center for Nursing Advocacy, 2006). Nurses can and have been found liable in courts of law for wrongdoings in patient care. Nurses also have and need liability insurance. All of this is a testament to the presence and recognition of nursing accountability and therefore, should also imply autonomy.

Finally, nurses must themselves have an understanding of what autonomy means to their practice and recognize their practice as autonomous. They need to be aware of their scope of practice as well as standards of practice. They need to know how their practice is delineated by the Board of Nursing and their own state legislature. As said previously, nurses need to have confidence in what they know and display that by exerting their professional expertise in patient care decision making and in all interactions with healthcare personnel. If nurses do not believe in and exhibit autonomous practice and professionalism, they cannot expect to be treated as an autonomous profession by other professions or by the general public.

PROFESSIONAL PRACTICE MODEL AND THEORETICAL FOUNDATIONS

What Is a Professional Practice Model?

As you begin your Magnet journey, you will need to visit your institution's professional practice model (PPM) for nursing care. This is a great time to evaluate the model you currently have and judge how well it fits your current practice environment, as well as if it can grow into your new Magnet environment. For the truly uninitiated, the first question is, "What is a professional practice model?" This is a very valid question. Many attempt to create a PPM without fully understanding its purpose and components. Hoffart and Woods (1996) define a PPM as

> a system (structure, process, and values) that supports registered nurse control over the delivery of nursing care and the environment in which care is delivered. A PPM has five subsystems: values, professional relationships, a patient care delivery model, a management approach, and compensation and rewards. (p. 354)

The American Nurses Credentialing Center (ANCC; 2008) defines the PPM as

> [t]he driving force of nursing care; a schematic description of a theory phenomenon, or system that depicts how nurses practice, collaborate, communicate, and develop professionally to provide the highest quality care for those served by the organization (e.g., patients, families, community). Professional practice models illustrate the alignment and integration of nursing practice within the mission, vision, and values that nursing has adopted. (p. 64)

From these two definitions, a picture appears of what a PPM should look like and the functions it should serve. In an institution, it is the foundation for nursing clinical care, defining the way nurses practice and how they interact with their environment to support the delivery of quality patient care in a professional, satisfying work environment. The PPM helps to professionalize the discipline of nursing.

What Is a Profession?

There has been and currently is much discussion as to the designation of the discipline of nursing as a profession. Nursing as a profession is relatively young, and continues to accumulate its own body of knowledge and develop theoretic frameworks to demonstrate its unique practice and contribution to society. It is difficult to state exactly what constitutes a profession. Much has been written, but many continue to cite Houle's (1980) 14 characteristics of a profession. They are the following: concept of a mission that is open to change, mastery of theoretic knowledge, capacity to solve problems, use of theoretic knowledge, continued seeking of self-enhancement by its members, formal training, credentialing system to certify competence, creation of subculture, legal reinforcement of professional standards, ethical practice, penalties against incompetent or unethical practice, public acceptance, role distinctions that differentiate professional work from that of other vocations and permit autonomous practice, and service to society.

Contemplating Houle's 14 characteristics, one sees the possible areas of controversy, especially in role distinctions that differentiate professional work from that of other vocations and permit autonomous practice and use of theoretic knowledge. These two characteristics are at the heart of what a PPM demonstrates. The former is constantly changing with the new roles nursing adopts as well as changes in state licensure and scope of practice. The latter, the use of theoretic knowledge, is the difficult one. Ask nurses about their use of theoretic knowledge and we would bet they would be hard pressed to tell you on what theory their practice is based, if any. As a clinical discipline with multiple educational points of entry (i.e., diploma, associate's degree, bachelor's degree), time to teach and understand the theoretic foundations of nursing practice are sometimes sacrificed in lieu of time spent mastering clinical practices.

Hoffart and Woods (1996) analyzed five PPMs described in the literature. They found that these PPMs showed that the professional values most often addressed were nurse autonomy, nurse accountability, professional development, and an emphasis on high-quality patient care. Approaches to enhance professional relationships were frequently described, such as teamwork, collaboration, and consultation. Within the PPMs are the defined care delivery systems used to deliver care to patients. There are a number of care delivery systems that have gone in and out of vogue throughout the years, such as team nursing, primary care nursing, etc.

These systems were many times driven by the skill mix available to deliver care as well as institutional culture (Seago, 2001).

Hoffart and Woods (1996) saw primary nursing and case management as the care delivery systems most often used in the PPMs they scrutinized. The PPMs also included decentralizing decision making, expanding the scope and type of unit nurse manager responsibilities, and instituting structural changes to support professional practice. There were incentive programs to recognize professional achievement and contributions made toward meeting organizational goals. The PPMs basically defined the practice environment and provided the organization with a defined structure to understand the components of the practice environment and how they interact to realize the goals of high-quality patient care in a satisfying, professional work environment.

Standards

The PPM should also be grounded in the American Nurses' Association (ANA) *Scope and Standards of Nursing Practice* (2004). This document delineates 15 standards for the professional practice of nursing. The first 6 standards focus on clinical practice, while the others focus on professional performance. They are as follows:

- Standards 1–6: Assessment, Diagnosis, Outcomes Identification, Planning, Implementation, and Evaluation respectively.
- Standard 7: "Quality of Practice – The registered nurse systematically enhances the quality and effectiveness of nursing practice" (2004, p. 33).
- Standard 8: "Education – The registered nurse attains knowledge and competency that reflects current nursing practice" (p. 35).
- Standard 9: "Professional Practice Evaluation – The registered nurse evaluates one's own nursing practice in relation to professional practice standards and guidelines, relevant statutes, rules, and regulations" (p. 36).
- Standard 10: "Collegiality – The registered nurse interacts with and contributes to the professional development of peers and colleagues" (p. 37).
- Standard 11: "Collaboration – The registered nurse collaborates with patient, family, and others in the conduct of nursing practice" (p. 38).
- Standard 12: "Ethics – The registered nurse integrates ethical provisions in all areas of practice" (p. 39).
- Standard 13: "Research – The registered nurse integrates research findings in practice" (p. 40).
- Standard 14: "Resource Utilization – The registered nurse considers factors related to safety, effectiveness, cost, and impact on practice in the planning and delivery of nursing services" (p. 42).
- Standard 15: "Leadership – The registered nurse provides leadership in the professional practice setting and the profession" (p. 44).

Some of these standards are delineated even further in other ANA publications, such as the *Code of Ethics for Nurses with Interpretive Statements* (2001) and *Nursing Administration: Scope and Standards of Practice* (2009).

Theoretical Foundations

Within the PPM, there needs to be some theory to guide your nursing practice.

Nursing theory is an organized and systematic articulation of a set of statements related to questions in the discipline of nursing. A nursing theory is a set of concepts, definitions, relationships, and assumptions or propositions derived from nursing models or from other disciplines and project a purposive, systematic view of phenomena by designing specific inter-relationships among concepts for the purposes of describing, explaining, predicting, and/or prescribing. (Current Nursing, 2010, para. 3)

You might ask why do we need to base our practice on theory. Well, again this is another valid question.

There are a many reasons. The article, *Application of Theory in Nursing Process* (2010) provides a number of reasons. Nursing theory

should provide the foundations of nursing practice, help to generate further knowledge and indicate in which direction nursing should develop in the future; theory is important because it helps us to decide what we know and what we need to know; it helps to distinguish what should form the basis of practice by explicitly describing nursing; the benefits of having a defined body of theory in nursing include better patient care, enhanced professional status for nurses, improved communication between nurses, and guidance for research and education, [and] the main exponent of nursing—caring—cannot be measured, it is vital to have the theory to analyze and explain what nurses do. As medicine tries to make a move toward adopting a more multidisciplinary approach to health care, nursing continues to strive to establish a unique body of knowledge. This can be seen as an attempt by the nursing profession to maintain its professional boundaries. (para. 4)

As Houle (1980) stated, one of the 14 characteristics of a profession is the use of theoretical knowledge. The use of theoretical knowledge in nursing practice is important in creating a common foundation. Nursing theory is used in practice to: ". . . (a)ssist nurses to describe, explain, and predict everyday experiences; (s)erve to guide assessment, intervention, and evaluation of nursing care; (p)rovide a rationale for collecting reliable and valid data about the health status of clients, which are essential for effective decision making and implementation; (h)elp to establish criteria to measure the quality of nursing care; (h)elp build a common nursing terminology to use in communicating with other health professionals. Ideas are developed and words defined; [and] enhance autonomy (independence and self-governance) of nursing by defining its own independent functions" (Current Nursing, 2010, para. 6). The use of theory in practice also just makes sense.

We bet you remember from the theory class in your nursing program the number of theories that have been proposed to help provide the profession of nursing with a common language and a common framework for research and practice. So, what theory should you use? Should you use more than one? Here is a bit of advice. Theories should be helpful, tools to help design a research study or a PPM. Most hospitals will adopt one main theory and a corresponding nursing theorist for the foundation of their nursing practice and their PPM. This theory and theorist might also be utilized as a framework for developing nursing research studies.

At one of the Magnet-designated hospitals we have had the privilege of working, the Neuman Systems Model (NSM) (Neuman & Fawcett, 2002) is utilized as the foundation of their nursing practice. The model is also used as the foundation for much of their nursing research. The NSM provides a framework that is easy to understand and a common language that is applicable to inquiry as well as practice. Nurses find the model a logical extension of the systems perspective they learned in anatomy and physiology and nursing curricula. The holistic perspective of nursing is also echoed in the model, and its concepts and propositions are general, applicable to the various nursing situations and specialties. Utilizing the NSM has been quite a benefit for this hospital, especially when they hosted a research conference with the keynote speaker none other than Betty Neuman, RN, PhD, herself. It was a surreal event, as nurses met the woman who developed the foundation for their nursing practice and whose theory has benefitted innumerable patients and practitioners; a woman who literally has made an indelible mark on nursing that will continue to contribute to excellence in patient care and the professionalism of nursing for years to come. Of course there are other nursing theories and theorists that might fit better with your institution's culture and practice environment. Let the nurses in your institution decide which nursing theory/theorist they believe is most in sync with your department. If you have a shared-governance structure, utilize it to have staff evaluate the current nursing theory and other possible theories to determine which they believe would be most useful to their practice.

Many institutions utilize Patricia Benner's novice to expert theory (1984) for their nursing education and professional development. Patricia Benner is a professor in the Department of Physiological Nursing in the School of Nursing at the University of California, San Francisco (Benner, n.d.). Benner used the model originally proposed by Dreyfus and Dreyfus (1980),

> and described nurses as passing through five distinct levels of development: novice, advanced beginner, competent, proficient, and expert. Each step builds on the previous one as abstract principles are refined and expanded by experience and the learner gains clinical expertise. (Dracup & Bryan-Brown, 2004, p. 449)

This theory has been instrumental in the development of stage-appropriate nurse education. One of the insights it uncovers is that a nurse can revert back to a novice from an expert if he or she transfers to a new area of nursing.

This insight has been quite valuable in understanding why nurses cannot perform at the same level in multiple specialties without experience, because experience is not transferrable. It has helped to define areas of nursing as specialized and in need of specific skills to achieve competence. Nursing is not completely generalized; skills and knowledge are specialty specific even though there are underlying foundational concepts. This is similar to the medical model, where physicians share a base of knowledge, but different specialties require specific knowledge and skills, seldom transferrable to other specialties. This theory has helped to change the paradigm that a nurse can be assigned to any area of nursing when staffing dictates the need, and has been fundamental in the closed-staffing model. Closed-staffing models have shown to improve patient outcomes. For example, closed-model intensive care units (ICUs) are associated with 33% reduced mortality of patients with acute lung injury (Treggiari et al., 2007).

What is important here is to realize the benefit of using theory in practice, and to use it as a tool. Remember, a tool is ". . . anything used as a means of accomplishing a task or purpose" ("Tool," n.d.), which means it should help you in your purpose, not become an effort in itself. There is no denying that it takes some initial effort to disseminate, educate, and enculturate theory into the clinical setting, but once accomplished, the theory can help provide a common and cohesive language and framework to better patient care and the work environment.

NURSING SHARED GOVERNANCE

Let us start with a definition of nursing shared governance from one of the gurus of nursing shared governance, Robert Hess.

> Governance is about power, control, authority, and influence. It answers the question in an organization, "Who rules?" Nursing shared governance extends that rule to nurses. It surfaced as a radical break from traditional hospital governance where nurses had little power within a rigid formal hierarchical bureaucracy. Nursing shared governance is a managerial innovation that legitimizes nurses' control over practice, while extending their influence into administrative areas previously controlled only by managers. (Hess, 1998; Hess, 2004, para. 2).

It sounds a bit ominous, but nursing shared governance is all about nurses having a voice in the decisions that affect their practice, the practice environment, and ultimately, patient care. It is sort of a no-brainer. How can nurses be professional if they cannot make decisions on how to provide patient care and how their care environment is structured? If we want accountability in practice, then we must provide a mechanism to determine practice. Nursing shared governance is that mechanism. Porter-O'Grady (2001) says that shared governance is a way of conceptualizing "empowerment and building structures to support it" (p. 470) and embodies four principles: partnership, accountability, equity, and ownership.

There are a number of models of shared governance. The structures are a bit different, but all should achieve the same purpose: providing nurses a voice in determining their practice and the characteristics of their practice environment. The different models allow you to determine what will work best in your institution, considering the culture, costs, and infrastructure already in place. Most institutions we have seen have some type of informal structure for addressing performance/quality improvement issues, utilizing teams or task forces to explore opportunities for improvement. Shared governance could be seen as an extension of this structure. The key to keeping shared governance to its intended purpose, is to give as much control to as many staff as possible. In other words, you want to give as many decisions related to nursing practice and the care environment to direct-care nurses as possible. You also want as many direct-care nurses participating in the decisions as possible. These are the two rules to live by: allowing nursing shared governance to fulfill its intended purpose and achieve its potential, realizing its contribution to excellence in patient care.

The Structures and Models and Which to Use

[S]hared governance, as an organizational form, has potential to bridge differences between the traditional bureaucratic models, characterized by centralized decision making, with professional models that are distinguished by independent authority for decision making. (Anthony, 2004, para. 7)

Four configurations of shared governance are described by O'May and Buchan (1999): unit-based systems, councilor models, administrative models, and congressional models. Unit-based systems are governance models specifically tailored to individual nursing units. Councilor models are designed using a number of department/system level councils to coordinate specific clinical and administrative activities. Administrative models demonstrate an executive level of coordination over smaller councils activities, establishing a council hierarchy. The congressional model is less popular in the literature, where all nursing staff belong, and work is given to cabinets.

Hess (2004) discusses three types of shared-governance structures:

The most common model is the Councilor Model in which a coordinating council integrates decisions made by managers and staff in subcommittees. A second model, the Administrative Model resembles a more traditional bureaucratic structure that splits the organizational chart into two tracks with either a management or clinical focus, although the membership in both tracks often encompass both managers and staff as implementation progresses. A third structure, the Congressional Model, relies on a democratic component to empower nurses to vote on issues as a group. (para 12)

Malleo and Fusilero (2009) describe their institution's experience implementing a shared-governance structure. Their structure is based on a senate model with elections held to determine representation. "The nursing senate represents all staff RNs within [their] health system, including nurses in inpatient, outpatient, and satellite units. Units [are] grouped by specialty, nominations and elections [are] held for representatives and alternates for each area, and meetings . . . begun" (p. 33). They have had successful growth for the past 8 years with some impressive accomplishments, including achieving Magnet designation.

Our experience is mostly with the councilor structure. It provides a relatively flexible structure with a degree of institutional individualization in the number and focus of councils. It also provides a good division of labor, and a specific focus and purpose to each council, allowing staff to determine which council they are most interested in based on its focus and purpose. Typically, within the council structure, you will see a coordinating council, which functions as the council that oversees the other councils. Other councils may focus on professional develop-ment, recruitment and retention, quality, research, clinical practice, informatics, patient education, staffing/budgeting, and rewards and recognition. You will need to determine what types of councils work best for your institution. We recommend at least a quality council, a professional development council, a research council, and a clinical practice council, along with the coordinating council. Structuring these councils is important and should be focused on the flow of communication. There also needs to be some type of nurse executive council where communication flows from nursing leadership to the other councils. Figure 9-1 shows the coun-cilor structure we helped to create at a Magnet-designated hospital in New Jersey.

Figure 9-1   Sample shared-governance councilor structure.

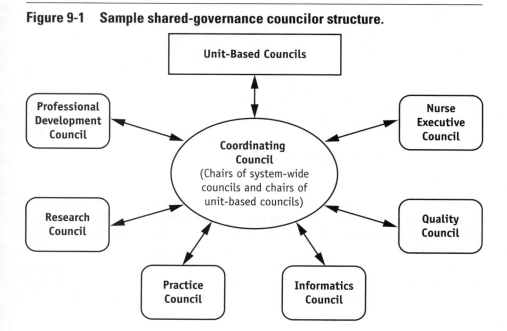

In our opinion, the unit-based practice councils (UBPCs) are crucial to getting both communication and shared-governance activity to the direct-care nurse. Each unit is charged with developing a UBPC with unit leadership acting as mentors. Each UBPC has a council chair, who by default is also a member of the hospital system's coordinating council. This integration allows a 2-way flow of communication and information. As the unit representative to the coordinating council, it is the UBPC chair's responsibility to bring the communication to everyone on his or her respective units. This occurs typically through presentations at unit staff meetings and in summary communication sheets, placed in binders on each unit and available to all unit staff.

Does it Work?

Although it is difficult to isolate and quantify directly, the anecdotal effects of a viable shared-governance structure can be impressive. The literature cites examples of benefits a shared-governance structure can bring: better decision making increased communication, collegiality, perceptions of autonomy, engagement, professional development, accountability, and satisfaction with work; and ultimately better patient outcomes. Remember, the impetus for initiating a shared-governance structure should, in some way, determine the purpose for the initiative, which in turn should be one of the ways you evaluate the success of your shared-governance structure. For example, if you are instituting a shared-governance structure because your nurse turnover rate is high when benchmarked nationally, then the purpose of the implementation is to decrease nurse turnover. Thus, evaluating nurse turnover after the shared-governance structure has been functioning for a bit of time will allow you to gauge its success. Of course there might be secondary benefits, such as those cited previously, that accompany your primary purpose. Measure everything you can to help you evaluate the benefits achieved through your shared-governance initiative. This will provide ammunition to defend this initiative to naysayers.

Considerations for Implementation

Purposeful Work

Make sure you are not establishing councils just to establish councils. Sure, the Magnet Recognition Program endorses nursing shared governance, but do not just establish the structure to fulfill a requirement; make the structure work for nursing and your institution. The councils need to be doing purposeful work. This will give the groups a mission and vision, demonstrating their contribution to the institution and their contribution to patient care and the work environment. Shared governance costs money; there is no denying it. Make it money well spent.

Authority of Group

Whatever you charge the group to do, make sure they have the authority to do it. There is nothing more disheartening than being given the responsibility for making a decision, only to be overturned after your decision has been made. It is as if your work on the issue was an effort in futility. If you give them the responsibility, give them the authority.

Administrative Liaison

You need an administrative liaison/mentor for each council. You may think this is contradictory to the shared-governance principles; that direct-care nurses should *own* the councils and not have interference from nursing leadership. Nurses can own the council and still have an administrative liaison/mentor. The liaison knows how to run meetings and can help guide the council, facilitating a productive meeting by keeping the council focused on its purpose. The liaison also knows what is plausible. For example, the nursing quality council is charged with reducing medication errors and decides the institution needs new intravenous pumps. The liaison knows there are no funds in this year's budget and that purchasing new pumps is not plausible. The liaison can speak up right away, instead of allowing the group to spend months formulating a recommendation that is not viable. You need to find the right balance. It is all about supporting the council and allowing nurses a voice. You also do not necessarily need to give councils decision-making authority. You can ask for recommendations on specific issues. This will ensure their voice is heard and accounted for when decisions are made. It also demonstrates that there are many factors to each decision, and direct-care nurses might not be knowledgeable in all of those factors (i.e., budgeting, necessary competencies, concordance with institutional culture, etc.). It is shared decision making, not staff decision making. Again, it is all about balance.

Develop Leaders

One of the benefits of a shared-governance structure is its ability to uncover and develop leaders. Councils should be chaired by direct-care nurses. This almost forces an institution to develop educational programs to teach council chairs and cochairs leadership skills: how to run a meeting, how to deal with conflict, and how to gain consensus. From this, the next generation of nurse leaders might be recognized and developed. It is all about personal and professional development and succession planning. At one institution, many of the unit-based council chairs were eventually promoted to assistant nurse managers, on track to become future nurse leaders. This was an effective way of evaluating nurses' leadership skills and desire to be administrators. It is not a fit for everybody. A great clinician does not necessarily make a great manager or leader, yet that is typically what happens. A nurse is recognized as a great clinician and is considered for a managerial or leadership position. Clinical skills do not necessarily transfer to leadership skills. Utilizing the council chair and cochair positions as trials for managerial positions is a cost-effective way to recognize the talent within your institution.

Education

Education will be necessary for all involved in the shared-governance structure. The education can basically be divided into three topics: general education on what shared governance is, its purpose, and its benefits for everyone involved; topics specific to staff participating in shared governance; and topics specific to management in shared governance. The general education is more of an introduction to the who, what, why, and how: the history and benefits of shared governance. The why is crucial. Make sure your argument for why shared governance is being implemented is strong, positive, and uses universal and unarguable benefits like better patient care and a better working environment. After general education is complete, you can target more specific education geared to your specific audiences: staff and management/leadership. We should comment here that senior leadership needs to be on board from the beginning with their endorsement, and should be educated on the general shared-governance stuff as well as the costs and benefits, so their decision to move forward with this initiative is based on knowledge and understanding. This needs to happen before any education for staff or management occurs.

Hess (2008) lists topics to consider for educating staff, such as: concepts of authority, responsibility, and accountability; assertiveness; decision making; leadership styles; negotiation and conflict resolution; team building and collaboration; delegation; time management; leading and participating in meetings; performance appraisal and peer review processes; interdisciplinary collaboration and collegiality; and the budget process. You might want to also consider evidence-based practice process, determination of cost vs benefit or cost-effectiveness, and data interpretation. "Staff nurses need to understand it is their right and professional obligation to participate in how decisions are made about nursing practice" (Brooks, 2004, para. 3).

Hess (2004) discusses five issues that need to be recognized and considered when implementing shared governance:

1. "Shared governance is a journey, not a destination" (para. 26). Do not expect to be finished. There are always more people to involve, and as the institution continues to grow, so does the shared-governance structure.

2. "The journey can be long and steep" (para. 27). There is a sharp learning curve with implementation. "[A]ttempts to elicit participation without allowing opportunities to acquire prerequisite skills can leave some people frustrated and others apathetic" (para. 26). Make sure there is education prior to implementation as well as leadership support.

3. "Not every environment is conducive to shared governance" (para. 28). Leadership needs to be ready to change its paradigm of "leading through control" to "leading through facilitation." Hess also cautions that due to regulatory or union requirements, shared governance may not be able to be implemented in all areas. As we have stated previously, and Hess reiterates, "committees must have legitimate organizational authority congruent with responsibility and accountability to carry out their decisions" (para. 30).

4. "Although not everyone might make the journey, it should be open to all" (para. 31). Eventually shared governance should include the entire institution as well as patient representation. Patient care and a positive work environment are interdisciplinary concerns, and models that restrict others, only inclusive of nursing, might not be effective.

5. "Is the journey worth the price?" (para. 32). Nursing research has to look at the relationship of shared governance with multiple possible correlates. Many of the studies show equivocal results. Some studies are small with others using flawed methodology. Other studies show cost-effectiveness and tangible benefits. These are usually case studies and are not necessarily replicable at other institutions. Shared governance does cost time, effort, and money, but if outcomes such as less nurse turnover can be realized, it will save money in the long run.

Hess also cautions that "[t]he implementation of shared governance is not easy. It can be riddled with conceptual ambiguity and resistance from the old bureaucratic guard and new professionals struggling to establish their skills. Not everyone will share the enthusiasm for this wonderful innovation" (para. 25).

Some of the skills necessary for staff to actively participate in shared governance are: the ability to engage in decision making about patient management issues; the ability to engage in the development of standards of practice; and the ability to engage in quality assurance (QA) monitoring, conflict resolution skills, and negotiation skills (Reeves, 1991). Staff council leadership (chairs and cochairs) will also need education in how to run a meeting, including the administrative tasks such as creating an agenda, taking minutes, documenting attendance, and the process of submitting issues for council consideration.

For management and leadership, the main education needed is how to become a facilitator instead of a director. For shared governance to be effective, managers must believe that staff can fulfill their responsibilities within the shared-governance framework if given the appropriate support. Instead of managers telling staff what to do, they need to ask what should be done to achieve this outcome, and how they can help. This is a major paradigm shift in most managers' thinking. Manager-as-director becomes manager-as-facilitator and mentor, authority-based governance becomes accountability-based governance, and top-down initiatives become bottom-up initiatives.

So let us be honest. What you are doing is asking managers to give up control for decision making to the staff. This is radical to many. They might manage a certain way and control might be a large part of their management style. However, as we have said before, management style should be flexible and individualized to each employee. Managers need to be able to assess the barriers preventing staff from participating in shared governance and use their legitimate institutional authority to eliminate these barriers. They are now working with staff instead of merely directing staff. It is a much more collegial approach and we believe it adds to development of managers as well as staff. It forces managers to recognize and evaluate their current management style and hopefully become more flexible in their style, enhancing mentoring skills while decreasing hierarchic divisions between staff and management.

Beth Brooks is a consultant working with healthcare providers on designing, implementing, and measuring the effectiveness of shared governance. She states, "[w]orking with managers so they understand their own change style, decision-making style, and leadership style is an important part of their journey of self-discovery. The journey from autocratic leader to democratic leader is not always an easy one" (2004, para. 5). Her insights might help you in preparing leadership to accept and support your shared-governance initiative.

At first, many institutions involve staff through a paradigm of invitation, allowing those who want to be part of it to join and those who do not want to be part of it to decline. At the beginning, this makes sense. It is not as radical as having everyone involved at once, disrupting all nurses while the bugs are still being worked out of the system. It allows those who are quick adopters to be brought in to help tweak the structure and make the processes run efficiently. After implementing a structure and establishing effective processes, however, we believe it is time to enculturate shared governance by getting everyone involved at some level. We believe this requires a paradigm shift from invitation to expectation. This expectation must be perpetuated by everyone, both leadership and staff. It needs to be worked into job descriptions, peer reviews, merit salary increases, performance reviews, incentives and goals; basically, anywhere you can incorporate the expectation for shared-governance participation. How you define participation is up to you. It can be anything from committee or council membership to participation in a shared-governance initiated project. Be creative; just set the expectation.

Bylaws

You will need bylaws for each of the system- or hospital-wide councils. These bylaws are similar to team charters you may be more familiar with. The bylaws for the council define the basic process of the council, discuss the membership of the council, outline the purpose of the council, the functions of the council; from these functions and the system's strategic goals, council goals can be established. The bylaws also define voting status and accountability of members and council leadership, and might define overall interactions with other councils or institutional groups. Do not reinvent the wheel. There are guidebooks and online references that can help you establish bylaws for each council, although the council needs to have input on their group's bylaws and be able to approve them. It is best to have a standard format for all council bylaws, so that you ensure the same topics are addressed for each group. In our practice environment, after each council approves their bylaws, the coordinating council must also approve them, as they are the oversight for the operational shared-governance structure. Revisit your bylaws either annually or biannually so that they remain fresh, usable, descriptive, and encultured. Following this section is a sample of a 3-hospital system's bylaws for their nursing practice council. Look at some Magnet-designated hospitals' nursing department Web sites, and you might find copies of their councils' bylaws to use for reference. Tweak them to your institution's needs and culture.

From these bylaws and the nursing department's strategic goals, you can develop the council's specific functions. From these functions, you can develop specific annual goals for each council to be evaluated for achievement at the end of the year.

Sample Bylaws

SHARED GOVERNANCE
NURSING PRACTICE COUNCIL BYLAWS

Purpose: To review and evaluate all changes affecting nursing practice in accordance with the Nurse Practice Act, revise and approve policies related to nursing practice using evidenced-based best practices, evaluate nursing care products and product failure data.

Functions of the Practice Council:

- Evaluates all proposed changes affecting nursing practice prior to implementation.
- Facilitates clinical competence by defining and revising clinical practice using evidence-based best practices, research outcomes, and standards of patient care including but not limited to: performance expectations and position descriptions.
- Evaluates impact of practice changes.

- Assesses staff practice needs, and develops, implements, and evaluates initiatives to meet these needs.
- Coordinates with other shared-governance councils to assist with nursing practice issues.
- Ability to grant additional powers to the chair as needed, or to remove the chair if necessary.

Membership:

1. Members will be 18 practicing licensed RNs (representation of all specialties and all three hospitals)

   1 Administrative advisor

   1 Nurse manager

   1 Nursing director

   1 Staff educator

   1 Clinical outcome advance practice nurse (APN)

   Patient/family/staff committee chair

   Ad hoc representation from nursing and other patient care disciplines will be added when deemed necessary

2. Responsibilities of members:
   - Must attend meetings regularly or appoint a surrogate to substitute, ensuring representation at all meetings.
   - Bring identified nursing practice issues to meetings.
   - Disseminate the information from practice council meetings to unit staff, manager, and director through staff meetings, leadership meetings, and other communication mechanisms.
   - Have an active voice in the council and participate in council activities.
   - Council decisions are approved through member consensus. All permanent members are considered voting members. If consensus cannot be achieved, majority vote will suffice.
3. Maintain a voting membership in the council with approximately 70% staff members (clinically based, which equates to 80% of their time spent on direct patient care activities).

Empowerment of the Chair:

- Represent the practice council to other councils/committees/groups.
- Represent the practice council at all coordinating council meetings.
- Make decisions on behalf of the practice council in the event the practice council cannot meet. Critical decision making will then be reviewed by the practice council.

- Chair will be responsible to communicate practice council activities and decisions to the executive council and communicate coordinating council information to the practice council members.
- Establish the agenda according to priority and ensure that minutes are recorded.
- Remove members from the practice council if the member:
  - Has had greater than 20% unexcused absences without surrogate representation.
  - Does not participate in practice council activities and initiatives.
  - Does not communicate effectively with peer group.
  - Has received previous notification of unmet responsibility by the chair.
- Facilitate decision making and reaching consensus

The Qualifications of the Practice Council Chair Person:

- Chair and cochair must be full-time/part-time staff RN who spends 80% of work time participating in clinical nursing practice.
- Chair is a member of the practice council for a minimum of 1 year.
- Chair will serve a term of no more than 2 years.

Recommended Guides

Tim Porter-O'Grady, DM, EdD, GCNS-BC, NEA-BC, FAAN is considered an expert in the topic of shared governance and has a consulting firm to assist with establishing its structure for those of you who want to go that route. If resources do not permit utilizing consultants, there are a number of resources available to guide you in the process. Porter-O'Grady has published a few books on shared governance, which will definitely be useful. *Implementing Shared Governance: Creating a Professional Organization* (2005) is available as a free download.

There are other venues to obtain assistance and advice (besides this book) that you can tap into. Take a look at other hospitals' nursing Web sites. You might find their models of shared governance displayed if they have one in place. You can get an idea of the structures used and the corresponding functions of each council. Also search the Web and nursing literature for stories and case studies of how other institutions implemented their shared-governance structures. You can learn a lot of things to do and things to avoid doing. When researching, note the hospital's demographics (i.e. bed size, geographic area, teaching status, and Magnet status). This will help you determine how similar your institution is to theirs, and what might be transferrable to your institution. We bet some of your peers came from other institutions where they had a working shared-governance model. Interview these individuals and find out about their experiences with shared governance and what their prior institution's model was like. Last but not least, we recommend that you find Magnet-designated hospitals in your area. Call and ask to speak with the

Magnet program director (MPD). Ask the MPD about his or her hospital's shared decision-making structure: the design of the structure, why the specific structure was chosen, the timeline for implementation, and anything else you feel might help you. Do not be shy. Ask for help. MPDs of Magnet-designated hospitals are typically willing to share, and can provide valuable insights for your initiative.

CERTIFICATION AND FORMAL EDUCATION

Briggs, Brown, Kesten, and Heath (2006) define certification as "a process by which a nongovernmental agency validates an individual's knowledge related to a specific area of practice. This process is based on certain predetermined standards. The focus is evidence-based practice and the application of clinical experience" (para. 4). We all pretty much know the standard format most professional organizations use for certification. The nurse typically must have either so many hours or years of experience in a certain specialty to qualify to sit for the certification exam. The nurse then schedules the exam, possibly taking a preparatory review course before the exam date. He or she then takes the proctored exam at a specific place. More and more certification exams are now computerized, some providing results minutes after exam completion. To receive accreditation to bestow certification from the National Commission for Certifying Agencies (NCCA), a certifying body must demonstrate that its examinations are based on current job analyses and accepted testing and measurement principles. Testing must reflect current practice in the specialty and must measure specified aspects of this practice appropriately (Briggs, Brown, Kesten, & Heath, 2006).

Reasons for Certification

The Institute of Medicine (IOM) recommends that healthcare providers be reevaluated and relicensed periodically, but there is currently no standard method in place for reevaluating registered nurses (Kohn, Corrigan, & Donaldson, 2000). It is thought that national specialty certification helps to fulfill this recommendation (Briggs, Brown, Kesten, & Heath, 2006). A study by Cary (2001) supported the association of certification with patient safety, finding that nurses who had been certified for 5 years or less reported that they made fewer errors in caring for patients than the overall group of nurses who responded. The American Board of Nursing Specialties (2009) states that specialty nursing certification is the main criterion used by the public to recognize quality nursing care. However, there is little data linking specific patient outcomes with national certification. Both the AACN's Beacon Award for Excellence in intensive care nursing and Magnet designation use national nursing specialty certification as one of their criteria in judging nursing excellence (Briggs, Brown, Kesten, & Heath, 2006).

Benefits of Certification

There are many benefits to national certification. Beyond the belief that it results in providing better patient care, 39% of respondents in a study of certified nurses indicated that recognition as an expert was one of the benefits of national specialty certification, 77% of certified nurses reported experiencing personal growth from obtaining national certification, and certified nurses also reported being more professionally satisfied (Cary, 2001). Many hospitals realize the benefits of national specialty certification both in patient care and professionalism. Obtaining national specialty certification satisfies two of Houle's (1980) 14 characteristics of a profession: the continued seeking of self-enhancement by its members and a credentialing system to certify competence. In our experience, those who seek and obtain national specialty certification see nursing as a profession, not just a job, and tend to be more involved in activities that advance the profession and better patient care.

National specialty nurse certification can be used to improve hospital recruitment and retention by demonstrating nursing excellence through a high proportion of certified nurses. This might provide a competitive advantage and be used as a marketing tool for hospitals, displayed in its advertisements, and on its Web site.

Incentives for Certification

First you need to recognize that, strategically and for many reasons, Magnet designation, promotes excellent patient care, promotes competitive advantage, decreases nurse turnover, increases nurse recruitment, advances the profession of nursing, and enables more knowledgeable staff. In seeking Magnet designation, your institution needs to encourage, promote, and incentivize the achievement of national nursing specialty certification. More certified nurses are to the institution's advantage. So, how much is the institution willing to pay for this advantage? This and your creativity will determine how you incentivize and promote national certification. We will share a few methods we observed.

Nearly all institutions we have observed pay the cost of the certification exam if the individual is successful; some pay up-front, some will reimburse. Paying for the exam up-front can have many benefits. Some individuals live paycheck to paycheck, and putting out the cost of the exam might be a hardship and act as a barrier to certification. Up-front payment may also demonstrate the faith the institution has in the individual's ability to successfully sit for the exam. If the individual is not successful, the cost of the exam can be reclaimed through incremental salary deductions to minimize the financial impact. Many institutions will also pay for review materials and review courses; again some with prepayment or reimbursement.

The cost-effectiveness of conducting your own in-house certification review course should be scrutinized. We have encountered various situations where the costs in personnel and media resources outweighed the benefits of producing an in-house course instead of sending individuals to an external established review class. You also need the necessary expert personnel to prepare individuals to sit for the exam, something your institution might be lacking.

Financial incentives are quite common. One institution, to the extreme as far as we can tell, provides a pay increase of $3.00 per hour to nationally certified nurses. We have not found another institution that matches this direct financial incentive. Some will give a one-time certification bonus, and others provide an hourly certification bonus. You will want to survey the staff and have them actively involved so that they have input on developing a meaningful incentive program. Many use national certification as a requirement within their clinical ladder, the program that recognizes the professional development of nurses. Some restrict the use of financial incentives to the support of educational endeavors, such as attending conferences or continuing education to maintain national certification. Others focus more on recognition to encourage certification, placing the names of certified nurses on a plaque in their specific unit, or publishing their achievements in an internal newsletter and possibly an external nursing publication.

Many institutions include the certification credentials on their individual name badges, both to let staff and the patients know which nurses have achieved national certification. Again, it is up to your institution and the nursing staff as to how the program is designed. Just make sure your program considers both incentives and recognition; not that they are mutually exclusive, just that it is good to have an awareness of both. Also realize that there are many inexpensive ways of incentivizing and recognizing. A hand written note from the chief nurse officer (CNO) recognizing the individual's achievement of national certification can go a long way.

Various Certifications

There are a number of different certifying agencies and a number of different certifications. As of this writing, the ANCC, one of the largest nursing certifying bodies, offers 42 distinct specialty nursing certifications (2009a). Now, extra knowledge is always beneficial, at least in our opinion. However, there might be minimal benefit for having a certified geriatric nurse who works in the pediatric unit. Certification should be meaningful to one's work, so you might want to restrict your institution's bonuses for obtaining national specialty certification to certifications that are beneficial to one's current area of nursing. The ANCC also publishes a list of acceptable nursing certifications when institutions are applying for Magnet designation, as the percentage of certified nurses in an institution is required for submission (ANCC, 2009b). Certifications listed are accredited by the American Board of Nursing Specialties or the National Commission for Certifying Agencies. There are actually three tiers of certification: The first tier includes accredited national RN certifications, the second tier includes nonaccredited national RN certifications, and the third tier includes national multidisciplinary certifications (ANCC, 2008). As you continue on your Magnet journey and develop incentive programs to encourage national nursing specialty certification, take a look at this list as a guide to validating appropriate certifications.

THE CLINICAL LADDER

The Nursing Clinical Ladder provides a framework for the promotion and recognition of excellence in nursing practice. The Ladder:

- Recognizes and rewards professional nurses who choose to develop excellence in direct patient care roles,
- Fosters professional growth and satisfaction for nursing personnel,
- Promotes recruitment and retention of nursing personnel,
- Encourages nursing and research with other nurses, disciplines, and institutions, [and]
- Improves the quality of patient/family care. (Seton Family of Hospitals, 2009, para. 1)

In general, a clinical ladder is a program that incentivizes and recognizes the professional development of direct-care nurses by promoting greater knowledge, professional growth, and engagement with the institution as well as with the profession of nursing. It is usually a hierarchic stepwise progression of projects, certification, and formal and informal education requirements, becoming more complex and encompassing greater skill as an individual ascends. Each step bestows a corresponding incentive and recognition, increasing as one climbs the ladder. There are a number of ways this program can be designed. We suggest utilizing the evidence-based practice process with direct-care nurses involved to develop the program. Search other institutions' programs and look at some of the commonalities with your clinical ladder development team. Determine through reviewing appropriate literature which incentives and recognition initiatives work and could be utilized in your own institution.

Use your local Magnet-designated hospitals as a resource for their structure and processes and note what has been most successful. Let your team design the program with your goals in mind. Do you want to increase certification, formal education, retention, or professionalism? Do you want the ladder to be exclusive, denoting achievement for just being in the program, or should everyone be on the ladder, allowing the different levels to differentiate achievements? From our experience, everyone should be a part of the clinical ladder, and should be eligible on the first day of hire, irrespective of degree or experience. Degree and experience should, however, determine the level or rung of the ladder. Exclusivity should come with the achievement of higher levels. The benefit is that everyone is now on the path to professional growth. There is no decision or barrier to getting on the path. It is now a matter of progression. Remember, your goal is to develop everyone, not just the motivated few.

CONTINUING AND FORMAL EDUCATION

Currently, 21 states require nurses to complete continuing education lessons to renew their licensure. The number and type of continuing education credits required varies from state to state (Career Toolkits, 2009). This need for continuing education can be a powerful motivator and incentive to encourage nurses to attend educational events. When we plan our annual Research Day, we always apply to receive continuing education credits through our state agency to encourage nurses to participate in the event. Many national specialty certifications can be renewed through proof of completion of specific continuing education programs after initial certification, eliminating the need to sit for another exam. Continuing education requirements might also be a part of your clinical ladder.

Formal education is important. Aiken, Clarke, Cheung, Sloane, and Silber, (2003) found that mortality rates for surgical patients in 168 Pennsylvania hospitals were nearly twice as high at hospitals where less than 10% of nurses had bachelor's degrees as they were at hospitals where over 70% did. They concluded that substantial improvements in patient care could be achieved by recruiting nurses from bachelor's degree programs rather than the 2-year associate's degree programs, arguing that nurses with more formal education tend to be better at critical thinking, a necessary skill in nursing. Formal education also fulfills many of Houle's (1980) characteristics of a profession: mastery of theoretic knowledge, capacity to solve problems, use of theoretic knowledge, continued seeking of self-enhancement by its members, and formal training.

New York and New Jersey state legislatures are considering bills requiring all newly licensed RNs to obtain a bachelor of science in nursing (BSN) within 10 years of initial licensure. These bills are in response to the profession's awareness of the increased complexity of patient care, as well as advocates for one mode of entry into the professional practice of nursing.

> Initiatives to raise the educational level of practice in nursing date back as early as 1965, when the American Nurses' Association voted to make the BSN the minimum for entry into practice. A similar initiative was proposed again in 1985. Although the proposal garnered support from some professional organizations, the initiative did not become law. (Boyd, 2009)

In 2007, in the United States, there were 1758 nursing programs, of which 683 were BSN, 1000 were associates degree in nursing (ADN), and 75 are diploma programs (National League for Nursing, 2007). At Kent State University (n.d.), a PowerPoint from a class titled Socialization to Professional Nursing Roles points out some of the drawbacks of multiple levels of entry into nursing that denigrates nursing's claim that it is a true profession, not merely a discipline:

- Only discipline that does not require at least a baccalaureate degree to be licensed.

- Practice of Nursing is not viewed as a career by some nurses.
- Nurses have the lowest educational requirements among professional health care providers. (n.d., slide 8)

There seems to be a push by nursing and the public simultaneously to require a high educational standard for entry into practice. The BSN requirement appears to be a first step in achieving this goal. The ANCC has a requirement that starting in 2011, to be eligible to apply for Magnet designation, an institution must have 75% of their nurse managers have a BSN, and by 2013, 100% must have achieved the BSN (ANCC, 2008). You can see the need to support, facilitate, promote, and encourage higher education in your institution.

Pragmatically, you want to have the highest proportion of BSN prepared nurses possible. So, how are you going to do this? First see what proportion of your nurses are already bachelor's degree prepared in nursing and compare it to a national benchmark to see where you compare. This will give you a reference for goal setting. It is not about having a certain percentage, though; it is about increasing your percentage and keep it growing. After determining a realistic goal, take it point by point:

Support: How much tuition reimbursement does your institution provide? Is it comparable to other institutions? Is it realistic considering the local cost of tuition? Do you have resources in your institution that can aid with school work questions?

Facilitate: Do you prepay tuition or reimburse? Do you pay for textbooks? Is there a program nearby? Do you have a relationship with a BSN-program school? Could they bring classes to your institution? Do you have someone acting as a guidance counselor for higher education? Do you schedule individuals according to their school schedule?

Promote: Do you disseminate a list of schools and programs? Do you disseminate school open-house events? Could you host a college fair for BSN/MSN/PhD nursing schools? Do you have BSN or higher nurse managers acting as role models for staff? Do you publicize when someone achieves an educational milestone?

Encourage: Do you have goals for managers to have a certain number of staff enrolled in classes? Do you have a reward or recognition program when someone achieves an educational milestone? Is the expectation for higher education enculturated through incorporation in your staff job descriptions, peer reviews, and performance evaluations?

Setting and enculturating the expectation for higher education in your institution is probably the most difficult, yet the most sustaining thing you can do. Be aware of the need to integrate this expectation and you will be surprised at how many opportunities there are. It will serve you well.

PROFESSIONAL ORGANIZATIONS AND CONFERENCES

The benefits of joining a professional organization are obvious: access to evidence-based best practices, networking with professionals from other institutions, opportunities for professional growth, opportunities for professional certification, and the ability to influence nursing policy. So why does everyone not belong to a professional organization and attend national conferences? There are many reasons. Some view nursing as a job, not a profession. Those individuals usually do not see the value in professional organizations and conferences. Of course, they typically have never been to a national conference. Your job is to entice these individuals to go and to facilitate their membership in these organizations.

We have seen individuals adopt a totally new view of nursing, understanding the contribution it makes to society and the contribution they can make from attending one conference. When we took a staff nurse to the international Magnet conference, she was affected so deeply, she became involved in shared governance as the cochair of a council, became the principal investigator of a nursing research study, and pursued a BSN with a vengeance. She was bitten by the bug and duly infected with the "I can make a difference" virus. There is no cure, but why would we want one? We just want to spread the infection. Get nurses involved. Facilitate their joining professional organizations and attending professional conferences. The payoff for your institution will be truly transforming.

AWARDS AND RECOGNITION

Everyone likes to be recognized, no matter how modest they are. Everyone wants to feel like they make a difference. Nursing is a profession that celebrates excellence. Many nursing organizations have awards for nurses in specific categories that recognize excellence in those categories. Why? Awards not only provide recognition, they also motivate individuals and set a definition of nursing excellence. They allow nurses to celebrate nurses, and for the chosen few, to realize how their contributions affect the profession of nursing as a whole, providing a broader view of what it means to make a difference in patient care and in the profession of nursing.

From our experience, it is truly essential that you strategically pursue nursing awards and professional recognition. We have seen firsthand how this recognition can transform an institution's staff, instilling the pride of knowing they are employed at the same institution where there is such nursing talent. It makes excellence real and achievable; not something others have, but something right here in your institution. It encourages others to strive for the same excellence. We have written many successful nomination. Following this section is an example of one that achieved national recognition for nursing excellence. Of course, you have to have excellence to write about, but excellence is truly everywhere. You just have to find it and promote it. Nursing awards are given by professional organizations, government agencies, and even nursing-related retail companies, such as uniform companies or promotional item companies.

Search these venues for nursing awards and ask staff and leadership to think of the individual who best exemplifies the award's criteria. Interview those who best know the nominee, and find a proficient writer to write up the nomination. You might want to tell the nominee of the impending nomination, and solicit information that only the nominee might know. From these interviews, create a nomination within the contest's guidelines. Submit the nomination and hope for the best. If the nominee is not chosen, do not fret. You might be able to use the nomination for another award. Just keep submitting. If your nominee is selected as the winner, publicize it in every internal and external venue possible. Let everyone know that your institution has someone of such caliber. It will elevate the staff, the public, and professional community's opinions of your institution's nursing workforce.

Sample Award Nomination

2009 Winner of Nursing Spectrum's National Nursing Excellence Award in the category of Teaching.

Question: Why should this nominee be selected as a winner? What sets the nominee apart from other nurses?

The nominee, with almost 40 years tenure at South Jersey Healthcare (SJH), plays a critical and integral role in the continued professional development and long-term learning of SJH nurses through education, mentoring, leadership, role modeling, and excellence in clinical nursing practice.

"Nurses strive to be like her. She makes you want to achieve, to be the best nurse you can be," says B.B., PhD, MBA, RN, CPHQ, the Director of Quality at SJH of the nominee. As the Clinical Specialist and Outcomes Manager for Cardiac Services at SJH's Regional Medical Center (RMC), the nominee is responsible for the continued education and professional development of approximately 80 registered nurses in three distinct cardiac units: acute, stepdown, and critical care. As a certified critical care registered nurse (CCRN) and a certified advanced practice nurse (APN)-C, the nominee recognizes the value of the American Association of Critical Care Nurses' (AACN) Beacon framework for excellence in critical care delivery as a means to professionally develop critical care nurses and demonstrate nursing quality. Working with the Director of Cardiac Service, the unit managers, and the unit-based practice councils, the nominee developed a plan to implement the AACN standards and apply for Beacon designation. She coordinated and presented CCRN review courses, critical care courses, dysrhythmia courses, and initiated daily interdisciplinary care rounds in all three units to support the educational needs of nurses and motivate and empower nurses to excel in patient care delivery. Extolling the benefits of national certification from both personal achievement and the research literature, the nominee motivated, educated, and mentored nurses throughout their quest for national certification, working one-on-one to provide both clinical expertise and emotional support. "[The nominee] doesn't just get educators to teach the certification review courses, she recruits certified staff members to teach and mentors them through the process. It makes the material so much more accessible and relevant. If that staff nurse can do it, then I can do it too!" says S.A., RN, BS, CCRN, the assistant nurse manager of the Cardiac ICU and Stepdown units at SJH. Concurrently, the nominee also collaborated with management, unit-based practice councils, Performance Improvement, and Quality to address opportunities for improvement in patient quality outcome indicators. Through her efforts, decreases in the rates of central line related bloodstream infections and ventilator-associated pneumonia were achieved, as well as increases in patient and staff satisfaction. The nurse turnover and vacancy rates have decreased in all three units, and national certification has increased by 33%. In 2007, the Cardiac ICU at SJH's RMC was awarded Beacon status. The initiatives launched by the nominee unified the staff and are enculturated in their practice.

The nominee continually looks to solicit for external resources to grow SJH nurses and enhance patient care. Providing inpatient nurses with a broader view of the continuum of care for SJH cardiac patients as well as a venue to impact cardiac patients' quality of life are goals of our nominee. She identified the need for more comprehensive cardiac care through admission and recidivism rates in SJH's high-minority, low socioeconomic status community. The nominee coordinated the application for a Robert Wood Johnson Foundation grant through the New Jersey Health Initiatives to develop solutions that improve the quality of health care to racial and ethnic minorities and reduce disparity in care. With a $180,000 grant awarded, the nominee, in coordination with senior management, unit managers, and SJH nurses, developed initiatives targeting the needs of the high-minority, cardiac patient population. The nominee hired a part-time APN to translate evidence-based initiatives into care plans, collecting and evaluating outcome data. A part-time registered nurse representing the minority culture was hired for community outreach, supplying education and raising awareness of cardiac care. This nurse acted as a liaison between SJH nurses and the minority community. The nominee developed and currently facilitates a heart failure support group for patients, their families, and all community members. Attendance continues to grow. Under the nominee's guidance, heart failure education was developed by SJH's nurses and is discussed with every heart failure patient. To help nurses remember the essentials of heart failure patient therapy, the nominee developed and implemented the WOW program, an acronym for Weigh, Output, Walk. In collaboration with management and staff, the nominee developed a new position, the Congestive Heart Failure (CHF) ambulator. This staff member focuses on increasing the ambulation of heart failure inpatients, stressing the importance of walking in preventing and ameliorating CHF symptoms. Acknowledging some patient resistance to ambulation, the nominee facilitated the pet therapy program, designed to encourage CHF patients to ambulate by walking the therapy dog. This program has spawned a nursing research project, currently in development, to determine if pet therapy is effective in encouraging and increasing the ambulation of CHF patients. As a member of SJH's Research Council and a voting member of SJH's Institutional Review Board, the nominee is mentoring staff nurses through this nursing research project. Through these initiatives, the nominee has educated and mentored the nursing staff, creating a staff of heart failure specialists, while bettering patient care. These initiatives, implemented by the nominee and SJH cardiac nurses, have reduced the length of stay for heart failure patients by 20% and decreased their readmission rate by 18%. The nominee attempts to integrate education into every interaction with nurses, making every moment a teachable moment. She provides the most current evidence-based research so that nurses can continually update their practice

The nominee's efforts were crucial to SJH's restructuring and subsequent journey for Magnet designation. Two hospitals were combining into one new facility as a four-hospital SJH system became a three-hospital system. The nominee facilitated this transition, unifying varying clinical practices and the most current evidence-based practice, ensuring nurses were educated and supported, achieving a seamless transition and uninterrupted quality patient care. At this time, senior nursing leadership began the Magnet journey. The nominee embraced this frame-work and was instrumental in educating staff about the Magnet standards and shared governance, helping to build its infrastructure at SJH. She is currently the mentor for the Practice Council and sits on both the Research Council and the Quality Council. She also educates and mentors the three unit-based practice councils from the Cardiac Care Center. She has recruited nurses to and mentored nurses through formal education programs to increase the percentage of bachelors and masters prepared nurses at the bedside. In February 2008, Magnet designa-tion was awarded to the SJH system, the first multihospital system to achieve this status in New Jersey and one of only 10% of Magnet designees that achieved this status as an entire healthcare system. But, she did not stop there. The nom-inee also saw initiatives to obtain The Joint Commission disease-specific certifica-tions in stroke and heart failure as an opportunity to develop nurses' skills even further. She educated nurses on The Joint Commission standards for care and their rationales, emphasizing the evidence behind the recommendations. She empow-ered staff nurses to take an active role in evaluating and developing processes to meet these standards. With the nominee's assistance and mentoring, staff nurses developed evidence-based policies and implemented practices to achieve The Joint Commission standards. In 2008, The Joint Commission certifications in stroke care and heart failure care were awarded to SJH. The nominee's contributions were essential to this achievement and elevated the nurses' confidence and the reputation of nursing within SJH to new heights.

Question: How has the nominee contributed to the nursing profession in general?

As a member of and ambassador for the AACN, a member of and previously on the Board of Directors of the Southern Shore chapter of AACN, and a member of and liaison to the Southeastern Pennsylvania (SEPA) chapter of AACN, the nominee works to provide nurses with a voice in national and local healthcare policy and guidelines. She is also leading the profession in creatively and practically educating nurses to develop professionally and impact patients' quality of life. M.Z., RN, BSN, CCRN, the Clinical Director of Cardiac Services at SJH, relates, "[The nominee] takes nurses under her wing and personalizes the education to meet their needs and our patients' needs, constantly pushing them to achieve more." She not only strives for personal professional growth, but also seeks to grow the profession through educating and mentoring nurses one by one. The nominee sees nursing as a collaborative act and the profession, only as strong as its weakest link. She strives to continually push for higher standards, higher education, and better patient outcomes. She is an active member of Sigma Theta Tau and attends many professional conferences, networking and exchanging best practices and creative solutions to educate and professionally develop nurses to achieve better patient outcomes. The nominee is also a member of the Ethics Committee at SJH, facilitates the Heart and Lung Support Group, is an advisor to the Value Analysis Committee at SJH, and facilitates the Code Blue Subcommittee at SJH.

Question: What else should the judges know about your nominee?

The nominee is an amazing role model for our culturally diverse workforce and actively participates in SJH's Cultural Heritage Day. E.T., RN, MSN, NEA-BC, the Administrative Director Education/The Joint Commission Coordinator at SJH says emphatically of the nominee "With her knowledge and expertise in a wide range of nursing experiences, she is known as the 'go-to person' at SJH to answer any practice question. Her approach to helping anyone with anything, at any time, is the consummate example of servant leadership." Every interaction with the nominee is an educational interaction. She creates a milieu of inquiry and debate, opening minds and empowering voices. In this changing healthcare environment, the nominee recognizes that nothing is absolute; there are no sacred cows. Everything must be questioned, so that we as nurses can ensure we are providing the best care to our patients and growing the profession of nursing.

CREATIVE SOLUTIONS

Creative Solution Title: *The Staff Peer Review*

Creative Solution Authors: Emily Turnure, RN, MSN, NEA-BC
Administrative Director Education/The Joint
    Commission Coordinator
South Jersey Healthcare, Vineland, NJ

Bruce Alan Boxer, PhD, MBA, RN, CPHQ
Director of Quality/Magnet Program Director
South Jersey Healthcare, Vineland, NJ

Purpose: The goal of this project is to establish a peer review process for staff RNs as part of the overall annual performance evaluation.

Legend

Overall Rating: **NOVICE**

Financial:

Time:

Personnel:

Other Resources: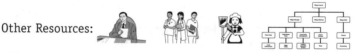

Efficacy: **A**

Transferability: **A**

Malleability/Adaptability: **A**

Ease of Implementation: **B**

Synopsis: Considered a best practice and an extension of the shared-governance structure, a peer review process was developed to better enable managers to evaluate direct-care staff's performance, as well as provide greater nurse autonomy and accountability to peers and colleagues through their participation in the process.

Description of Organization: South Jersey Healthcare (SJH) is a Magnet-designated, multiple-hospital system. The health system encompasses two full service inpatient hospitals consisting of approximately 350 inpatient beds, comprehensive health centers, and outpatient and specialized services such as a Bariatric Center of Excellence, Wound Care Center, Sleep Center, and Balance Center. In 2008, SJH performed over 18,700 surgeries and the emergency department visits topped

97,400. The system contains an inpatient behavioral health facility, Bridgeton Health Center. The health system also serves as a clinical site for nursing students from a number of local colleges and maintains a professional relationship with Cumberland County College, which is adjacent to the RMC campus.

The Case Study: The 360-degree performance review process existed for some time at SJH for those in a leadership position. The next step was to bring this process to the direct-care staff so that they might benefit from and contribute to their colleagues' growth in the nursing profession. A task force of direct-care nurses led by the Director of Education and the Magnet Program Director was charged with the development of the peer review tool and process. Relevant literature was searched and a template was found that was in accordance with the contents of the current performance evaluation, incorporating SJH's and the nursing department's values and expectations. The tool was tweaked to make it more in tune with SJH's culture. The task force then took to developing the process to roll out the peer review tool and integrate the process into the current performance evaluation process. They utilized the existing shared-governance structure, giving accountability for the process to the Coordinating Council since they had representation from every nursing unit and were considered the overseer in the councilor structure. After developing the process and the tool, the task force brought them to the Nursing Executive Council for leadership input and approval, Coordinating Council for direct-care staff input and approval, to Human Resources for input and approval, and to each of the remaining shared-governance councils for input and approval. The tool utilized was adapted from the tool used at Johns Hopkins University Hospital in Baltimore, MD, keeping the same major evaluative sections: Clinical Practices, Team Contribution, and Service Standards (The Advisory Board Company, 2006).

The original tool remained mostly intact with a few modifications and suggestions incorporated. The process was guided by the idea that a staff member should be evaluated by a peer working the shift before, a peer working the same shift with the staff member, and a peer working the shift after, someone who would possibly follow the staff member's assignment. In this way, a more complete and holistic picture of the staff member is developed, looking at how he or she performs when giving and taking report, when working as a team member, and when performing patient care activities. Of course, this level of coordination is not always achieved, but it is a guide and a goal.

The tool and the process were promoted at every venue possible for 3 months before the rollout occurred to get everyone comfortable with the process. The process assured the anonymity of the evaluators, essential in the peer review process. Special considerations were made for units with few staff members, where anonymity might be jeopardized. The first year of the staff peer review process was a little chaotic, but a terrific learning experience. The process was tweaked for the second year, and went much more smoothly. Since its implementation, the staff peer review process has become an essential part of the staff's performance evaluations, giving direct-care staff an active role in evaluating colleagues' contributions to nursing care—the mark of a true profession.

With the evolution and professional growth of our nursing staff, it became evident that there were key areas that were missing from the peer review tool. The following sections listed in Table 9-1 were added with shared governance council approval. We believe this addition is necessary to enculturate the expectations for professional development.

Table 9-1　Addition to Peer Review Tool

IV. PROFESSIONAL DEVELOPMENT
A. Knowledge Acquisition (has national certification, advances the profession of nursing through presentations/publications, participates in formal and informal continuing education, and participates in research and evidence-based practice projects)
B. Knowledge Dissemination (plays an active role in nursing shared governance, attends professional conferences and/or presents information to peers, and participates in initiatives to educate peers)

The tool continues to be a flexible document, reviewed annually by members of the Nurse Executive Council and the Coordinating Council.

Outcome Measures:

Formative/Compliance: Compliance with the process is nearly 100% for staff RNs and 100% of managers utilize the peer reviews in their performance evaluations of direct-care staff.

Summative/Outcome: Anecdotal reports from Coordinating Council representatives are overwhelmingly positive in relaying that the peer review process has added value to the performance evaluation process. Managers at the Nurse Executive Council concur. Employee opinion survey results seem to bear this out.

Evidence Supporting this Creative Solution: The tool was adapted from *Unlocking clinical excellence. Embedding quality standards at the front line* (The Advisory Board Company, 2006). Harrington and Smith (2008) provides the benefits of and more instruction on establishing a nursing peer review process. The peer review process is utilized by journals to establish the credibility and validity of submissions and published content. The information in a peer reviewed journal is seen as more credible than a journal not using the peer review process (Steinbach, 2009).

The Advisory Board Company (2006). *Unlocking clinical excellence. Embedding quality standards at the front line.* Washington, DC: Author.

Harrington, L. C., & Smith M. (2008). *Nursing peer review: A practical approach to promoting professional nursing accountability.* Marblehead, MA: HCPro, Inc.

Steinbach, L. (2009). *Periodicals explained: Scholarly, peer reviewed or not?* Available at: http://lib.tcu.edu/www/eref/tutorials/periodicals_explained.html. Accessed December 24, 2009.

Recipe for: *The Staff Peer Review*

Ingredients:

> CNO/Director support
>
> Staff buy-in
>
> Management support
>
> Human resource department support
>
> Shared-governance structure
>
> Literature search/process and tool development skills
>
> Paid time for staff to develop tool and process and complete assigned reviews
>
> Peer review tool that demonstrates the institution's and the nursing department's values and expectations
>
> Process that works within your institution's structure and culture

Step-by-Step Instructions (see Figure 9-2 for Step-by-Step Instruction Timeline):

Step 1: Obtain support from CNO/directors, management, human resources department, and direct-care staff.

Step 2: Establish task force of nurse leaders and direct-care staff with literature search/process and tool development skills.

Step 3: Find and develop tool and process that works with your current performance evaluation process. Integrate the new peer review process into the current performance evaluation process.

Step 4: Obtain feedback for tool and process from leadership, human resources department, and direct-care staff utilizing the shared-governance structure.

Step 5: Tweak tool and process as necessary to obtain a consensus of support.

Step 6: Promote the tool and inform the staff at every venue possible before rolling out the process. Ensure anonymity.

Step 7: Roll out the tool and process noting opportunities for improvement in both the tool and the process.

Step 8: Improve the tool and process for the next scheduled peer review. Survey staff and management as to the satisfaction for the tool and process.

Establish a regular interval and determine who is responsible to review the tool and process. (See sample process following this Creative Solution.)

Step 9: Continue utilizing the tool and process with each scheduled performance evaluation. Eventually link the results from the peer review tool and process to salary increases or bonuses.

Figure 9-2   Timeline for "The Staff Peer Review."

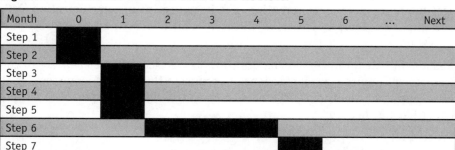

Month	0	1	2	3	4	5	6	...	Next
Step 1									
Step 2									
Step 3									
Step 4									
Step 5									
Step 6									
Step 7									
Step 8									
Step 9									

Additional Outcomes to Consider Measuring:

Formative/Compliance: No additional measures.

Summative/Outcome: Formally survey staff and management to obtain metrics for satisfaction with process and tool.

Insights from Original Implementation:

- Link money to metrics. Eventually link the peer review process and performance evaluation to staff's merit raise/bonus. This will help to enculturate the process and demonstrate its importance, possibly incentivizing teamwork and excellent nursing care.
- Ensure anonymity. Be conscious of the fears of staff. If they do not believe the process is anonymous, they will likely not be as honest as they might otherwise be when completing the reviews.
- Tweak as institution grows. The staff peer review tool should be designed to incorporate the institution's and the nursing department's values and expectations. These values and expectations might change as the institution and nursing department grows. Reevaluate the tool periodically to ensure it fulfills your needs.

GUIDELINES FOR RN PEER INPUT TOOL – SAMPLE PROCESS

Purpose: Peer review is a component of professional practice. It provides an opportunity for professionals in common practice areas to assess, monitor, and provide feedback to peers by comparing actual practice to established standards. It is considered *one part* of the RNs overall annual performance appraisal process.

Expected Outcomes: This peer review process will become part of the professional nursing practice model and allows for the increase in professionalism, accountability, autonomy, retention, and improvement in communication skills and quality outcomes. The goal will be to continue with an annual RN peer review process.

Responsibilities: Unit Based Practice (UBP) leaders/council members are to collaborate with nurse manager/designee to complete the RN peer input tool for all RNs working on their units. The nurse manager/designee will provide a current list of RNs for their unit.

Procedure:

- The UBP Leader will obtain a list of RNs who work on their unit from their nurse manager/designee.
- At each UBP/staff meeting, members will use the list of RNs to complete an RN peer input tool until all RNs on that unit have been completed.
- It is suggested that a minimum of three RN peer input tools be completed per RN.
- The evaluators must be RNs and can be UBP council members or other RNs on the unit. If the size of UBP council membership is small, then evaluators can be rotated to maintain anonymity.
- The size of RN staff on your unit will determine the numbers of RN peer input tools that must be completed at each meeting to complete the list by the end of 2008.
- The UBP Council leader will work with the unit's nurse manager/designee to devise an implementation plan that will accommodate the size of RN staff on your units and meet the completion deadline.
- The three RN peer input tools are completed during the meeting and are *anonymously* placed in a sealed envelope and returned to your nurse manager/designee.
- The nurse manager/designee records/tracks the numbers of received RN peer input tools/nurses and guides the UBP leader's compliance to complete all peer evaluations for the RN staff in your units by end of 2008.
- The nurse manager/designee will utilize the RN peer input tool information for constructive feedback to the employee.

Tips to Remember:

You are reviewing the performance of your peer as a nurse, not as a friend or a foe.

Base the review on the nurse's daily performance, not just one incident.

Speak from personal experience, not hearsay.

Thank you for helping to achieve the goal of recognizing nursing excellence at the bedside.

For Further Guidance Contact:

Emily Turnure, RN, MSN, NEA-BC
Administrative Director Education/The Joint Commission Coordinator
turnuree@sjhs.com

Bruce Alan Boxer, PhD, MBA, CPHQ
Director of Quality/Magnet Program Director
boxerb@sjhs.com

Creative Solution Title: *Pressure Ulcer Prevalence and Prevention*

Creative Solution Author: **Bonnie Michaels, RN, MA, NEA-BC, FACHE**
Vice President, Chief Nursing Officer
Mountainside Hospital, Montclair, NJ

Purpose: The goal of this project was to create a new nursing care model to monitor and prevent the occurrence of pressure ulcers in the named hospital. This was a nursing initiative undertaken in an effort to adhere to The Joint Commission's Nursing Sensitive Care Performance measures and the National Quality Forum's Developing a Framework for Measuring Quality for Prevention and Management of Pressure Ulcers project as well as Centers for Medicare and Medicaid Services' (CMS) charge for hospitals to reduce the number of nosocomial pressure ulcers.

Legend

Overall Rating: **COMPETENT**

Financial: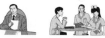

Time:

Personnel:

Other Resources: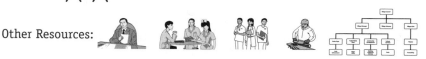

Efficacy: **A**

Transferability: **A**

Malleability/Adaptability: **A**

Ease of Implementation: **C**

Synopsis: To meet that need for a means of tracking the occurrence of inpatient pressure ulcers and a mandate to prevent such nosocomial ulcers, the CNO in discussion with her Nurse Executive Council and Nurse Practice Councils initiated a new nursing care model that included expanding the role of the Wound Care Nurse (WOCN) specialist, daily Braden Scale assessment of all patients, and a team of unit-based resource nurses that receive extensive training quarterly by the inpatient certified WOCN.

Description of Organization: Mountainside Hospital is a 364-bed for-profit community teaching suburban hospital, owned by Merit Health System. A 2-hospital system operates as a stand alone institution. Mountainside hospital has been on the journey to Magnet for approximately 4 to 5 years.

The Case Study: In January 2007, The Joint Commission initiated a 24-month project to field test the Nursing Sensitive Care (NSC) performance measures endorsed by the National Quality Forum in January 2004. In November 2008, The Joint Commission convened a panel of experts to review the results of the testing and suggested modifications to these measures based on the field testing. One of those measure specifications and descriptive information originally endorsed in January 2004 and updated in February 2009 was pressure ulcer surveillance. These modifications are currently being reviewed by the National Pressure Ulcer Advisory Panel (NPUAP) and the National Quality Forum's Developing a Framework for Measuring Quality for Prevention and Management of Pressure Ulcers project.

In addition, all hospitals have been charged by CMS to reduce the number of nosocomial pressure ulcers and aggressively address skin breakdown during hospitalization. Medicare and Medicaid added pressure ulcers to their list of reasonably preventable illnesses, which will no longer be covered beginning in 2008. The Institute of Health Improvement predicted that the United States spends as much as $11 billion per year treating this ailment. In addition, the New Jersey Patient Safety Act of 2004 required stage 2 or higher hospital-acquired pressure ulcers as a state reportable event.

To address the issue of pressure ulcer occurrence in Mountainside Hospital, the CNO in discussion with her Nurse Executive Council and Shared Governance Nurse Practice Councils, initiated a new nursing care model. A certified inpatient WOCN was hired to lead this effort. The model included daily Braden Scale assessment of all patients, and a team of unit-based resource nurses that receive extensive training quarterly by the inpatient WOCN. This team conducts prevalence studies quarterly that is reported to the division of nursing front line staff. Team members also receive quarterly education to update their knowledge base on evidence-based wound care practice. The resource nurses are also seen as the unit-based expert/champion and assist in mentoring their peers and providing nurse-to-nurse consultations, recommending interventions resulting in early detection, and referrals to the wound care specialist nurse. Since inception of the program, the prevalence studies reflect a decrease in hospital acquired pressure ulcers from 20.72% in April 2008, to 4.68% in February 2009, a 442% improvement in less than 1 year. This improvement has been sustained, decreasing the number of pressure ulcer cases, decreasing length of stay (LOS), improving patient safety, increasing service quality and nursing expertise at the front line, limiting complications and reducing costs by contributing to the length of stay decrease realized by Mountainside Hospital.

Data is now shared at the unit level, making the outcomes transparent. The unit-based champions, the provision of wound care education, the use of evidenced-based practice protocols, and new devices to use in aggressive interventions has changed and improved nursing clinical practice. This creative solution is a pristine example of how nursing can independently execute an initiative that affords patient outcome improvements and cost reduction. The use of a nurse specialist to educate and promote peer education allows professional development of nurses as the patient care initiative is enforced. This initiative exemplifies nursing autonomy and professional development.

Outcome Measures:

Formative/Compliance: Consistency with quarterly team meetings and daily wound care rounds.

Summative/Outcome: Quarterly prevalence studies.

Evidence Supporting this Creative Solution: Pressure ulcers are a preventable cause of patient morbidity and mortality as well as a very expensive illness to treat. The incidence and prevalence of pressure ulcers are also indicators of nursing care quality. The Institute for Healthcare Improvement challenges clinicians and administrators to raise care quality through its 5 Million Lives Campaign, a sequel to the 100,000 Lives Campaign. An area for recommended improvement is pressure ulcer prevention, which is a constant nursing challenge (Griffin, Cooper, Horack, Klyber, & Schimmelpfenning, 2007). As nursing is charged with pressure ulcer prevention, this is an area for nurses to exert their autonomy and evaluate and improve their practice.

Reducing health care-associated pressure ulcers is both a Joint Commission National Patient Safety Goal and a goal for Healthy People, 2010. Pressure ulcer prevalence is number two on the National Quality Forum's 15 National Voluntary

Consensus Standards on Nurse-Sensitive Care (Stokowski, 2008). It also now has a price tag as CMS has introduced the pay for performance initiative and will not pay for pressure ulcer care if the ulcer was not present on hospital admission (Landro, 2007). So, although the care of pressure ulcers is a multidisciplinary issue, nurses as the front line caregivers need to implement evidence-based practices as well as be inventive in finding new means of prevention. It appears that all of the pressure ulcer prevention devices and products have not lowered the national pressure ulcer rate, but nursing quality improvement projects implementing best practices have successfully lowered pressure ulcer incidence rates in some facilities. This creative solution, when evaluating the pressure ulcer prevalence rates prenursing and postnursing intervention, seems to have followed suit.

Griffin, B., Cooper, H., Horack, C., Klyber, M., & Schimmelpfenning, D. (2007). Reducing harm from pressure ulcers, *Nursing Management, 38*(9), 29–32.

Landro, L. (2007, September 5). Hospitals combat dangerous bedsores. *The Wall Street Journal.* Available at: http://online.wsj.com/article/SB118894998795817515.html. Accessed December 29, 2009.

Stokowski, L. A. (2008*). A closer look at pressure ulcers* (MedscapeCME). Available at: http://cme.medscape.com/viewprogram/12612. Accessed December 29, 2009.

Recipe for: *Pressure Ulcer Prevalence and Prevention*

Ingredients:

> 1 CNO
>
> 1 Certified WOCN
>
> Wound care team
>
> Unit-based resource nurses

Step-by-Step Instructions (see Figure 9-3 for Step-by-Step Instruction Timeline):

Step 1: CNO initiated plans for hospital wide pressure ulcer prevalence study.

Step 2: Clinical wound care nurse specialist hired.

Step 3: Prevalence study conducted. Pressure ulcer rate was 20.72%

Step 4: Discussions with Nursing Executive Council and Practice Council, model identified using hospital unit-based RN champions.

Step 5: Education of identified resource nurses provided by nurse educators and wound care specialist.

Step 6: Quarterly team meetings and daily wound clinical specialist rounds initiated.

Step 7: CNO shared initiative with medical staff.

Step 8: Second prevalence study conducted, rate decreased to 14.03%.

Step 9: Third prevalence study conducted with improvement to 5.26%.

Step 10: Fourth prevalence study conducted with improvement to 4.68%.

Step 11: CNO reported outcomes to the medical staff, nurse executive and practice councils, performance improvement committee, and graphic charts of outcomes were distributed and posted for front line staff.

Step 12: Continue quarterly prevalence studies, outcomes sustained between 4% and 5%.

Figure 9-3   Timeline for "Pressure Ulcer Prevalence and Prevention."

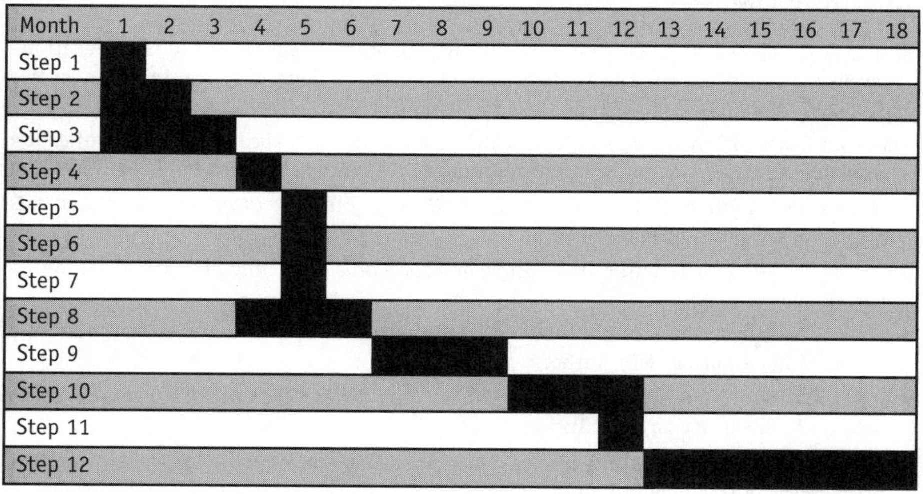

Month	1	2	3	4	5	6	7	8	9	10	11	12	13	14	15	16	17	18
Step 1	■																	
Step 2	■																		
Step 3	■	■																
Step 4				■														
Step 5					■													
Step 6					■													
Step 7					■													
Step 8				■														
Step 9							■	■										
Step 10										■	■	■						
Step 11												■						
Step 12												■	■					

Additional Outcomes to Consider Measuring:

Formative/Compliance: No additional measures.

Summative/Outcome: Evaluation of patient outcomes with pressure ulcer treatment if they occur, rate of morbidity and mortality related to pressure ulcers and change in length of stay. Nursing knowledge of, motivation for, and compliance with pressure ulcer prevention and treatment activities can also be measured to evaluate how the initiative promoted education and professional development and autonomous nursing actions in pressure ulcer prevention.

Insights from Original Implementation: This program was achieved through the interest of the staff nurses to increase quality outcomes, sharing evidence-based practice and data, giving front line nursing staff opportunities to learn and improve their skills, support by nurse managers to release nurses from direct-care to support educational and team meetings, sharing nurse sensitive positive and negative data, and highlighting and recognizing nurses' achievements.

For Further Guidance Contact:

Bonnie Michaels, RN, MA, NEA-BC, FACHE
Vice President, Chief Nursing Officer
Mountainside Hospital
1 Bay Avenue, Montclair, NJ 07042
bonnie.michaels@mountainsidehosp.com

REFERENCES

Aiken, L. H., Clarke, S. P., Cheung, R. B., Sloane, D. M., & Silber, J. H. (2003). Educational levels of hospital nurses and surgical patient mortality. *Journal of the American Medical Association, 290*(12), 1617–1623

American Board of Nursing Specialties. (2009). *Promoting excellence in nursing certification.* Available at: http://www.nursingcertification.org/index.html. Accessed December 23, 2009.

American Nurses Association. (2001). *Code of ethics for nurses with interpretive statements.* Silver Spring, MD: Author.

American Nurses Association. (2004). *Scope and standards of nursing practice.* Silver Spring, MD: Author.

American Nurses Association. (2009). *Nursing administration: Scope and standards of practice.* Silver Spring, MD: Author.

American Nurses Credentialing Center. (2008). *Application manual. Magnet recognition program®.* Silver Spring, MD: Author.

American Nurses Credentialing Center. (2009a). *ANCC nurse certification.* Available at: http://www.nursecredentialing.org/Certification.aspx. Accessed December 13, 2009.

American Nurses Credentialing Center. (2009b). *Magnet Recognition Program. Download tools. ANCC Magnet accepted national certifications.* Available at: http://www.nursecredentialing.org/Magnet/ApplicationProcess/MagnetReconitionProgramDownloadForms.aspx. Accessed December 13, 2009.

Anthony, M. K. (2004). Shared governance models: The theory, practice, and evidence. *Online Journal of Issues in Nursing, 9*(1).

Benner, P. (n.d.). *Patricia Benner.* Available at: http://home.earthlink.net/~bennerassoc/patricia.html. Accessed December 7, 2009.

Benner P. (1984). *From novice to expert: Excellence and power in clinical nursing practice.* Menlo Park, Calif: Addison-Wesley.

Boyd, T. (2009, September 7). N.Y. and N.J. consider BSN requirement. *Nursing Spectrum.* Available at: http://news.nurse.com/article/20090907/NATIONAL02/309070028/-1/frontpage. Accessed December 13, 2009.

Briggs, L. A., Brown, H., Kesten, K., & Heath, J. (2006). Certification: A benchmark for critical care nursing excellence. *Critical Care Nurse, 26*, 47–53.

Brooks, B. (2004). Measuring the impact of shared governance. *Online Journal of Issues in Nursing, 9*(1).

Career Toolkits. (2009). *Nursing continuing education.* Available at: http://www.careertoolkits .com/nursing/nursing-continuing-education.html. Accessed December 13, 2009.

Cary, A. H. (2001). Certified registered nurses: Results of the study of the certified workforce. *American Journal of Nursing, 101,* 44–52.

Current Nursing. (2010). *Application of theory in nursing process.* Available at: http:// currentnursing.com/nursing_theory/application_nursing_theories.htm. Accessed April 18, 2010.

Dracup, K., & Bryan-Brown, C. W. (2004). From novice to expert to mentor: Shaping the future. *American Journal of Critical Care, 13,* 448–450.

Dreyfus, S. E., & Dreyfus, H. L. (1980). *A five-stage model of the mental activities involved in directed skill acquisition.* University of California, Berkeley. Unpublished report supported by the Air Force Office of Scientific Research, USAF (contract F49620-79-C0063).

Hess, R. G. (1998). Measuring nursing governance. *Nursing Research, 47*(1), 35–42.

Hess, R. G. (2004). Bedside to boardroom: Nursing shared governance. *Online Journal of Issues in Nursing, 9*(1).

Hess, R. (2008). *Essential education for sharing governance.* Available at: http://www .sharedgovernance.org/educationessentials.htm. Accessed December 11, 2009.

Hoffart, N., & Woods, C. Q. (1996). Elements of a nursing professional practice model. *Journal of Professional Nursing, 12*(6), 354–364.

Houle, C. O. (1980). *Continuing learning in the professions.* San Francisco: Jossey-Bass.

Kent State University. (n.d.). *Socialization to professional nursing roles* (PowerPoint). Available at: www.library.kent.edu/files/Week2_Intro.ppt. Accessed December 13, 2009.

Kohn, L., Corrigan, J., & Donaldson, M. (Eds.) (2000). *To err is human: Building a safer health system.* Washington, DC: National Academies Press.

Kramer, M., & Schmalenberg, C. E. (2003). Magnet hospital staff nurses describe clinical autonomy. *Nursing Outlook, 51*(1), 13–19.

Maas, M., Specht, J., & Jacox, A. (1975). Nurse autonomy: Reality or rhetoric. *American Journal of Nursing, 75*(12), 2201–2208.

MacDonald, C. (2002). Nurse autonomy as relational. *Nursing Ethics, 9*(2), 194–201.

Malleo, C. & Fusilero, J. (2009). Shared governance: Withstanding the test of time. *Nurse Leader, 7*(1), 32–36.

National League for Nursing. (2007). *Basic RN programs by type of program, region and state: 2007.* Available at: http://www.nln.org/research/slides/pdf/AS0607_T01b.pdf. Accessed December 13, 2009.

Neuman, B., & Fawcett, J. (Eds.) (2002). *The Neuman Systems Model* (4th ed.). Upper Saddle River, NJ: Prentice Hall.

O'May, F., & Buchan, J. (1999). Shared governance: A literature review. *International Journal of Nursing Studies, 36,* 281–300.

Porter-O'Grady, T. (2001). Is shared governance still relevant? *Journal of Nursing Administration, 31*(10), 468–473.

Porter-O'Grady, T. (2005). *Implementing shared governance: Creating a professional organization.* Available at: http://www.tpogassociates.com/SharedGovernance.htm. Accessed December 11, 2009.

Reeves, S. (1991). *Professional governance: Assessing readiness of an organization for change* (Unpublished master's thesis). University of New Hampshire, Durham.

Schutzenhofer, K. K. (1987). The measurement of professional autonomy. *Journal of Professional Nursing, 3*, 278–283.

Seago, J. A. (2001). Nurse staffing, models of care delivery, and interventions. In *Making health care safer: A critical analysis of patient safety practices* (Chapter 39). Available at: http://www.ahrq.gov/clinic/ptsafety/chap39.htm. Accessed December 6, 2009.

Seton Family of Hospitals. (2009). *Nursing education and professional development. Clinical ladder.* Available at: http://www.seton.net/employment/nursing/nursing_education__ professional_development/. Accessed December 13, 2009.

The Center for Nursing Advocacy. (2006). *Are you sure nurses are autonomous? Aren't physicians calling the shots?* Available at: http://www.nursingadvocacy.org/faq/ autonomy.html. Accessed November 28, 2009.

Tool. (n.d.). In *Dictionary.com unabridged.* Available at: http://dictionary.reference.com/ browse/tool. Accessed December 8, 2009.

Treggiari, M. M., Martin, D. P., Yanez, N. D., Caldwell, E., Hudson, L. D., & Rubenfeld, G. D. (2007). Effect of intensive care unit organizational model and structure on outcomes in patients with acute lung injury. *American Journal of Respiratory and Critical Care Medicine, 176*, 685–690.

Wade, G. H. (1999). Professional nurse autonomy: Concept analysis and application to nursing education. *Journal of Advanced Nursing, 30*(2), 310–318.

## CHAPTER 10

What Now?

"Whatever you want to do, do it now! There are only so many tomorrows."
—POPE PAUL VI

"Don't wait. The time will never be just right."
—NAPOLEON HILL

HOW TO BEGIN

So you are ready to start the Magnet journey. You want to make the commitment. What do you do first? Well if the decision is solely up to you, then it is easy. Go straight to the Gap Analysis and start building your infrastructure for your processes to obtain your desired outcomes. If the decision rests with other leaders in your institution, it is a bit more complex. We recommend first obtaining leadership approval for the Gap Analysis. This could be done by a consultant or by in-house personnel, but we believe a consultant would provide you with a more comprehensive account of what you need to implement and possibly assist you in a timeline or budget. It is probably a worthwhile investment. As we said before, make sure the consultant has experience with assisting institutions in the Magnet journey. Look at his or her credentials and references. Make sure you will get the deliverables you want, whether it is a formal written report for senior leadership or an estimated timeline and budget for the journey.

To get approval for the Gap Analysis, be ready to provide the cost of the consultant and the scope of their commitment for senior leadership. Call local Magnet-designated hospitals and ask who they utilized as a consultant, or go on the American Nurses Credentialing Center (ANCC) Web site and request a consultant through their service. You will also need to educate senior leadership on the Magnet program, what it is and its benefits to your institution. It is unlikely that they will not have heard of the program, but might not be well versed in its requirements, costs, time frame, and outcomes. Be ready to provide as much as you can. We hope this book helped to prepare you.

After you have approval for the Gap Analysis, secure your consultant. If you are using in-house people, gather as much information about the Magnet program requirements that you can. Purchase the application manual from ANCC. Look at the information on the ANCC Web site and evaluate their products for your use. Have internal people familiar with doing a Gap Analysis assist, if available. You may want to coordinate a team for the Gap Analysis, possibly contacting an area Magnet-designated hospital and obtaining assistance from their Magnet Program Director (MPD).

Complete the Gap Analysis and from this, estimate a timeline for implementing the necessary structures and processes and perform a cost analysis/estimate. The cost analysis/estimate should coincide with your institution's budgeting process, which is typically an annual event. Do not forget to include the cost of data collection and dissemination, as well as staff recognition and incentives. Refer to this volume to help recognize what will be needed and what you will need to budget for. This is not an exact budget. This is a realistic estimate of what costs you will incur. It is somewhat futile to use budgeting data from other institutions, since your budget is dependent on what you need, as determined by your Gap Analysis. And your Gap Analysis is unique, unlike any other institution. Your Gap Analysis depends on what you already have in place, what your organizational structure is like, and what internal resources you have. Possibly the only standardized cost is the application to ANCC for Magnet consideration. Beyond that, your budget will be your own. You might want to ask area Magnet-designated hospitals about their budget to get a rough idea. It has been our experience that financial information is not something many institutions like to share.

Now you will want to submit your Gap Analysis, your estimated timeline, and your budget to senior leadership for approval. With these, we recommend submitting a list of expected benefits, both tangible and intangible from the Magnet journey and possible Magnet designation. Even better would be a cost-savings/ profit-enhancing estimate from these tangible and intangible benefits to make your proposal that much more desirable. Quantify benefits as much as possible, such as: decreased nurse turnover, better patient outcomes, better staff satisfaction, better patient satisfaction, increased professional and public status, etc.

Well, you have got the go-ahead! Senior leadership realizes that the Magnet journey is an opportunity to enhance the quality of care, the autonomy of nursing, and the reputation of the institution. It is time to form your steering committee and start educating everyone on the Magnet framework. Make sure everyone on your committee has a copy of this volume to better understand the skills and activities that will be needed on the journey (yes, an unscrupulous plug to sell more books!). Truly, we hope this book can be used as both a primer for the journey as well as a reference as you travel nearer and nearer toward Magnet designation and redesignation. It is all about moving forward and embracing change, the change that makes a difference in the profession of nursing and in the care of patients.

WHY MAGNET?

Why Magnet? Why Grade A? Because we all want the best. The best quality food, the best quality health care, and all else that is important in our lives. Magnet status was originally introduced and sought by hospitals to increase nurse job satisfaction and retention. Today, it is primarily to gain and retain the best quality nurses and attain the best nursing quality to achieve the best quality patient care. So, why not Magnet?

When deciding to begin the journey, you must evaluate your institution's reasons for striving for Magnet designation. It is a journey, one that is meant to be continuous. To ensure sustainability, you need to be passionate about the goals you are working to achieve. What do you think Magnet status will do for you, for your institution, and for your institution's nurses and patients?

Magnet is a symbol of nursing quality and a prestigious achievement in the healthcare world. It is a label that enables nurses to decide the best places to work and offers guidance to the public in choosing quality hospital care. The label is not quality; quality achieves the label. If you provide an environment that allows for, promotes, and provides quality, you can achieve Magnet designation. Although there is some controversy over the effect of Magnet status on patient outcomes, several studies favor Magnet hospitals as being superior and producing better patient outcomes than their non-Magnet counterparts. A recent article by Aiken, Havens, and Sloan (2009), states that the organizational attributes of Magnet hospitals have been associated with better patient outcomes in contrast to non-Magnet comparisons. In one of their own studies, they showed the Medicare mortality rate to be significantly lower in Magnet hospitals and the other showed AIDS patients to have a lower chance of dying in Magnet hospitals than any other setting (2009). Despite the debate regarding the overall effects of Magnet status, we know the goals of Magnet designation are good. We must evaluate and work to improve the individual aspects of nursing that Magnet highlights in our own institutions.

Magnet promotes a culture of professionalism and excellence in practice. This is attractive to nurses and patients regardless of the label it is given. The 14 forces of Magnetism are characteristics that should be core to all nursing practice. Higher education, quality nursing leadership, autonomy in practice, professional development, these are goals we must all strive for in our daily practice, putting it all together for Magnet recognition should just be a formality. Rather than an award, we must think of Magnet as a standard. Magnet is simply a systematic and evidence-based framework designed to enhance nursing quality and patient care. Do not be intimidated by Magnet. No matter how big or small your institution, you can do it. You might just need to be more creative when resources are not abundant. As we said before, why reinvent the wheel. The Magnet program will keep your wheel spinning and we hope we have given you the impetus and guidance needed to get the wheel started. Enjoy the journey to being the best you can be.

REFERENCES

Aiken, L. H., Havens, D. S., & Sloane, D. M. (2009). The Magnet nursing services recognition program: A comparison of two groups of Magnet hospitals. *Journal Of Nursing Administration, 39*(7/8), 5–13.

Glossary

Adaptability – the quality of being easily assimilated

Algorithm – "(a) step-by-step problem-solving procedure, especially an established, recursive computational procedure for solving a problem in a finite number of steps" ("Algorithm," 2010, para. 1)

Anecdotal – "based on or consisting of reports or observations of usually unscientific observers" ("Anecdotal," 2010, para. 1)

Believability – the confidence one has that the evidence is valid and reliable based on specific objective criteria. Consider it as believability $= -($chance $+$ bias$)$. This equation is conceptual, not literal; meant to demonstrate that believability decreases as chance and bias increase.

Benchmarking – "the process of identifying, understanding, and adapting outstanding practices and processes from organizations anywhere in the world to help your organization improve its performance" (American Productivity & Quality Center, 2008, para. 3)

Bias – "systematic error introduced into sampling or testing by selecting or encouraging one outcome or answer over others" ("Bias," 2010, para. 1)

Bottom-up approach – goals and action plans are developed by direct care and midlevel leadership and communicated to those higher in the authority hierarchy

Buy-in – engagement; belief in

Causation – "(r)elation that holds between two temporally simultaneous or successive events when the first event (the cause) brings about the other (the effect)" ("Causation," n.d. "Britannica Concise Encyclopedia: causation," para. 1)

CEU – continuing education unit; typically needed for relicensure or recertification of professional nurses

Chi square – "a statistical method used to test whether the classification of data can be ascribed to chance or to some underlying law" ("Chi square," 2009); Chi-square test is analogous in purpose to the t test, but used for discrete data instead of continuous data.

Clinical ladder – program with a progressive series of levels denoting progressive levels of expertise that is utilized in developing direct-care nurses professionally by incentivizing the achievement of successive levels with progressively more valuable incentives

Cookbook medicine or nursing – medical or nursing interventions that are the same for everyone with a specific diagnosis; a recipe for care of a patient with a specific diagnosis without individualizing the care

Core measures – "developed by The Joint Commission, the nation's predominant standards-setting and accrediting body in health care, to improve the quality of health care by implementing a national, standardized performance measurement system. The Core Measures were derived largely from a set of quality indicators defined by the Centers for Medicare and Medicaid Services (CMS). They have been shown to reduce the risk of complications, prevent recurrences and otherwise treat the majority of patients who come to a hospital for treatment of a condition or illness" (Baylor Health Care System, n.d., para. 2)

Correlation – a measure of the degree to which two things are related

Creative solution – an evidence-based intervention that innovatively translates an effective practice to meet the specific needs of the environment where there is a noted opportunity for improvement

Curriculum vitae (CV) – "a written description of your work experience, educational background, and skills . . . it is more detailed than a resume and is commonly . . . used by someone looking for an academic job, i.e. in a college or university" (McKay, 2010, para. 1).

Dashboard – a graphic chart that typically presents data in comparison with a benchmark and possibly a goal

Database – an ongoing collection of information or metrics

Debriefing – the process of gathering information related to a specific incident or situation and providing those involved with the opportunity for self-reflection and verbalizing emotions

Disseminate – to circulate information as widely and appropriately as possible

DMAIC – define, measure, analyze, improve, control; a process improvement strategy

Double-blind – who receives experimental treatment and who receives placebo is unknown by the subject as well as the investigator

Efficacy – "the power to produce an effect" ("Efficacy," 2010, para. 1)

80/20 rule – posits, with respect to a situation, that 80% of the problem is caused by 20% of the causes

Enculturate – the process by which a practice or process is assimilated into the institutional culture and becomes "the way it is done here"

Evidence based – "Evidence based clinical practice (EBCP) is an approach to healthcare practice in which the clinician is aware of the evidence that bears on her clinical practice, and the strength of that evidence" ("Definitions of Evidence-based Practice," n.d., para. 1)

Exemplar – "one that serves as a model or example" ("Exemplar," 2010, para. 1)

Feedback loop – "The section of a control system that allows for feedback and self-correction and that adjusts its operation according to differences between the actual output and the desired output" ("Feedback loop," n.d., para. 1)

Gantt chart – a graphic timeline of events and actions necessary to reach a specific goal

HCAHPS – "The HCAHPS (Hospital Consumer Assessment of Healthcare Providers and Systems) survey is the first national, standardized, publicly reported survey of patients' perspectives of hospital care" (HCAHPS, 2009, para. 1)

Impetus – "Something that incites; a stimulus" (Impetus, n.d.)

Incentivize – to provide a positive reinforcement for

Indicator – a metric that provides a measure of how well or how poorly the corresponding efforts are working to achieve the desired outcome

Infrastructure – the basic physical resources, processes, and procedures, used as a foundation for an organization or system

Insider bias – the phenomenon that an external source is given greater credibility than an internal source in identifying and addressing opportunities for improvement

Intangible – something that is not physical, and thus not easily valued fiscally, (e.g., satisfaction, creativity)

Journey to nursing excellence – See Magnet Journey

Likert scale – "A scale, usually of approval or agreement, used in questionnaires. The respondent is asked to say whether, for example, they 'Strongly agree,' 'Agree,' 'Disagree,' or 'Strongly disagree' with some statement" ("Likert scale," 2010, para. 1)

Magnet designation – acknowledgment from the American Nurses Credentialing Center that an institution meets the criteria for nursing excellence as defined by the Magnet Recognition Program

Magnet framework – the evidence-based structure and requirements underlying the Magnet Recognition Program

Magnet journey – the interventions, activities, and culture change that culminate in the achievement of Magnet designation; the Magnet journey is an incremental adoption of and adaptation to the evidence-based Magnet program framework for nursing excellence

Magnet program – See Magnet recognition program

Magnet program director – the person responsible for coordinating and facilitating the institutional efforts to meet the Magnet program requirements

Magnet recognition program – "The Magnet recognition program was developed by the American Nurses Credentialing Center (ANCC) to recognize healthcare organizations that provide nursing excellence. The program also provides a vehicle for disseminating successful nursing practices and strategies. The Magnet recognition program is based on quality indicators and standards of nursing practice as defined in the newly revised 3rd edition of the *ANA Nursing Administration: Scope & Standards of Practice"* (ANCC, 2010)

Magnet redesignation – acknowledgment from the ANCC that an institution continues to meet the criteria for nursing excellence as defined by the Magnet recognition program. Magnet redesignation is required every 4 years to assure continued compliance with the Magnet recognition program.

Malleability – the quality of being able to be molded to accommodate various differences in culture, location, etc. without losing its inherent efficacy

Mean – the average

Median – the 50th percentile

Operationalize – to make measurable

Paradigm – "A set of assumptions, concepts, values, and practices that constitutes a way of viewing reality for the community that shares them, especially in an intellectual discipline" ("Paradigm," 2002)

Pareto chart – is a graphic designed to look at the many causes of a specific problem and help you determine which causes, if rectified, would take care of most of the problem in a specific situation

Perception – a wholly subjective meaning created by the individual receiving the stimulus based on the individual's beliefs, values, prior and current experience, and culture

PR – public relations; used to designate the promotional activities necessary to achieve awareness and engagement

Prescriptiveness – directing explicit actions to be taken, restricting the variability in a process or procedure

Quasi-experimental – this research design is similar to a true experimental design but lacks randomization; the lack of randomization makes it harder to rule out confounding variables and introduces threats to internal validity; conclusions of causal relationships are difficult to determine because the experimenter does not have total control over the extraneous variables (Gribbons & Herman, 1997)

Query letter – a preliminary letter typically inquiring if an idea has merit according to what the receiver desires; used, for example, to inquire if an idea for an article is viable for a specific journal

Rapid-cycle PDSA (PDCA) – "is applying the recurring sequence of PDCA (plan, do, study/check, act) in a brief period of time to solve a problem or issue facing a team or organization that will achieve breakthrough or continuous improvement results quickly" (Duffy, Moran, & Riley, 2009, para. 1)

Reliability – in statistics, this is precision of a measurement, as determined by the variance of repeated measurements of the same object

Run chart – a graphic that communicates data, showing the trending over time and shows how a process is operating

Shared decision making – is the main goal of the shared governance structure; it posits that more effective decisions are made when as many of those involved as possible contribute to the decision, especially those affected, closest to where the decision will be implemented; it also may encourage engagement and ownership of the decision by those affected

Shared governance – "Shared governance is an organizational innovation that gives healthcare professionals control over their practice and extends their influence into administrative areas previously controlled only by managers" (Hess, 2009, para. 6)

Site visit – "a visit in an official capacity to examine a site to determine its suitability for some enterprise" ("Site visit," 2010, para. 1)

Six sigma black belt – "Six Sigma team leaders responsible for implementing process improvement projects . . . within the business—to increase customer satisfaction levels and business productivity. Black Belts are knowledgeable and skilled in the use of the Six Sigma methodology and tools" (Coarde, 2003, para. 1)

Slippery slope – "a fallacy in which a course of action is objected to on the grounds that once taken it will lead to additional actions until some undesirable consequence results" (Nordquist, 2010, para. 1)

Stakeholder – "One who has a share or an interest, as in an enterprise" (Answers Corporation, 2010, para. 1)

Standard Deviation – "(a) statistic used as a measure of the dispersion or variation in a distribution" (American Heritage Dictionary of the English Language, n.d.)

Syntax – "pattern of formation of sentences or phrases in a language" (Answers Corporation, 2010, para. 1)

Tangential – superficially relevant to the topic under discussion

Tangibles – material things; things able to be touched, and in this circumstance, able to be valued fiscally

TCAB – transforming the care at the bedside; an initiative, a national program of the Robert Wood Johnson Foundation (RWJF) and Institute of Healthcare Improvement (IHI), to improve care on medical and surgical units in participating hospitals; an estimated 35 to 40% of unexpected hospital deaths occur on medical and surgical units. RWJF and IHI created, tested, and implemented changes to dramatically improve care on medical and surgical units, and improve staff satisfaction (IHI, n.d., para. 1–2)

Top-down approach – goals and action plans are created by senior leadership and communicated to those lower in the authority hierarchy

Transactional leadership – "transactional leadership is based on a transaction or exchange of something of value the leader possesses or controls that the follower wants in return for his/her services" (Homrig, 2001, para. 4)

Transferability – the quality of being exchangeable to a different location, a different time, and/or a different culture

Transformational leadership – "transformational leaders have internalized a sense of commitment to their goals and articulate this in such a way to their followers so as to convert their followers to a high level of commitment as well" (Homrig, 2001, para. 10)

Trending – graphically plotting data and noting tendencies in the data over time

t test – a statistical test to determine if there is a difference in the means of two groups' scores

Validity – the quality of credibility determined through evaluating various attributes of the item under scrutiny

Work-around – "a plan or method to circumvent a problem (as in computer software) without eliminating it" ("Work-around," 2010, para. 1)

Worker bees – those who perform the tasks of a specific initiative

REFERENCES

Algorithm. (n.d.). In *The American Heritage® Dictionary of the English Language, Fourth Edition*. Retrieved January 30, 2010, from Answers.com Web site: http://www.answers.com/topic/algorithm

American Productivity & Quality Center. (2008). *Glossary of benchmarking terms*. Available at: http://www.apqc.org/portal/apqc/ksn/Glossary%20of%20Benchmarking%20Terms.pdf?paf_gear_id=contentgearhome&paf_dm=full&pageselect=contentitem&docid=119519. Accessed December 28, 2009.

American Nurses Credentialing Center. (2010). *Magnet recognition program overview*. Available at: http://www.nursecredentialing.org/Magnet/ProgramOverview.aspx. Accessed January 20, 2010.

Anecdotal. (2010). In *Merriam-Webster online dictionary*. Available at: http://www.merriam-webster.com/dictionary/anecdotal. Accessed January 30, 2010.

Answers Corporation. (2010). *Stakeholder.* Available at: http://www.answers.com/topic/stakeholder. Accessed January 30, 2010.

Answers Corporation. (2010). *Syntax.* Available at: http://www.answers.com/topic/syntax. Accessed January 30, 2010.

Baylor Health Care System. (n.d.). *Core measures.* Available at: http://www.baylorhealth.com/About/FactsStats/QualityData/Pages/Default.aspx. Accessed January 30, 2010.

Bias. (2010). In *Merriam-Webster online dictionary.* Available at: http://www.merriam-webster.com/dictionary/bias. Accessed January 31, 2010.

Causation. (n.d.). In *Britannica concise encyclopedia.* Retrieved January 31, 2010, from Answers.com Web site: http://www.answers.com/topic/causation

Chi-square. (2009). In *Webster's new world college dictionary.* Cleveland, OH: Wiley Publishing, Inc.

Coarde, G. (2003). *Black belt.* Available at: http://www.isixsigma.com/dictionary/Black_Belt-62.htm. Accessed January 30, 2010.

Definitions of Evidence-Based Practice. (n.d.). Available at: http://www.shef.ac.uk/scharr/ir/def.html. Accessed January 30, 2010.

Duffy, G., Moran, J., & Riley, W. (2009). *Rapid cycle PDCA.* Available at: http://www.phf.org/pmqi/Rapid-Cycle-PDCA.pdf. Accessed January 30, 2010.

Efficacy. (2010). In *Merriam-Webster online dictionary.* Available at: http://www.merriam-webster.com/dictionary/efficacy. Accessed January 30, 2010.

Exemplar. (2010). In *Merriam-Webster online dictionary.* Available at: http://www.merriam-webster.com/dictionary/exemplar. Accessed January 30, 2010.

Feedback loop. (n.d.). In *The American Heritage dictionary of the English language, Fourth Edition.* (2003). Retrieved January 31, 2010, from http://www.thefreedictionary.com/feedback+loop

Gribbons, B., & Herman, J. (1997). True and quasi-experimental designs. *Practical Assessment, Research, and Evaluation, 5*(14). Available at: http://PAREonline.net/getvn.asp?v=5&n=14. Accessed January 31, 2010.

HCAHPS. (2009). *Fact sheet.* Available at: http://www.hcahpsonline.org/files/HCAHPS%20Fact%20Sheet,%20revised1,%203-31-09.pdf. Accessed January 30, 2010.

Hess, R. (2009). *Forum for shared governance.* Available at: http://www.sharedgovernance.org/. Accessed January 30, 2010.

Homrig, M. A. (2001). *Transformational leadership.* Available at: http://leadership.au.af.mil/documents/homrig.htm. Accessed January 30, 2010.

Impetus. (n.d.). In *American Heritage dictionary of the English language* (4th ed.). Available at: http://dictionary.reference.com/browse/impetus. Accessed January 31, 2010.

Institute for Healthcare Improvement. (n.d.). *Transforming care at the bedside.* Available at: http://www.ihi.org/IHI/Programs/StrategicInitiatives/TransformingCareAtTheBedside.htm. Accessed January 30, 2010.

Likert scale. (n.d.). In *A Dictionary of Statistics.* Retrieved January 30, 2010, from Answers.com Web site: http://www.answers.com/topic/likert-scale

McKay, D. R. (2010). *Curriculum vitae*. Available at: http://careerplanning.about.com/od/resumewriting/g/def_vitae.htm. Accessed January 31, 2010.

Nordquist, R. (2010). *Slippery slope*. Available at: http://grammar.about.com/od/rs/g/slipslopeterm.htm. Accessed January 30, 2010.

Paradigm. (2002). In *American Heritage dictionary of the English language* (4th ed.). Orlando, FL: Houghton Mifflin Company.

Site visit. (n.d.) In *WordNet 3.0, Farlex clipart collection*. (2003-2008). Retrieved January 30, 2010, from http://www.thefreedictionary.com/Site+visit

Standard Deviation. (n.d.). In *American Heritage dictionary of the English language*, Fourth Edition. Retrieved January 31, 2010, from Answers.com Web site: http://www.answers.com/topic/standard-deviation

Work-around. (2010). In *Merriam-Webster online dictionary*. Available at: http://www.merriam-webster.com/dictionary/work-around. Accessed January 30, 2010.

Index

Note: Page numbers followed by *f* indicate figures and those followed by *t* indicate tables.